EPILEPSY:
THE EIGHTH INTERNATIONAL SYMPOSIUM

EIGHTH INTERNATIONAL SYMPOSIUM ON EPILEPSY

ORGANIZERS

Epilepsy International
  International League Against Epilepsy
  International Bureau for Epilepsy
Irish Epilepsy Association

PRESIDENT

Cearbhaill O'Dalaigh, *President of Ireland*

VICE-PRESIDENTS

D. D. Daly, *Dallas*
President, International League Against Epilepsy

E. Grass, *Quincy, Massachusetts*
President, International Bureau for Epilepsy

M. Lindsay, *Dublin*
Honorary Secretary, Irish Epilepsy Association

P. A. McNally, *Dublin*
President, Irish Epilepsy Association

J. N. Moore, *Dublin*
Medical Director, St. Patrick's Hospital

SCIENTIFIC COMMITTEE

D. D. Daly, *Dallas (Chairman)*
G. Burden, *London (Secretary)*
G. Fenton, *Belfast*
E. A. Martin, *Dublin*
N. O'Donohoe, *Dublin*
J. K. Penry, *Bethesda*
M. Swallow, *Belfast*

LOCAL COMMITTEE

R. Holmes *(Secretary)*
J. Kirker
J. B. Lyons

Epilepsy:
The Eighth International Symposium

Editor

J. Kiffin Penry, M.D.
Chief, Epilepsy Branch
National Institute of Neurological
and Communicative Disorders and Stroke
National Institutes of Health
Bethesda, Maryland
and
Secretary-General
International League Against Epilepsy

Raven Press ■ New York

Raven Press, 1140 Avenue of the Americas, New York, New York 10036

Made in the United States of America

Library of Congress Cataloging in Publication Data

International Symposium on Epilepsy, 8th, Dublin, 1976.
    Epilepsy.

    Includes index.
    1. Epilepsy-Congresses.   I. Penry, J. Kiffin,
1929-   II. Title.
RC372.I47   1976   616.8'53   76–58059
ISBN 0–89004–190–3

Preface

The Eighth International Symposium on Epilepsy, hosted by the Irish Epilepsy Association in Dublin, September 12–15, 1976, provided an excellent opportunity for participants from communities around the world to learn more about epilepsy. In the atmosphere of the traditional Irish welcome, *Céad Mile Failte,* a hundred thousand welcomes, the Symposium was initiated by the presentation of a new national program on epilepsy, a lecture on the impact of computerized axial tomography of the brain—a revolutionary technical advance—and a social reception to continue the exchange of new ideas. In the scientific program, 64 papers were presented and discussed. New therapeutic agents, new diagnostic and therapeutic instruments, new books and periodicals, and new films were exhibited. Medical and rehabilitative facilities were visited to learn how Ireland helps people with epilepsy.

The themes of the Eighth International Symposium on Epilepsy not only reflect the current frontiers of research and problems of international interest, but they have also evolved from the two previous annual symposia. The program of the Sixth International Symposium on Epilepsy concentrated on the problems of people suffering from the more severe varieties of epilepsy, and compared the methods and results of multidisciplinary teams located in five different national centers. The function of special centers in providing treatment to inpatients was described. The Seventh International Symposium on Epilepsy emphasized the treatment and rehabilitation of outpatients with epilepsy, further defining a multidisciplinary approach. It became apparent that better methods were needed to bring relief to the patient with severe epilepsy. Moreover, long-term seizure control was required, because even minor relapses would undermine the rehabilitative efforts. Consequently, the themes of the Eighth International Symposium on Epilepsy centered on long-term control of seizures, intensive monitoring of the patient with severe epilepsy, and behavior modification and rehabilitation. In addition, the international variation in the availability of care for patients with epilepsy made it necessary to consider the needs of developing countries. Each of the four themes was introduced by a keynote speaker during plenary sessions.

This volume comprises 65 chapters, with 159 contributors representing 24 countries. Each chapter presents the essence of the subject without the details of methodology and complete discussion that would preempt the publication of a full-length scientific paper. It is hoped that each contribution represents an abbreviated account of the essentials commensurate with the quality of the usual scientific literature. The reader should have enough information to comprehend the significance of the research findings or theses presented and the author, although presenting more than a brief abstract, should not be precluded from publishing a complete report. The discussions and comments following each paper were not included, and the transactions of business meetings were also omitted. It was considered more important to bring rapidly and inexpensively to interested parties the essence of the new ideas and research findings presented at the meeting.

This volume, then, should make available to individuals who were unable to attend the Symposium the important contributions of that meeting, a valuable collection for study and review. For those who attended the Symposium, the volume presents a clear and complete record of those presentations not heard in parallel sessions.

J. Kiffin Penry
Bethesda, May 1977

Contents

Introduction

1   Opening Address
    Marjorie Lynch

5   Computerized Axial Tomography in Epilepsy
    Henri Gastaut and Jean-Louis Gastaut

Long-Term Control of Seizures

17   Long-Term Control of Seizures
     H. Meinardi, M. W. van Heycop ten Ham, J. W. A. Meijer, and E.
     Bongers

27   Implications of Long-Term Follow-Up Studies in Epilepsy: With a Note
     on the Cause of Death
     D. C. Taylor and S. M. Marsh

35   Experience in the Long-Term Use of Carbamazepine (Tegretol ®) in the
     Treatment of Epilepsy
     M. N. Hassan and M. J. Parsonage

45   A Comprehensive Interdisciplinary Approach to the Care of the Institu-
     tionalized Person with Epilepsy
     Brian P. O'Neill, Barbara Ladon, Linda M. Harris, Harold L. Riley, III,
     and Fritz E. Dreifuss

47   Anticonvulsive and Psychotropic Effects of Carbamazepine in Hospitalized
     Epileptic Patients: A Long-Term Study
     Amarendra Narayan Singh, Bishan M. Saxena, and Marcel Germain

57   Long-Term Treatment in Severe Epilepsy (Institutionalized Patients): II.
     Retrospective Evaluation of Carbamazepine
     H. Schneider

63   Therapy-Resistant Epilepsies with Long-Term History—Slow Spike-and-
     Wave Syndrome

T. Osawa, M. Seino, M. Miyokoshi, K. Yamamoto, N. Kakegawa, K. Yagi, T. Hirata, T. Morikawa, and T. Wada

69　Clinical, Therapeutic, and Social Status of Epileptic Patients Without Seizures for More than Five Years
L. Oller-Daurella, L. Oller F-V, and R. Pamies

77　Long-Term Combination Therapy with Phenytoin and Phenobarbital-Evaluation of Serum Levels
F. O. Müller, H. K. L. Hundt, A. K. Aucamp, L. Olivier, W. Wessels, and J. M. Steyn

81　The Middle Age of Epilepsy
A. Earl Walker

87　Chromosomal Damage in Patients with Epilepsy: Possible Mutagenic Properties of Long-Term Antiepileptic Drug Treatment
Jan Herha and Günter Obe

Intensive Monitoring

95　Intensive Monitoring of Patients with Intractable Seizures
J. Kiffin Penry and Roger J. Porter

103　Antiepileptic Drugs in Human Cerebral Cortex: Clinical Relevance of Cortex:Plasma Ratios
A. L. Sherwin, C. D. Harvey, and I. E. Leppik

109　Prolonged Monitoring of the EEG in Ambulatory Patients
J. F. Woods and J. R. Ives

115　Evaluation of Reliability in Determination of Antiepileptic Drug Levels
Alan Richens

119　A Prospective Longitudinal Study of Serum Levels of Sulthiame and Phenytoin, Together with an Evaluation of Seizure Control
N. Callaghan, M. Feely, M. O'Callaghan, and B. Duggan

125　Long-Term Intensive Monitoring of Epileptic Patients
M. J. O'Kane and R. Sauter

131　Long-Term Monitoring of Antiepileptic Drugs in Patients with the Lennox-Gastaut Syndrome
F. Viani, G. Avanzini, A. Baruzzi, B. Bordo, L. Bossi, R. Canger, G. Porro, A. Riboldi, M. E. Soffientini, P. Zagnoni, and P. L. Morselli

139   Precise Adjustment of Phenytoin Dosage
      Alan Richens

143   Has Carbamazepine-10, 11-Epoxide an Independent Antiepileptic Effect
      in Man?
      Mogens Dam, Janne Sury, and Johannes Christiansen

147   Influence of Phenobarbital on the Serum Level of Phenytoin and Effect
      of Phenytoin on Primidone Metabolism
      P. Ruf and R. Sauter

151   Automated Analysis of Prolonged EEG Recordings in Epileptic Patients
      H. H. von Albert

153   Relationship Between Quantitative EEG Measurements and Clinical State
      in Epileptic Patients
      Peter Kellaway and James R. G. Carrie

Antiepileptic Drugs

159   A Trial of Clonazepam in the Treatment of Severe Epilepsy in Infancy
      and Childhood
      N. V. O'Donohoe and B. A. Paes

163   Treatment of Chronic Epilepsy for 1 to 2 Years with Clonazepam
      *R. N. Nanda, R. H. Johnson, H. J. Keogh, D. G. Lambie, I. D. Melville,
      and R. A. Shakir*

169   Clinical Observations on Clonazepam in Intractable Epilepsy
      A. D. Gregoriades and E. G. Frangos

177   Clinical Experience with Clonazepam in the Treatment of Posttraumatic
      Epilepsy
      T. Syz and U. Spieler

181   Comparison of Sodium Valproate (Epilim®) and Clonazepam (Rivotril®)
      in Intractable Epilepsy
      *R. A. Shakir, R. H. Johnson, H. J. Keogh, D. G. Lambie, and R. N.
      Nanda*

187   Sodium Valproate in Treatment of Children with Refractory Epilepsy
      Ingrid Gamstorp

191   Elimination of Carbamazepine in Children after Single and Multiple Doses
      S. Pynnönen, M. Sillanpää, E. Iisalo, and H. Frey

199   Effectiveness of Daily Phenobarbital in the Prevention of Febrile Seizure
      Recurrences in "Simple" Febrile Convulsions and "Epilepsy Triggered
      by Fever"
      Sheldon Mark Wolf

203   Phenytoin-Induced Salivary IgA Deficiency and Gingival Hyperplasia
      Johan A. Aarli

209   The Influence of Phenytoin and Carbamazepine on Endocrine Function:
      Preliminary Results
      K. Lühdorf, P. Christiansen, J. M. Hansen, and M. Lund

215   Effect of Diphenylhydantoin on Serum Cholesterol and Triglyceride Levels
      in Patients with Epilepsy
      Mauri I. Reunanen and Eero A. Sotaniemi

219   Variation of Therapeutic Plasma Concentrations of Phenytoin and Pheno-
      barbital with the Type of Seizure and Co-Medication
      D. Schmidt

223   WODADIBOF III: Third International Workshop on the Determination
      of Antiepileptic Drugs in Body Fluids
      Christopher Gardner-Thorpe

Behavior Modification and Rehabilitation

225   Behavior Modification and Rehabilitation of Patients with Epilepsy
      Olaf Henriksen

235   Psychological Intervention with Parents of Children with Epilepsy
      J. Clausen

239   Behavior Therapy for Seizure Control
      D. I. Mostofsky

245   Behavior Disturbance and Type of Epilepsy in Children Attending Ordi-
      nary School
      G. Stores

251   Long-Term Casework Support with Epileptic Patients
      Rachel Tavriger

257 Personality Traits in Epilepsy
P. Bech, K. Kjaersgärd Pedersen, N. Simonsen, and M. Lund

265 The Concept of Preventive Rehabilitation in Childhood Epilepsy: A Plea Against Overprotection and Overindulgence
P. Lerman

269 How Doctors "Manage" Epilepsy
Anthony Hopkins and Graham Scambler

277 Pilot Study on Theme-Centered Interaction Groups with Epileptic Patients
Brunhilde Mayer and Leopold Gutjahr

285 Operant Conditioning for Behavior Modification in Institutionalized Retarded Children
Ulrike Zöllner-Breusch

291 A Study of Intellectual Function in Children with Epilepsy Attending Ordinary Schools
D. H. Mellor and I. Lowit

295 Progressive Aphasia and Epilepsy with a Self-Limited Course
Hans C. Lou, Sven Brandt, and Peter Bruhn

305 Aphasia and Seizure Disorders in Childhood
Christoph Foerster

307 Epilepsy and Driving in Israel
Sonia Laks and Amos D. Korczyn

Other Aspects of Epilepsy

313 Cerebrospinal Fluid Cyclic AMP and Epilepsy
V. V. Myllylä, E. Hokkanen, H. Nousiainen, E. R. Heikkinen, and H. Vapaatalo

317 HL-A Antigens in Primary Generalized Epilepsy
Raffaella Scorza Smeraldi, Carlo L. Cazzullo, Giovanna Fabio, Claudio Rugarli, Enrico Smeraldi, and Raffaele Canger

325 Temporal Lobe Epilepsy: On Whom to Operate and When
Inge Jensen

333 Chronic Cerebellar Stimulation in the Treatment of Epilepsy: A Prelimi-
nary Report
*G. W. Fenton, P. B. C. Fenwick, G. S. Brindley, M. A. Falconer, C. H.
Polkey, and D. N. Rushton*

341 Multiple Sclerosis and Seizures
Marta Elian and Geoffrey Dean

345 Epileptic Seizures During Sleep in Children
*C. A. Tassinari, G. Terzano, G. Capocchi, B. Dalla Bernardina, C. Valladier,
F. Vigevano, O. Daniele, C. Dravet, and J. Roger*

The Needs of Developing Countries

355 Epilepsy in Developing Countries
C. L. Bolis

359 Epilepsy in India
G. Arjundas

365 Epilepsy in the African Continent
B. O. Osuntokun

379 Epilepsy, Health, and Underdevelopment
R. Rada

385 Sociocultural and Economic Implications of Epilepsy in India
Vimla Virmani, V. Kaul, and S. Juneja

393 The Epilepsies: Clinical and Epidemiological Aspects/Availability and De-
sirability of Services
Tarik I. Hamdi, Ala A. Al-Husaini, and Faiq Al-Hadithi

401 Problems of Epilepsy in Rhodesia
Laurence F. Levy and William C. Auchterlonie

405 Index

Contributors

A

J. A. Aarli, 203
F. Al-Hadithi, 393
A. Al-Husaini, 393
G. Arjundas, 359
A. K. Aucamp, 77
W. C. Auchterlonie, 401
G. Avanzini, 131

B

A. Baruzzi, 131
P. Bech, 257
C. L. Bolis, 355
E. Bongers, 17
B. Bordo, 131
L. Bossi, 131
S. Brandt, 295
G. S. Brindley, 333
P. Bruhn, 295

C

N. Callaghan, 119
R. Canger, 131, 317
G. Capocchi, 345
J. R. G. Carrie, 153
C. L. Cazzullo, 317
J. Christiansen, 143
P. Christiansen, 143, 209
J. Clausen, 235

D

B. dalla Bernardina, 345
M. Dam, 143

O. Daniele, 345
G. Dean, 341
C. Dravet, 345
F. E. Dreifuss, 45
B. Duggan, 119

E

Marta Elian, 341

F

G. Fabio, 317
M. A. Falconer, 333
M. Feely, 119
G. W. Fenton, 333
P. B. C. Fenwick, 333
C. Foerster, 305
E. G. Frangos, 169
H. Frey, 191

G

I. Gamstorp, 187
C. Gardner-Thorpe, 223
H. Gastaut, 5
J. L. Gastaut, 5
M. Germain, 47
A. D. Gregoriades, 169
L. Gutjahr, 277

H

T. I. Hamdi, 393
J. M. Hansen, 209
L. M. Harris, 45

C. D. Harvey, 103
M. N. Hassan, 35
O. Henriksen, 225
E. R. Heikkinen, 313
J. Herha, 87
T. Hirata, 63
E. Hokkanen, 313
A. Hopkins, 269
H. K. L. Hundt, 77

I

E. Iisalo, 191
J. R. Ives, 109

J

I. Jensen, 325
R. H. Johnson, 163, 181
S. Juneja, 385

K

N. Kakegawa, 63
V. Kaul, 385
P. Kellaway, 153
H. J. Keogh, 163, 181
K. Kjaersgärd Pedersen, 257
A. D. Korczyn, 307

L

B. Ladon, 45
S. Laks, 307
D. G. Lambie, 163, 181
I. E. Leppik, 103
P. Lerman, 269
L. F. Levy, 401
H. C. Lou, 295
I. Lowit, 291
K. Lühdorf, 209
M. Lund, 257
M. Lynch, 1

M

S. M. Marsh, 27
B. Mayer, 277
J. W. A. Meijer, 17
H. Meinardi, 17
D. H. Mellor, 291
I. D. Melville, 163
M. Miyokoshi, 63
T. Morikawa, 63
P. L. Morselli, 131
D. I. Mostofsky, 239
F. O. Müller, 77
V. V. Myllylä, 313

N

R. N. Nanda, 163, 181
H. Nousiainen, 313

O

G. Obe, 87
M. O'Callaghan, 119
N. V. O'Donohoe, 159
M. J. O'Kane, 125
L. Olivier, 77
L. Oller F-V, 69
L. Oller-Daurella, 69
B. P. O'Neill, 45
T. Osawa, 63
B. O. Osuntokun, 365

P

B. A. Paes, 159
R. Pamies, 69
M. J. Parsonage, 35
J. K. Penry, 95
C. H. Polkey, 333
G. Porro, 131
R. J. Porter, 95
S. Pynnönen, 191

R

R. Rada, 379
M. I. Reunanen, 215
A. Riboldi, 131
A. Richens, 115, 139
H. L. Riley III, 45
J. Roger, 345
P. Ruf, 147
C. Rugarli, 317
D. N. Rushton, 333

S

R. Sauter, 125, 147
B. M. Saxena, 147
G. Scambler, 269
D. Schmidt, 219
H. Schneider, 57
R. Scorza Smeraldi, 317
M. Seino, 63
R. A. Shakir, 163, 181
A. L. Sherwin, 103
M. Sillanpää, 191
N. Simonsen, 257
A. N. Singh, 147
E. Smeraldi, 317
M. E. Soffientini, 131
E. A. Sotaniemi, 215
U. Spieler, 177
J. M. Steyn, 77
G. Stores, 245
J. Sury, 143
T. Syz, 177

T

C. A. Tassinari, 345
R. Tavriger, 251
D. C. Taylor, 27
G. Terzano, 345

V

C. Valladier, 345
M. W. van Heycop ten Ham, 17
H. Vapaatalo, 313
F. Viani, 131
F. Vigevano, 345
V. Virmani, 385
H. H. von Albert, 151

W

T. Wada, 63
A. E. Walker, 81
W. Wessels, 77
S. M. Wolf, 199
J. F. Woods, 109

Y

K. Yagi, 63
K. Yamamoto, 63

Z

P. Zagnoni, 131
U. Zöllner-Breusch, 285

INTRODUCTION

Epilepsy, The Eighth International Symposium,
edited by J. K. Penry. Raven Press, New York
© 1977.

Opening Address

The Honorable Marjorie Lynch

Undersecretary of Health, Education, and Welfare, Washington, D.C. 20201

The conquest of epilepsy is a problem best solved by the family of nations working together. We in America have much to learn from this organization, and we have some experiences that we hope to share with you at this gathering. As some of you may know, our national program for medical research is carried out at the National Institutes of Health in Bethesda, Maryland, a suburb of Washington, D.C. The National Institutes of Health is the federal government's primary health research agency and is part of the Department of Health, Education, and Welfare, one of the major departments in the President's Cabinet. America's epilepsy research effort has gathered excellent momentum these past 8 years under the dedicated and able direction of two men well known to this audience: Dr. Donald Tower, Director of the National Institute of Neurological and Communicative Disorders and Stroke, which is within the National Institutes of Health, and Dr. J. Kiffin Penry, Director of the Institute's Neurological Disorders Program, who as you know also serves as Secretary-General of the International League Against Epilepsy—the scientific co-sponsor of this conference. You will be hearing of the work they are directing later.

All of us here are aware of the problems of an individual who has epilepsy. But in most countries, the general public is ignorant as to the causes of the disorder. Many people have the false notion that epilepsy is inherited, but in most instances epilepsy is a result of injury or disease of the nervous system. Relatively few people outside of this gathering realize, for example, that seizures often lessen as a person gets older, and the average individual is frightened when he sees a seizure and has never received any instruction as to what to do when it happens. Unfortunately, because of the public's genuine ignorance, many children and adults with epilepsy are made to feel different, and it becomes difficult for them to live like other people. Declared one authority, "Epilepsy is the only common disorder I know where the sufferer is more handicapped by the attitude of society than by his disability."

Certainly, attitudes must be changed internationally and nationally so that people with epilepsy have the same rights as all citizens. In the United States, we are attempting to change such viewpoints in several ways. One of the ways we are doing this is through legislation. Recently Congress passed the Health Services Act of 1975, which created a nine-member commission on epilepsy to conduct a 1-year study on epilepsy in America. The resulting comprehensive

1

national plan will go to Congress. The report will contain specific recommendations for research, treatment, and rehabilitation efforts for the control of epilepsy
and its consequences. Members of the Commission represent both the research
and the service arms of epilepsy control. Several of its members are well known
to you here: Dr. David Daly, its Chairman; Dr. Richard Masland, its Executive
Director; and Mrs. Ellen Grass, who as you know is President of this symposium's co-sponsor, the International Bureau for Epilepsy. As you also know, the
Bureau is the voluntary arm of the international epilepsy control movement.

Through the years, volunteer organizations have played an important role in
the United States. It is illustrated in the fact that the National Epilepsy Foundation of America inspired our Congress to establish the Commission for the
Control of Epilepsy. Volunteer organizations have always been in the vanguard
of national social programming, and I venture to say that without voluntary
organizations in epilepsy, we would still be in the dark ages of epilepsy research
and services.

Another piece of legislation recently passed by our Congress is not only for
citizens with epilepsy but for all handicapped individuals. The Rehabilitation Act
protects the rights of every handicapped citizen whose employer receives any
federal financial assistance. We expect this law to have a far-reaching impact on
the opportunity of every handicapped person in America to obtain a job and to
be able to participate on an equal basis. A recent Congressional study indicates
they have not had the same opportunities in employment. Only about 800,000
of America's 25 million handicapped people have jobs, and according to the
National Epilepsy Foundation of America, 15 to 25% of the 4 million people
with epilepsy are unemployed. From those statistics, one can correctly assume
there has been discrimination against handicapped citizens and, more specifically,
people with epilepsy. Hopefully, the Rehabilitation Act will help eliminate the
employment barriers.

At the present time, the regulations to implement the legislation are being
reviewed, and the final regulation will be published later this year. During the
writing of the regulations, we had a 30-day public comment period in which town
meetings were held throughout the United States so that as many people as
possible would have an opportunity to voice their opinions. We listened to the
handicapped individuals, the employers, the educators, and service providers.
Some of the key provisions of the proposed legislation are: schools and colleges
must make their programs accessible to handicapped students; all new construction should be free of barriers to handicapped people; employers must not refuse
to hire qualified persons because they are handicapped; and employers must make
reasonable accommodation to a person's handicap, unless they can prove that
to do so would impose an undue hardship. As you can imagine, this legislation
is a valuable contribution to the rights of all handicapped individuals, including
those people with epilepsy.

Also, there has been some expansion in our legislation. In 1970, the Mentally
Retarded Facilities and Construction Act was expanded to include people with

epilepsy and cerebral palsy, as well as mentally retarded persons. This legislation then became the Developmental Disability Services and Facilities Construction Act. It provides for a council in every state to coordinate a program of service for people with long-term disabilities. Grants are authorized to states for planning, administration, services, and construction of facilities for developmentally disabled persons, and it supports 35 university programs that provide training facilities for health and health-related education in the area of developmental disabilities.

In addition to the legislative action, the government has supported research and job projects for people with epilepsy. Just recently, the Department of Labor awarded a grant for $625,000 to conduct training projects in five cities. The purpose of this endeavor is to train and place young people with epilepsy who are high school graduates, high school dropouts, or seniors in high school. This project is the first of its kind and could lead to more programs of significant nature in the future.

Epilepsy research has been an important part of our efforts in the United States. The National Institute of Neurological and Communicative Disorders and Stroke conducts much basic and clinical research aimed at finding more effective and less toxic anticonvulsant drugs. This year, the Institute implemented two new concepts for making that research pay off faster. Comprehensive Epilepsy Centers were contracted at five important medical centers for the primary purpose of getting research results to the patients who need them. In addition, a new anticonvulsant drug screening project was added to the Antiepileptic Drug Development Program to study more drugs. The Institute supports 65 epilepsy research projects throughout the United States and two in foreign countries. We have six research centers at major universities throughout the United States that focus on specific research aspects, new knowledge about brain mechanisms and functions, and the development of new treatment techniques. Also, there is an epilepsy program within the Bethesda laboratories of the National Institutes of Health. That center has been designated by the World Health Organization as one of their collaborating international centers on epilepsy. Within this program, the United States federal government is supporting fellowships for scientists to receive special training about research on epilepsy.

Another measure to advance the needs of all handicapped citizens in America is the White House Conference on Handicapped Individuals to be held in May of next year. We realize that there must be a change in the attitudes of the general public toward all handicapped persons. Hopefully, the conference will point out and help erase the attitudinal barriers that separate man from man and man from things. Authorized by Congress, the conference will assess the needs and potentials of the physically and mentally handicapped people of all ages, races, ethnic backgrounds, and both sexes, and we are involving many people throughout the United States. In fact, issues and recommendations from meetings now being held in all of our 50 states will serve as the agenda for the conference. Approximately 2,500 persons will attend and they will include voting delegates, 50% of whom will be handicapped individuals, alternates, and observers. Conference delegates will recommend what programs need to be expanded or begun and will describe how these recommendations are to be implemented. In addition, the conference will focus attention on the contributions that handicapped individuals can make to our society, given opportunities, understanding, and support. Specific foreign visitors will be invited to participate and contribute their expertise concerning specific White House Conference topics.

Before closing, I want to mention one exciting project we are just beginning —our Vinland National Center for Handicapped Individuals, which will be patterned after the work of that marvelous blind Norwegian, Mr. Stordahl. The main emphasis of the center will be physical fitness to enhance the personal growth and development of the individual. Mr. Stordahl has done incredible work with handicapped individuals in Beitostolen, Norway, and we hope to have similar accomplishments at our center in Minnesota. Also, I want to take this opportunity to thank Norway for their generous contribution to this center, and I want you to know that your country has been most helpful in our progress with handicapped individuals, as have many other countries participating in this conference.

I think we need more cooperation and exchange of ideas, as you will have here during the next few days. By having input from many different countries, we are able to learn which projects are feasible and which are not, and through the generous cooperation of many countries here today, as well as the dedication of many Americans, we in the United States have made significant progress in our efforts to ensure that people with epilepsy are given the same opportunities. We intend to continue this endeavor. It is not a task that can be accomplished immediately but will require the continued determination of many people; nevertheless, I am confident we will accomplish our goal of providing equal opportunities to people with epilepsy so that they can have the rewarding and content life that they have a right to.

Epilepsy, The Eighth International Symposium,
edited by J. K. Penry. Raven Press, New York
© 1977.

Computerized Axial Tomography in Epilepsy

Henri Gastaut and Jean-Louis Gastaut

*Department of Clinical Neurophysiology Medical Faculty of Marseille,
Hopitâl de la Timone, 13385 Marseille, Cédex 4, France*

Two series of 500 epileptic patients have been investigated with an EMI Scanner in the Hopitâl de la Timone, Marseilles, after neuropsychiatric examination and electroencephalographic recording, and 832 of them were assessed into one or the other category of the International Classification of the Epilepsies (Gastaut, 1969). The results of these two studies were presented at the 21st and 22nd Marseilles Colloquium (September, 1975, and September, 1976), along with the results of 2,200 epileptics investigated in the same conditions by Moseley and Bull (Great Britain), Collard et al. (Belgium), Von Gall et al. (Germany), Scollo-Lavizzari et al. (Switzerland), Caille et al. (France), Angeleri et al. (Italy), and Munari et al. (Italy).

These results can be classified under two major headings depending on (1) the proportion and the type of cerebral lesions discerned by computerized axial tomography (CAT) in the different electroclinical types of epilepsy, and (2) the etiology of these lesions.

PROPORTION AND TYPE OF CEREBRAL LESIONS IN THE DIFFERENT ELECTROCLINICAL CATEGORIES OF EPILEPSY

Primary Generalized Epilepsy

There were 80 patients in this group corresponding roughly to essential, idiopathic, or genuine epilepsy: 71 (89%) with a normal CAT and 9 (11%) with atrophic lesions. Since 89% of patients had a normal CAT, the conclusions can be drawn that (1) this form of epilepsy is usually not caused by a cerebral lesion but is due to a constitutional predisposition to epilepsy, either acquired or genetic, and (2) tonic-clonic seizures of primary generalized epilepsy (grand mal) and absence seizures (petit mal) do not cause deterioration, except perhaps when they recur frequently over years or decades.

The distribution of the lesions according to the type of primary generalized epilepsies is shown in Table 1.

Such figures agree with the clinical prognosis, which is the best for idiopathic grand mal and the worst for complex typical absences (chiefly myoclonic absences) and mixed grand mal and petit mal seizures.

TABLE 1. *Findings on CAT in 80 patients with primary generalized epilepsy*

Seizures	No. of patients	No. with abnormal CAT
Grand mal (with or without epileptic myoclonies)	28	1 (3.5%)
Petit mal		
Simple absences	15	1 (7%)
Complex absences	6	1 (17%)
Grand mal and petit mal	25	6 (24%)
Other forms (chiefly hyperthermic clonic seizures)	6	0 (0%)

Secondary Generalized Epilepsy

There were 160 patients in this group, which corresponds roughly to the malignant epileptic encephalopathies of infancy (West syndrome) and childhood (Lennox-Gastaut syndrome). A cerebral lesion was found on CAT in 85 (53%) of the patients, confirming the "secondary" nature of this type of epilepsy, which is usually accompanied by mental retardation.

Of the 30 infants or children with an evolutive West syndrome or an encephalopathy secondary to West syndrome, 23 (77%) had abnormal findings on CAT (Table 2). Of the 94 patients with a Lennox-Gastaut syndrome, 49 (52%) had an abnormal CAT (Table 3). Of the 36 patients with a secondary generalized epilepsy which could not be classified as West or Lennox-Gastaut syndrome, 14 (39%) had atrophy and/or malformation on CAT.

In all of the 160 cases, there was no relationship between the existence of atrophy of the brain and the age of the patients or the duration of their illness. For instance, in people with West syndrome or an encephalopathy consecutive to West syndrome, the average duration of the illness was 23 months and 3 days in children with a normal CAT and 27 months in children with brain atrophy. There was, however, a relative but positive relation between the existence of brain atrophy and the mental condition. For instance, in the same population, the development quotient was 0.62 in children with a normal CAT and 0.35 in children with brain atrophy.

TABLE 2. *Findings on CAT in 30 patients with West syndrome*

Normal		7 (23%)
Abnormal		23 (77%)
Tumor	1 (4%)	
Atrophy and/or malformation	22 (96%)	
Atrophy (cortical or corticosubcortical)	12	
Atrophy + calcifications	4	
Calcifications	1	
Atrophy + agenesis of corpus callosum	2	
Agenesis of corpus callosum	2	
Porencephaly	1	

TABLE 3. *Findings on CAT in 94 patients with Lennox-Gastaut syndrome*

Normal		45 (48%)
Abnormal		49 (52%)
Tumor	2 (4%)	
Leukoblastic infiltrate	1 (2%)	
Focal lesion (type unknown)	3 (6%)	
Atrophy and/or malformations	43 (88%)	
Atrophy (cortical, corticosubcortical, or subcortical)	29	
Atrophy + calcifications	5	
Calcifications	2	
Atrophy + agenesis of corpus callosum	2	
Porencephaly (encephaloclastic)	5	

Because of these data we may assume that:

1. The lesions responsible for the secondary generalized epilepsies are always quite atrophic and often characterized by a generalized corticosubcortical atrophy with a frontotemporal predominance.

2. Such characteristic lesions, with a possible common mechanism, if not a common etiology, are acquired before the beginning of the affection (before, during, or after birth) and are not dependent on the duration of the illness, the number of seizures, and the importance of the brain dysrhythmia.

3. The generalized character of the seizures and of the EEG patterns of such epilepsies are due not to the lesions *per se* (which are lacking or, eventually, focal in one-half of the cases) but to some secondary factors, metabolic, immunologic, or viral.

Partial Epilepsies

There were 490 patients in this group, with an abnormal CAT in 308 (63%). Such percentage differs little from the one found by Collard et al. (53%) and by Scollo-Lavizzari et al. (62.5%). The types of lesions shown by the CAT are described in the section devoted to the etiology of the epilepsies.

These lesions were focal in 78% of the cases but diffuse in 22%, confirming the possibility that certain diffuse lesions cause partial attacks because of the predominance of histological lesions in certain areas with a particularly low convulsive threshold. The 22% of diffuse lesions were due in part to the relatively few focal lesions in patients with seizures of complex symptomatology. Either CAT is not reliable in demonstrating temporal lobe pathology or some diffuse lesions cause partial attacks because temporolimbic structures have a low convulsive threshold.

Epilepsy with symptoms due to rolandic discharges (somatomotor and somatosensory) had the highest proportion of focal lesions, although the lesions affected rolandic cortex in only half the cases. The mechanism by which subcortical (central gray matter) or cortical lesions that do not impinge on the rolandic area cause rolandic symptoms is not known.

Other Types of Epilepsy

Apart from the generalized and partial types of epilepsy, which are well described in the International Classification of the Epilepsies (Gastaut, 1969), we have studied the groups described below.

Benign Epilepsy with Rolandic EEG Paroxysms

The 17 children with this type of epilepsy had a normal CAT, confirming other evidence that this syndrome is not organic but is a functional epilepsy similar to generalized primary epilepsy.

Grand Mal Generalized Epilepsy of Late Onset

Of 65 patients with grand mal seizures of late onset (the clinical and EEG findings did not justify including them in the group of primary grand mal or of partial epilepsy with secondary generalized seizures), 26 were normal on CAT and 39 had diffuse atrophic lesions. Such findings confirm the existence (which we suspected in 1974) of secondary generalized epilepsy in adults and particularly in old people, depending on involutional or arteriopathic encephalopathy.

Epilepsy with Unilateral Seizures

Of 20 cases with hemiclonic seizures, involving only one side or, alternatively or independently, both sides, only 2 were abnormal on CAT.

Hemiconvulsion-Hemiplegy-Epilepsy Syndrome

From the 490 patients with partial epilepsy, 18 presented with a hemiconvulsion-hemiplegy-epilepsy (H-H-E) syndrome. From these 18 cases, 3 were normal

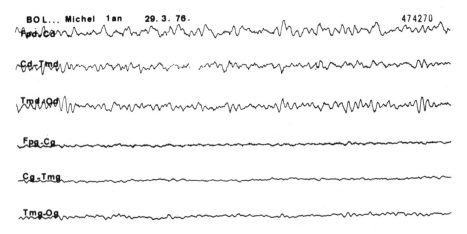

FIG. 1. EEG showing depression of left hemisphere electrical activity.

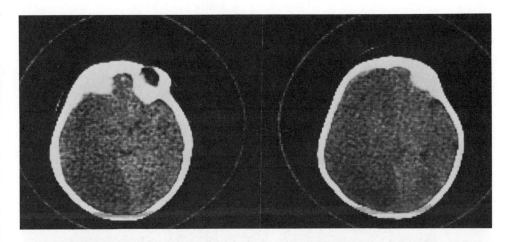

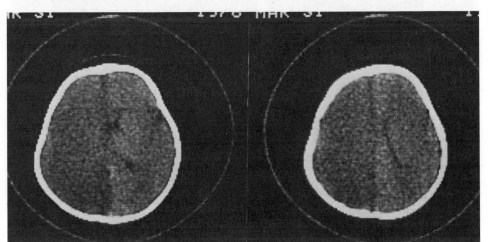

FIG. 2. CAT showing left hemispheric edema and hypodensity.

on CAT, 9 had diffuse or unilateral atrophic lesions, and 5 had parenchymal changes in the sylvian area, with or without cysts. From these findings, the conclusion can be drawn that the H-H-E syndrome is the result of not only venous thrombosis, as some have contended, but also arterial thrombosis or, independent of the etiology, the hemiconvulsive status epilepticus itself.

Status Epilepticus

In 20 children, CAT was performed immediately after status epilepticus and again a few weeks later, showing in 7 of them and in such a short interval of time the succession of brain edema and brain atrophy. Since the edema and the atrophy were unilateral or bilateral and related to the localization of the convulsions

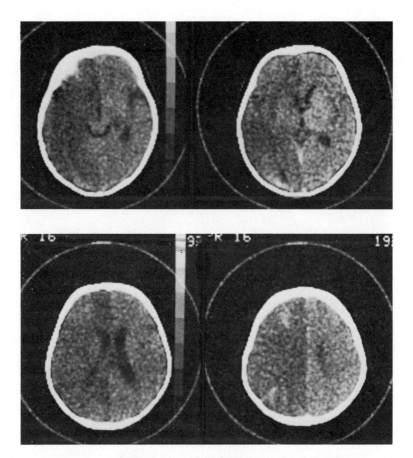

FIG. 3. Persistent left hemisphere edema in CAT performed 16 days after that in Fig. 2.

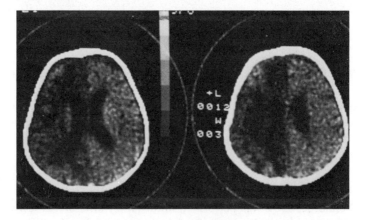

FIG. 4. Final CAT 35 days after that in Fig. 3. Edema has regressed, but a slight bilateral ventricular dilatation and extensive cortical atrophy are apparent, especially in the left hemisphere.

(unilateral or bilateral clonic seizures), the conclusion can be drawn that the atrophic process depends on the epileptic process and not on the cause of the status (see Figs. 1–4).

COMPUTERIZED AXIAL TOMOGRAPHY AND ETIOLOGY OF THE EPILEPSIES

This section deals only with the 401 classified epileptic patients of our first study, the results of which were presented in September, 1975, at the 21st Marseilles Colloquium.

Epilepsy Secondary to Brain Tumor

In 53 of 401 patients CAT showed an expansive intracranial lesion, but in 10 of these cases the diagnosis had been established by X-ray or after surgery. In 20 patients, clinical and/or EEG findings made tumor likely. In 17 patients who had infrequent seizures, most of late onset, tumor was not suspected, and the diagnosis had even been excluded by X-ray in 6 patients. Thus, CAT has discovered a tumor in 10.7% of our patients of all ages. This agrees with the figures reported by Collard et al. (8.3%), Von Gall et al. (10%), and Moseley and Bull (10%) and gives a total figure of 9.8% for the 1,500 epileptic patients studied by the four teams, a figure which is considerably higher than the one reported before the use of CAT, from 1% (Krohn, 1961) to 5% (Gudmundsson, 1966).

The distribution of tumors following the type of epilepsy is shown in Table 4.

TABLE 4. *Findings on CAT and seizures of 53 patients with brain tumor*

Number of patients	53
Previously diagnosed	10
Previously undiagnosed	43
Incidence in epilepsy (undiagnosed cases only)	
All 401 patients	43 (11%)
222 patients with late onset	36 (16%)
Repartition following the type of epilepsy (all 53 cases)	
Partial epilepsy	47 (89%)
Generalized epilepsy	4 (8%)
Unilateral seizures	2 (4%)

CAT is by far the best method of diagnosing brain tumors in patients with epilepsy, since tumors were found in all our patients and in 23 of the 24 in the series of Payan and Gawler (1975). The yield of various methods, including CAT, for the diagnosis of tumoral etiology in our epileptic patients is shown in Table 5.

TABLE 5. *Diagnostic yield of various methods in 47 patients with epilepsy secondary to tumor*

Clinical	
Progressive neurological deficit and/or intracranial hypertension	10 (21%)
EEG	
Continuous focal polyrhythmic delta or "projected" monorhythmic delta	14 (30%)
Neuroradiology (in only 32 patients)	
Arteriogram and/or pneumogram	19 (59%)
CAT	47 (100%)

Posttraumatic Epilepsy

There were 27 patients (7%) with posttraumatic epilepsy established by a history of prolonged coma, depressed fracture, fracture of the base of the skull, or neuropsychiatric sequelae. In 23 patients (85%), CAT revealed focal lesions in 19 (83%) and diffuse lesions in only 4. The site of the focal lesion was frontal or temporal or both in 17 (90%) and parieto-occipital in only 2 patients. These lesions varied from simple, fairly focal cortical atrophy to parenchymal affection of a whole lobe (or more) with ventricular dilatation and cortical atrophy. In most patients, the latter type of lesion, probably cortical scarring and subjacent demyelination, leads to parenchymal resorption and subsequent formation of an arachnoid cyst or to porencephaly, with or without communication to the ventricle.

Fronto-orbital and temporal posttraumatic "coup" or "contrecoup" lesions, which have long been recognized by pathologists (Courville, 1945), can also be confirmed by CAT. This precise visualization of a posttraumatic lesion can be extremely important for forensic medicine.

The clinical and EEG findings in patients with posttraumatic epilepsy are shown in Table 6.

TABLE 6. *Findings in 27 patients with posttraumatic epilepsy*

CAT findings		
Normal		4 (15%)
Abnormal		23 (85%)
Focal lesion	19 (83%)	
Diffuse lesion	4 (17%)	
Clinical findings		
Primary generalized epilepsy		0 (0%)
Secondary generalized epilepsy		4 (15%)
Partial epilepsy		23 (85%)
EEG findings		
Normal		6 (22%)
Focal paroxysms		11 (41%)
"Secondary bisynchronism"		10 (37%)

Postischemic Epilepsy

Twenty epileptics (5%) appeared in this category and were divided into two very different groups according to the lesions detected by the CAT.

Epilepsy after Occlusion of the Sylvian Artery or Its Branches

Epilepsy in this group is seen at all ages, but particularly in children with congenital hemiplegia or after H-H-E syndrome and chiefly in patients over 61 years. In this group, CAT showed parenchymal changes in the superficial and/or deep sylvian area, with or without cysts.

Epilepsy after Occlusion of the Posterior Cerebral Artery

Epilepsy is frequent in the syndrome of posterior cerebral artery occlusion occurring at birth or resulting from a brain insult in infancy. Although it is fairly frequent, it has not hitherto been recognized. We found nine patients less than 20 years old, often mentally retarded, often with hemiplegia and/or hemianopsia or quadrantanopsia, who had secondary generalized epilepsy or, more often, partial epilepsy with complex symptomatology of the temporal lobe. CAT demonstrated smooth porencephalic cysts communicating with the lateral ventricle; the cysts occupied the occipital lobe and sometimes also the parietal or temporal lobe supplied by the posterior cerebral artery. Only Remillard et al. (1974) reported eight similar lesions in patients with temporal lobe epilepsy and with hemianopsia or quadrantanopsia. That such lesions have not been recognized more often is explained by the large volume of the porencephaly and the small amount of air injected in fractionated pneumoencephalography.

Postinfectious Epilepsy

In our first series, there were only seven such patients, and CAT showed parenchymal changes after purulent meningitis or presuppurative meningoencephalitis due to otitis media in five patients, empyema in one patient, and abscess in another. In our second series, the number with abscess increased to seven.

Epilepsy of Other Etiology

Several case reports are selected from our two series to illustrate the fact that CAT provided the diagnosis.

CAT demonstrated lesions with moderate calcium deposits that had not been picked up by X-ray in: (1) 14 patients with the syndrome of Bourneville, (2) 3 patients with the Sturge-Weber-Krabbe syndrome, and (3) 3 patients with Fahr syndrome.

CAT showed in patients with blood diseases: (1) intraparenchymal leukoblastic infiltration in three patients with acute lymphoblastic leukemia, (2) cerebral hemorrhage in a patient with acute myeloblastic leukemia, (3) meningeal granulomatosis in two patients with Hodgkin disease, (4) subdural hematoma in a patient with polycythemia vera, and (5) intracerebral hematoma in a patient with idiopathic thrombocytopenic purpura.

CAT showed external hydrocephalus and frontotemporal hydroma in a patient with Menkes syndrome; triventricular hydrocephalus due to benign stenosis of the aqueduct of Sylvius in three patients, with epilepsy as the only symptom in two patients, so pronounced as to simulate hydranencephaly in the last patient; and two postoperative epileptogenic lesions.

DISCUSSION AND CONCLUSIONS

Computerized axial tomography is of prime importance for the etiologic diagnosis of epilepsy. In the past, when such a diagnosis was made on the basis of the patient's history, clinical findings, and the methods available (EEG, scintigraphy, angiography, and pneumoencephalography), the proportion of established cerebral lesions was at most 30% (30%, Juul-Jensen, 1965; 30%, Roger and Brichler, 1965; 17%, Gudmundsson, 1966). In the study reported here, the proportion of cerebral lesions discerned by CAT is 50%, a finding that agrees with those reported by Von Gall et al. (51%), Caille et al. (47%), Collard et al. (47%), and Scollo-Lavizzari et al. (34%). Indeed, in 81 (20%) of our patients, CAT revealed a cerebral lesion which had been missed in the other examinations and had merely been suspected from the history. One of the best examples of the superiority of CAT is perhaps the diagnosis of Bourneville disease in 88% of cases in infants and young children before the appearance of specific clinical symptoms.

It is, therefore, likely that physicians who treat epilepsy will request CAT as often as EEG. After examination of the patient, they will request an EEG in order to establish a positive diagnosis, to classify the patient according to the International Classification of the Epilepsies (Gastaut, 1969), and to identify those patients with primary generalized epilepsies that are mainly functional. They will then request CAT to ascertain or rule out an organic lesion. Other methods of examination will be reserved for such special problems as demonstrating vascular malformations by angiography.

CAT is also of theoretical interest since it allows an anatomical study of the brain in living persons and thus opens a new era in the study of epilepsy. One may even suppose that the present-day electroclinical classification of the epilepsies will become an anatomoelectroclinical classification because of the use of CAT.

CAT IN STATUS EPILEPTICUS

Having published two comprehensively illustrated articles on the CAT method (Gastaut, 1976; Gastaut et al., 1976), we will restrict the illustration of this chapter to a CAT study of the particular condition of status epilepticus. Not only has the CAT method not been used before in this way, but we believe the results we have obtained are indispensable for an understanding of some of the anatomical consequences of status epilepticus.

On March 28, 1976, Michel, 1 year of age, had hemiclonic epileptic status on the right side, which after several hours was replaced by right hemiplegia associated with coma that persisted for 2 days. An EEG obtained the next day (March 29) showed a depression of left hemisphere electrical activity (Fig. 1), which was still present 4 months later when the last control EEG was made. The CAT performed 3 days after the seizure (March 31) showed a left hemispheric edema with characteristic hypodensity. This edema was most marked in the posterior area and was accompanied by a severe collapse of the left ventricular system (Fig. 2).

Another CAT performed 16 days later (April 16) showed the left hemisphere edema persisting in all sections (Fig. 3). The final CAT 35 days later (May 21), or 54 days after the status epilepticus, showed regression of the edema, which at this stage affected only the left hemisphere white matter. At the same time, a slight bilateral ventricular dilatation and widespread cortical atrophy could be seen, particularly in the left hemisphere (Fig. 4).

Thus, for the first time, by the use of CAT, it has been possible to show a succession, in less than 2 months, of edema, followed by cortical and subcortical atrophy in a hemisphere which had, for several hours, epileptic discharges responsible for hemiclonic contralateral status epilepticus.

REFERENCES

Courville, C. B. (1945): *Pathology of the Central Nervous System.* Pacific Press Publishing Association, Mountain View, California.

Gastaut, H. (1969): Classification of the epilepsies, proposal for an international classification. *Epilepsia [Suppl.]*, 10:514–521.

Gastaut, H., and Gastaut, J. L. (1976): Computerized transverse axial tomography in epilepsy. *Epilepsia,* 17:325–336.

Gastaut, H., Gastaut, J. L., Regis, H., Raybaud, C., Farnarier, P., Michotey, P., and Michel, B. (1976): Etude des épilepsies par la tomographie axiale commandeé par ordinateur. *Nouv. Presse Med.,* 5:481–486.

Gudmundsson, G. (1966): Epilepsy in Iceland. *Acta Neurol. Scand. [Suppl.* 25], 43.

Juul-Jensen, P. (1965): Epilepsy. A clinical and social analysis of 1,020 adult patients with epileptic seizures. *Acta Neurol. Scand. [Suppl.* 13], 41.

Krohn, W. A. (1961): A study of epilepsy in Northern Norway. *Acta Psychiatr. Scand. [Suppl.],* 150:215–227.

Payan, J., and Gawler, J. (1975): E.E.G. and E.M.I. scan: early results of a comparative study. *Electroencephalogr. Clin. Neurophysiol.,* 38:212.

Remillard, G. M., Ethier, R., and Andermann, F. (1974): Temporal lobe epilepsy and perinatal occlusion of the posterior cerebral artery. *Neurology (Minneap.),* 24:1001–1009.

Roger, J., and Brichler, C. (1965): In: Contribution a l'Étude du Pronostic Éloigne de l'Épilepsie, edited by C. Brichler. Thesis, Rennes.

LONG-TERM CONTROL OF SEIZURES

Epilepsy, The Eighth International Symposium,
edited by J. K. Penry. Raven Press, New York
© 1977.

Long-Term Control of Seizures

H. Meinardi, M. W. van Heycop ten Ham, J. W. A. Meijer, and
E. Bongers

Instituut voor Epilepsiebestrijding, Heemstede, The Netherlands

The long-term control of seizures is a primary goal of therapy. It is hoped that the natural course of epilepsy will terminate in a complete remission, but not everyone is convinced that this will be the case. Rodin (1968) has summarized the points on which the majority of authors appear to agree in regard to the chance of epileptic patients achieving at least 2 years of terminal remission. Terminal remission of at least 2 years occurs in 33.3% of all epilepsies, in about 50 to 60% of patients with generalized tonic-clonic seizures only, and in about 20 to 30% of those with partial complex seizures only. Furthermore, there was agreement that (1) the percentages of patients who are regarded in terminal remission stand in marked indirect relationship to the length of follow-up; (2) the longer the illness has lasted, the less likely it is that control will be achieved; (3) the more seizures the patient has experienced prior to his first visit to the physician, the less likely will be complete control; (4) the more different seizure types a given patient has experienced, the less likely control; (5) the more abnormal the neurological examination and mental status examination and the lower the IQ, the more difficult it will be to control the seizures; (6) the younger the patient at the time of onset of the illness, the less likely it is that complete control will be achieved; but some authors feel that age at time of onset is not a good prognostic indicator.

ANTIEPILEPTIC DRUGS AND SEIZURE CONTROL

Van Heycop ten Ham studied a group of patients who had been free from seizures on medication for at least 5 years. Medication was withdrawn gradually. The results are presented in Table 1. The findings in primary generalized epilepsy are similar to those reported by Oller-Daurella et al. (1976) and also by Janz and Sommer-Burkhardt (1976).

Data on seizure control by drugs also vary (Table 2). It has to be kept in mind that investigators rarely cover the overall population of epileptics. At the time of our survey of the province of Zeeland in 1973, the general practitioners reported 835 cases of epilepsy. Of these, 448 (53%) were seizure-free.

Is it possible to increase seizure control by monitoring levels of antiepileptic

TABLE 1. *Consequences of cessation of antiepileptic medication after remission of at least 5 years*

Diagnosis	> 2 years free of seizures without medication	Relapses after reduction or withdrawal of drugs
Primary generalized epilepsy	26	10
Secondary generalized epilepsy	1	2[a]
Focal epilepsy	21	2
Benign epilepsy in childhood	7	—
Unclassified	11	1
Total	66	15[a]

[a] Includes one patient who had only an "EEG-relapse."

drugs in serum? Dawson and Jamieson (1971) studied 30 children on phenytoin therapy. At the onset of the trial, three-fourths had phenytoin levels of less than 10 mg/liter. With the aid of monitoring serum levels, it was possible to reduce this number to one-fifth. Thirteen of the children with inadequate levels had seizures; after correction of the dosage, eleven became seizure-free. Of 100 patients first seen at an outpatient department of our Institute, 56 had very low serum levels of one or more antiepileptic drugs, in particular phenytoin, and 13 had levels in the toxic range.

Buchthal et al. (1960) published a short-term prospective study on the value of measuring diphenylhydantoin (DPH) levels. Their findings have been corroborated by Lund (1974) in a 3-year study. The mean plasma DPH level during the first year of observation was 6.1 ± 2.9 mg/liter, and the mean number of generalized tonic-clonic seizures during that year was 5.8 per patient. The corresponding figures for the second year were 11.7 ± 3.3 mg/liter and 4.1 generalized tonic-clonic seizures, and for the third year 15.0 ± 2.5 mg/liter and 1.6 generalized tonic-clonic seizures.

Sherwin et al. (1973) noticed that monitoring of the level of ethosuximide increased the percentage of control to 81%, whereas without this help only 64%

TABLE 2. *Percentage control of seizures with antiepileptic medication*

Source	Complete control (%)	Partial control (%)	No control (%)
National Epilepsy League (1955)	50	35	15
Justis (1962)	48	37	15
Thomas (1962)	50	30	20
Lundervold and Jabbour (1962)	——83——		17
Fukuyama et al. (1963)	53	36	12
Bratanov and Kerekovski (1970)	70	14	16
1972 NINDS Research Profiles	60	——40——	

From Epilepsy Foundation of America (1975).

TABLE 3. *Comparison of seizure-free and uncontrolled patients on phenytoin therapy*

	Seizure-free	Uncontrolled
Patients	34 (13 F, 21 M)	38 (14 F, 24 M)
Mean age	34.9 years	35.0 years
Mean age at onset of epilepsy	18.7 years	25.6 years
DPH mg/kg ± SD	5.2 ± 1.5	4.9 ± 1.4
Etiology	26 cryptogenic	24 cryptogenic
	8 symptomatic	14 symptomatic
Seizures	20 focal	22 focal
	14 generalized	16 generalized
Serum level ± SD (mg/liter)	20.6 ± 11.0	19.7 ± 12.0
Patients	10/34 (3 F, 7 M)	23/38 (10 F, 13 M)
Serum level	< 15 mg/liter	> 15 mg/liter

From E. Dörrscheidt (1973).

had achieved freedom from seizures. On the other hand, in the case of sodium valproate, Meinardi et al. (1974) found a wide range of serum levels in patients who had achieved a 50% reduction in seizures after the addition of sodium valproate. Elisabeth Dörrscheidt (1973) found no significant differences between two groups of patients who were, respectively, seizure-free and still suffering from seizures (Table 3).

In fact, to quantify the epilepsies would require individualized studies, each patient serving as his own control. However, the period since the introduction of the determination of antiepileptic drugs in body fluids has also seen the adoption of other approaches toward the management of the epilepsies.

The average patient under our care still takes three drugs. The usual annual cost per patient on an average medication of three drugs and a bimonthly evaluation of serum levels amounts to Dfl. 360.-. The annual cost of the medication itself, if phenobarbital, phenytoin, and carbamazepine are given, is approximately Dfl. 500.-, whereas a combination of carbamazepine, sodium valproate, and primidone requires an annual expenditure of approximately Dfl. 1,200.-. It is therefore debatable whether it would be ethically possible to start a prospective study with alternate allocation of patients to a group managed without information about serum levels and to one with regular monitoring.

It is usually stated that information to the patient about serum level monitoring increases compliance. Of 367 patients seen at one of our outpatient clinics regularly, 4 had very low or unestimable serum levels. Three of these refused hospitalization for further analysis, even though they continued to visit the clinics and reported frequent seizures. It is under consideration whether a pharmacologically indifferent marker may perhaps be added to the medication. A low dose of lithium carbonate would offer a solution.

Even though achievement of seizure control is a primary goal for the epileptologist, there are clear indications that for the well-being of the patient this is a necessary but not sufficient condition.

LONG-TERM CARE OF THE EPILEPSIES

Many studies (Table 4)—and to the ones presented here may be added the epidemiological studies of Zieliński (1974) and the one by Hakkarainen (1973) —have stressed the fact that the situation with respect to seizures does not correlate with the social status of the patient. Perhaps we should therefore speak not of long-term control of seizures but of long-term care of the epilepsies. On the other hand, it might be argued that to speak of long-term care of the epilepsies is in fact a pleonasm, as all care for people with epilepsy is a long-term proposition. Even further objections can be raised against such a statement. Isn't it rather archaic and prepossessing to state that care is taken of people with epilepsy? Haven't we evolved sufficiently to realize the deleterious effect of the passivity to which the ailing person is reduced if the professionals insist on caretaking from the first encounter of the patient with the caretaker until the undertaker takes over? Briefly, "long-term help" for people with epilepsy is, we think, the most appropriate connotation.

One might ask: If I were suffering from epilepsy, what type of help would I be looking for? First, I would want to be sure of the diagnosis and possible etiological factors. Second, I would like to know the consequences of this affliction, both now and in the long run. Third, I would insist on receiving the best treatment available with a minimum of inconvenience.

Diagnosis and Etiology

At first sight, the establishment of the diagnosis seems a matter of immediate help. However, it is well known that among patients first booked as suffering from idiopathic epilepsy an appreciable number are, unfortunately, found to have a cerebral tumor. Müller (1965) claimed that 123 of 346 patients suffering from tumors with seizures had been diagnosed as having idiopathic epilepsy for over a year. Among 280 people with epilepsy, Huber and Eichenberger (1963) found a tumor in 12 patients with a history of epilepsy over 3 years. Loiseau and co-workers (1976) recently subjected 200 people with partial epilepsy to computerized tomography and revealed 20 tumors, of which 13 were astrocytomas. It is not always the obvious case with evident partial epilepsy. Gall and co-workers (1976) found 8.3% malignancies in 120 patients with different types of epilepsy.

Case Report

Miss v. d. O., a schoolteacher with a fairly strict Roman Catholic upbringing, went to Uganda at the age of 30 as a Peace Corps volunteer. She had been in Uganda for only a few months when she fainted during church services. It is not

TABLE 4. *The relationship of selected variables to successful employment*

Source	Intel-ligence	Psycho-motor skills	Social attitudes (mental) health	EEG abnor-mality	Age of onset	Frequency of seizures	Special or normal education	Other disabil-ities	Success-ful work history	Seizure type
Rodin et al. (1972)	+	+	+	−	−				+	
Michigan Epilepsy Center (Rodin, 1968)	+	+		−		0	+		+	0
Juul-Jensen (1963)			+			0				
Schwartz and Dennerll (1966)			+			0	+ +			0
Schlesinger (1966)	+	+	+			+	+ +			
Dennerll et al. (1966)	+	+	+ +	−			+ +	−	+ +	
Dennerll (1970)	+	+	+ +	−		0	+	−	+ +	0
De Torres et al. (1962)						+ +				0
Goodglass et al. (1963)				0		+				0

+ indicates a positive relationship; − indicates a negative relationship; 0 indicates no relationship.
From Epilepsy Foundation of America (1975).

known whether she had a generalized tonic-clonic seizure or not. Anyway, she did bite her tongue and remembers that she recovered but a few hours after the event. There was no reason to suspect a hypoglycemic seizure as she had had an adequate breakfast. A similar episode occurred once more. She returned to the Netherlands and saw a general neurologist. About a year later she took a job as a teacher in a school for gypsies and vagabonds in The Hague and came under our care. The EEG, apart from some diffuse irregularities, was essentially normal. Psychological testing showed her to be of an adequate intelligence with respect to her job. Her personality, however, appeared to be dysharmonic, with certain infantilistic traits and emotional ambiguities. She could be expected to create for herself situations in life with which she could not cope. Conversion hysteric reactions might ensue. At her visits to the outpatient clinic, she complained about occasional brief lapses of consciousness. She was not sure whether the children at school noticed them; anyway, they did not tell her so. Then she reported another "fainting" spell and it was decided to take her in for a full analysis.

General neurological examination, including fundoscopy, was without abnormalities, cerebrospinal fluid findings were normal, and EEGs with sleep provocation presented sharp waves and steep slow waves in the left temporal region. A pneumoencephalogram showed enlarged frontal horns, the left frontal horn being also flattened and displaced toward the right. This was about 2 years after the initial seizure. She was referred to the neurosurgeon.

On operation an astrocytoma, grade II, was found in the left temporal region and was partly excised. Within a year a second operation was necessary, which the patient did not survive.

Immediate and Long-Term Consequences

This case history takes us to the second question: What are the immediate and long-term consequences of being afflicted with seizures? It is obvious that it is almost impossible to answer this question. Yet each doctor has to meet this challenge to the best of his ability. Of course, the answer is related to the age of the patient at the onset of the epilepsy as well as to its etiology, its severity, and the socioeconomic circumstances.

There is a dictum that primary generalized epilepsy carries a favorable prognosis; nonetheless, we all know the cases that Gastaut so aptly describes as *petit mal qui tourne mal*. There is some indication that this group is characterized at a later stage by having both generalized and focal irritative activity in the EEG, the focal activity localized in one or both temporal lobes. There is still no consensus whether these cases present primary generalized epilepsy with secondary focalization or whether they are in fact cases with secondary bilateral synchrony.

From the data on the incidence of epilepsy, nearly half of the epilepsies have their onset before the age of 20. If all cases of febrile convulsions are also taken into consideration, this number is greatly increased. Hartlage and co-workers (1972) discussed the impression shared by many professionals that epileptic children are typically more dependent than children with other types of disability, even though some of the other disabilities were experienced as more handicapping than epilepsy (Barsch, 1968). Their own data supported the greater dependency, but no correlation with parental or clinical variables emerged from this study. Nevertheless, several authors (Harlin, 1965; Ounsted, 1970) feel the oversolicitous family to be an important factor. Ounsted succinctly expresses the situation as hyperpedophilia. Taylor (1976) recently explained that Ounsted did not imply over- or hyperreactivity of the parents toward their child's disorder. The reaction in itself is normal. He most vividly described the shock to the uninitiated parents when confronted with the first seizure of their child.

Both Sedman (1966) and Oostdam and van Zijl (1971) found considerable emotional reaction of adults with epilepsy toward their affliction. The reaction was not so much fear of having seizures as it was a sense of loss of their former expectations and the shattering of their plans for the future. The women in particular, but also the men, experienced fear of the attitudes of their environment toward epilepsy. Studies have been published about the change in attitudes toward epilepsy by Caveness et al. (1974). Nevertheless, apart from more subtle mechanisms, there is sufficient reason for an epileptic to become depressed and doubt the future. So many books—especially books that are relatively accessible to the layman, such as encyclopedias and textbooks on nursing—still quote the concept of an "epileptic character."

Epileptologists have not sufficiently clarified this point. It is one thing to analyze the different factors at play (Fig. 1), another to estimate the importance of each factor in the final result. Only then can a strategy be developed to remedy or prevent an undesirable outcome.

Drugs do have side effects, both dose-related toxic effects and idiosyncratic reactions. Some toxic effects are quite insidious, such as the influence of antiepileptic drugs on steroid metabolism due to induction of the mixed oxidase enzyme system, as witnessed, for example, by disturbance of calcium metabolism. Even if one maintains optimal drug therapy and avoids intoxication by adequate monitoring of serum levels, unwanted side effects may accumulate over the years. Thus, a patient would like to be convinced of the *necessity* to take the drugs his physician prescribes for him. He would like to know whether the benefits and the side effects of anticonvulsant drug combinations are greater or less than those of single-drug therapy. Indeed, will the benefits of therapy outweigh the *hazards* of chronic side effects, not to mention the inconvenience of taking pills daily for many years? As it is, we find ourselves embarrassed to discover that these questions cannot be answered adequately.

In *Meyler's Side Effects of Drugs,* Mindham (1975) has recently reviewed the literature on anticonvulsant drug side effects, contained in 81 articles published from 1971 to 1975. Female patients will be disappointed to learn that the effects of anticonvulsant drugs on the fetus are still not understood. They should, however, be informed that barbiturates can stimulate the inactivation of estrogenic and progestational hormones, including oral contraceptive agents.

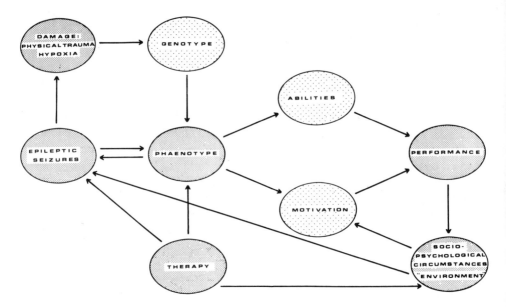

FIG. 1. Interaction of seizures and performance.

Long-term side effects are associated with phenobarbital and phenytoin therapy and include connective tissue changes such as Dupuytren contracture, coars-
ening of the features, gingival hyperplasia, and osteopathic changes, osteoporosis,
and rickets. There have been reports of cerebellar atrophy, lymphoid reactions,
raised serum copper levels, and increased plasma cholesterol in association with
phenytoin therapy.

The newer anticonvulsant drugs, such as the benzodiazepines, carbamazepine,
and sodium valproate, are felt by many to have fewer untoward effects than the
drugs we have discussed. However, a longer experience is clearly needed before
we can say what the chronic toxic effects may be. Blood dyscrasias, skin reactions,
and vasopressin-like actions have already been reported for carbamazepine, and
gastrointestinal disturbances, diminished aggregation of thrombocytes, and alo-
pecia areata have been observed in the case of sodium valproate.

The interaction of anticonvulsant drugs has been recognized recently as an
important factor that complicates polytherapy. Interactions between barbiturates
and hydantoinates are widely recognized. Other studies report increased break-
down of hydantoinates after the addition of carbamazepine (Hansen et al., 1971)
and precipitation of hydantoinate toxicity by diazepam (Valjda et al., 1971).

Surgical Treatment

If one would like to receive the best treatment of one's epilepsy with the least
inconvenience, one is apt to ask the epileptologist what chances there would be

TABLE 5. *Comparison of the outcome of various neurosurgical techniques*

Technique	No. of patients	Seizure-free (%)	Improved		Unchanged/worse (%)	Success rate (%)
			Greatly (%)	Moderately (%)		
Temporal lobectomy	> 2,034	36	26	9	29	62
Local excision in focal epilepsy	841	38	21	9	32	59
Hemispherectomy	155	68	7	6	19	75
Amygdalotomy	150	36	18	19	27	54
Campotomy	85	33	23	22	17	61
Methods Bancaud and Talairach	?	?	?	20	20	60
Combined techniques	77	24	35	25	16	59
Fornicotomy	36	14	39	11	36	53

From Sonnen (1971).

of an operation. A few years ago, Sonnen (1971) collected data from the literature, which are stated in Table 5.

Three neurosurgical centers in the Netherlands and the special centers for epilepsy have established a preview committee to assess the indications for operation. In its first year, 1972, three cases were presented, of which one was accepted for operation and became seizure-free. In 1973, six cases were presented and three accepted; one became seizure-free. In 1974, eight were presented, five accepted, and two became seizure-free. In 1975, five were presented and none was accepted. The reason is quite clear. The present attitude of epileptologists is: no operation before all pharmacotherapeutic possibilities have been tried and have failed.

CONCLUSION

In summary, when one has one's first seizure, one will receive few or no satisfactory answers to the four basic questions that one is going to ask: What exactly is the matter with me? What are the consequences? What is the best treatment available? How can I cope with my new phenotype?

The lack of answers will be an additional stress and one will expect from one's doctor that, even though he does not know the exact answers, he should at least be well trained in neurology, psychiatry, clinical pharmacology of antiepileptic drugs, clinical neurophysiology, and neurochemistry. In fact, "the lack of knowledge about epilepsy calls for the training of epileptologists."

REFERENCES

Barsch, R. H. (1968): *The Parent of the Handicapped Child*. Charles C Thomas, Springfield, Ill.

Buchthal, F., Svensmark, O., and Schiller, P. J. (1960): Clinical and electroencephalographic correlations with serum levels of diphenylhydantoin. *Arch. Neurol.*, 2:624–630.

Caveness, W. F., Merritt, H. H., and Gallup, G. H., Jr. (1974): A survey of public attitudes toward epilepsy in 1974. With an indication of trends over the past twenty-five years. *Epilepsia,* 15:523–536.
Dawson, K. P., and Jamieson, A. (1971): Value of blood phenytoin estimation in management of childhood epilepsy. *Arch. Dis. Child.,* 46:386–388.
Dörrscheidt, E. (1973): Ueber die Serumkonzentration von Diphenylhydantoin in der Epilepsiebehandlung. Thesis, Heidelberg.
Epilepsy Foundation of America (1975): *Basic Statistics on the Epilepsies.* F. A. Davis, Philadelphia.
Gall, M. v., Becker, H., Hacker, H., and Maxion, H. (1976): Computerized tomography in epilepsy diagnosis. In: *Epileptology,* Proceedings of the Seventh International Symposium on Epilepsy, Berlin (West), June 1975, edited by D. Janz, pp. 357–363. Thieme/PSG, Stuttgart.
Hakkarainen, H. (1973): Rehabilitation of patients with epilepsy. *Acta Univ. Ouluensis,* Series D, Medica 5, Oulu.
Hansen, J. M., Siersbaek-Nielsen, K., and Skovsted, L. (1971): Carbamazepine-induced acceleration of diphenylhydantoin and warfarin metabolism in man. *Clin. Pharmacol. Ther.,* 12:539.
Harlin, V. (1965): Experiences with epileptic children in a public school program. *J. School Health,* 35:20–24.
Hartlage, L. C., Green, J. B., and Offutt, L. (1972): Dependency in epileptic children. *Epilepsia,* 13:27–30.
Huber, P., and Eichenberger, M. (1963): Die Indikation zur neuroradiologischen Untersuchung von Patienten mit langdauerndem Anfallsleiden. *Schweiz. Med. Wochenschr.,* 93:616–620.
Janz, D., and Sommer-Burkhardt, E.-M. (1976): Discontinuation of antiepileptic drugs in patients with epilepsy who have been seizure free for more than two years. In: *Epileptology,* Proceedings of the Seventh International Symposium on Epilepsy, Berlin (West), June 1975, edited by D. Janz, pp. 228–234. Thieme/PSG, Stuttgart.
Loiseau, P., Caille, J. M., Jallon, P., and Constant, P. (1976): L'encéphalotomographie axiale transverse traitée par ordinateur dans les épilepsies partielles. *Rev. Neurol. (Paris),* 132:363.
Lund, L. (1974): Anticonvulsant effect of diphenylhydantoin relative to plasma levels. *Arch. Neurol.,* 31:289–294.
Meinardi, H., Hanke, N.F.J., and van Beveren, J. (1974): Sodium di-*n*-propylacetate: Estimation of effective serum levels. *Pharm. Weekbl.,* 109:45–47.
Mindham, R. H. S. (1975): Anticonvulsants. In: *Meyler's Side Effects of Drugs,* edited by M. N. G. Dukes, pp. 99–113. Excerpta Medica, Amsterdam.
Müller, N. (1965): Die Bedeutung des epileptischen Anfalles für die Diagnose einer organischen Hirnerkrankung. *Dtsch. Med. Wochenschr.,* 90:1852–1855.
Oller-Daurella, L., Pamies, R., and Oller F. V. L. (1976): Reduction or discontinuance of antiepileptic drugs in patients seizure-free for more than 5 years. In: *Epileptology,* Proceedings of the Seventh International Symposium on Epilepsy, Berlin (West), June 1975, edited by D. Janz, pp. 218–227. Thieme/PSG, Stuttgart.
Oostdam, E. M. M., and van Zijl, C. H. W. (1971): Epilepsie: Meningen van epileptici. Internal report, Heemstede.
Ounsted, C. (1970): Hyperpaedophilia. The reaction of normal families to children with epilepsy and associated handicaps. 3rd European Symposium on Epilepsy, Marienlyst, Denmark.
Rodin, E. (1968): *The Prognosis of Patients with Epilepsy.* Charles C Thomas, Springfield, Ill.
Sedman, G. (1966): Being an epileptic. A phenomenological study of epileptic experience. *Psychiatr. Neurol. (Basel),* 152:1–16.
Sherwin, A. L., Robb, J. P., and Lechter, M. (1973): Improved control of epilepsy by monitoring plasma ethosuximide. *Arch. Neurol.,* 28:178–181.
Sonnen, A. E. H. (1971): De operatieve behandelingen van epilepsie. Internal report, Breda.
Taylor, D. (1976): The developmental psychiatry of epilepsy. Paper read at the Oxford meeting "Children with Epilepsy," March, 1976.
Valjda, F. J. E., Prineas, R. J., and Lovell, R. R. H. (1971): Interaction between phenytoin and benzodiazepines. *Br. Med. J.,* 1:346.
Zieliński, J. J. (1974): Epidemiology and medical-social problems of epilepsy in Warsaw. Psychoneurological Institute, Warsaw.

Epilepsy, The Eighth International Symposium,
edited by J. K. Penry. Raven Press, New York
© 1977.

Implications of Long-Term Follow-up Studies in Epilepsy:
With a Note on the Cause of Death

D. C. Taylor and S. M. Marsh

*Human Development Research Unit, Park Hospital for Children,
Headington, Oxford OX3 7LQ, England*

Follow-up studies of particular groups of patients are devices that help to clarify the effects of treatments and elucidate the natural history of a disorder. The group under study can be very closely defined; the continuing need for analysis keeps a strong rapport between patient and researcher, which improves the quality of the data; any classification errors in the material are made plain; useful classifications emerge. Personal experience of several long-term follow-up studies of patients with epilepsy has raised issues that relate to prevalence studies, incidence studies, and attrition rates as well as to methodological issues in follow-up studies themselves. These will be discussed in relation to a recent study of deaths following anterior temporal lobectomy.

This study was undertaken to determine whether the lobectomy operation itself was related to subsequent deaths or whether any of the variables of powerful effect, such as age at onset, age at operation, side, or pathological changes in the resected lobe, had any value in postoperative prognosis. In particular, it was concerned with the suicide rate which had previously been estimated at 5% per mean 5 years of follow-up (Taylor and Falconer, 1968). There were suggestions early in this work that depressive episodes often followed lobectomy (Hill et al., 1957) and theoretical reasons to believe this might be worse after nondominant temporal lobectomy (Flor Henry, 1974).

METHOD

At the close (with his retirement) of Murray Falconer's series of patients at the Guys Maudsley Neurosurgical Unit, 296 patients had undergone anterior temporal lobectomy between 1951 and 1975. This study started during 1974 and proceeded until the series closed. Routine follow-up procedures in the unit were tight so that the review concentrated on patients not seen since 1970 for whatever reason. Thirty patients who were abroad were excluded from further consideration, and nine patients could not be traced. The 193 patients who were operated before 1970 and who had a potential survival of at least 5 years form the main group under study.

Hospital and general practitioners' records were used to ascertain the causes of death, but recourse was taken to death certificates and to the findings of Coroner's Courts when necessary. The "official" explanation of death was considered in the light of its probability.

Six categories of death emerged:

1. Death as a late effect of the small tumor found by chance in the resected lobe.
2. Death by natural causes unrelated to the epilepsy.
3. Death in epilepsy.
4. Death in "unclear" circumstances.
5. Death by suicide.
6. Postoperative death and accident.

RESULTS

A total of 39 deaths were known, so the minimal death rate would be 39 of 296 patients. However, 39 patients were excluded, giving 39 deaths in 269 patients. Of the 193 patients operated before 1970, 37 had died. Only these 37 deaths are analyzed further.

Tumors (N = 4)

Two patients, 35 and 36 years of age, died 8 and 7 years after their lobectomy, but another patient 51 years of age at operation survived 15 years and another 56 years of age survived 19 years before late death due to tumor invasion.

Natural Causes (N = 7)

All these deaths took place under the age of 55 years, the youngest being at the age of 37, of respiratory disease. Cancer and heart disease were the usual causes of death.

Death in Epilepsy (N = 8)

All eight deaths occurred from uncontrollable status epilepticus. One death occurred in a children's home, one in a prison, the remainder in hospitals.

Death in "Unclear" Circumstances (N = 6)

Although the coroner or the attending doctor was satisfied that there was an explanation for the death other than suicide, patients were placed in this category when the circumstances of their deaths were anomalous or the evidence equivocal. These patients were found dead in bed, drowned at sea, and in the bath. There was no evidence given in regard to poisoning.

Death by Suicide (N = 9)

In nine cases the cause of death was unequivocally suicide. Six of the nine poisoned themselves.

Postoperative Deaths and Accidents (N = 3)

These were two postoperative deaths and one death by accident in which the circumstances were clearly known.

Age

The patients' ages at the onset of epilepsy and at operation have been previously shown to be strongly associated with outcome. In this analysis the year in which the operation was performed and the age at death were also considered. Only statistically significant results are mentioned. After 1960, during a period lasting about a decade, there were more deaths by suicide and in "unclear" circumstances. Patients who died in epilepsy or by suicide were more likely to be aged under 35 at operation. These patients died younger than those dying of tumors or by natural causes. The interval between operation and death was shorter for those dying by suicide or in "unclear" circumstances than from tumors or natural causes. Patients who died by natural causes experienced more years of preoperative epilepsy (27.0 years) than other groups, "unclear" circumstances (15.9 years); suicide (12.6 years); epilepsy (11.6 years); and tumors (5.5 years).

One-third of the population, 64 patients, underwent operation under 20 years of age, of whom 12 (18.8%) died; 63 patients underwent operation between the ages of 21 and 30, of whom 5 (7.9%) died; and 66 patients were over 30 at operation, of whom 20 (30.3%) died.

The age at onset of epilepsy was without notable effect.

Length of Follow-up

Of the 37 deaths, 11 occurred within 2 years of operation and 27 within 10 years. The mortality of the first 2 postoperative years was nearly double that in any subsequent 2 years.

Side Operated

The side operated was without effect.

Pathological Findings

Apart from the tumor group, no other type of pathological changes had an effect on the mode of death.

Age at Death and Mode of Death

The purpose of Fig. 1 is to illustrate some of the many complexities in the analysis of this type of material. First, the age of the patients at operation ranged from 2.5 to 58 years, and the potential length of follow-up from 5 to 24 years. The study cases were assembled over a 19-year period, and selection criteria changed with experience over that time in ways that were, at the time, not always obvious. It is difficult to know how to express or interpret "risk."

The two vectors age at operation and survival allow for a resultant which is natural aging. Age at the time of follow-up or at death can be determined in "bands" on the figure.

Death Under 20 Years

Three impulsive suicides, the one known accident, and one death in epilepsy 7 years after operation occurred under the age of 20.

Death Between 20 and 30 Years

Seven of the eight "epilepsy" deaths occurred in this decade. Four of these patients underwent operation under 20 years of age and survived into this decade. No patient over 30 died of status epilepticus.

Death Between 30 and 40 Years

All six remaining suicides occurred in patients aged between 30 and 40. The total suicide risk is about 50 times the expectation and is at its peak in the decade prior to its peak in the general population. This might be due to their being an extremely disturbed group aggregating high loadings of "suicide factors" such as isolation, bereavement, divorced or single status, physical illnesses, or aging. Bitter disappointment at a failed operation or "loss of an old friend" (Ferguson and Reyport, 1965) with its success should be considered. Half the patients who died by suicide had had no fits since their operation.

Even so, some "organic" basis in the sense suggested by earlier studies is not ruled out.

Deaths over 40

The causes of most of these deaths were understandable.

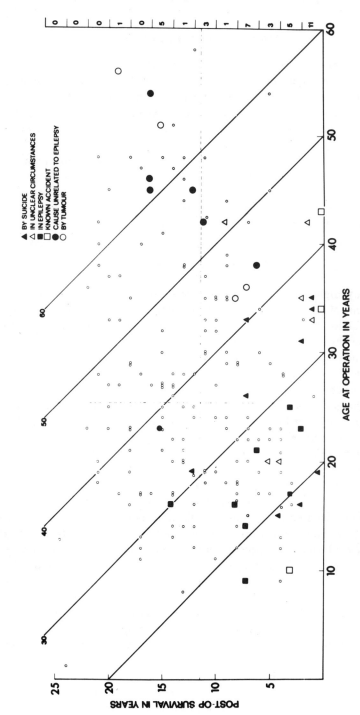

FIG. 1. Survival after temporal lobectomy showing age at operation and death.

Deaths in Unclear Circumstances

These deaths can now be looked at in the light of the above analyses. Two patients who underwent operation at 20 died 4 and 5 years after operation. No mode of death other than death by epilepsy occurred during that decade. One boy was found dead in bed and one drowned at sea. Although the young man who drowned had been incautious, in neither case was there any reason not to believe that a fit might have caused the deaths.

Two deaths in the 30 to 40 band were more doubtful. One man, grossly mother-attached to an increasingly frail woman, had just taken out life and funeral insurance. The other was a priest whose sudden mysterious renal failure might have been induced by drug overdosage.

The two later deaths were mysterious in any terms.

DISCUSSION

The study might simply be viewed as a necessary stage in following the outcome of treatment of temporal lobe epilepsy by lobectomy. As such, it suggests first the vulnerability to lethal status of those patients who came to require the treatment under the age of 25. In addition, it highlights the serious psychiatric states found in such a population and the need for a psychiatrist in their management. Indeed, those patients who survived 2 years before their suicide were all maintained in psychiatric care.

But perhaps some general lessons can be learned from the practice of following patients carefully over long periods of time to see the unfolding of their disorder. Experience of a follow-up of children with epilepsy over 25 years undertaken at the same time (Harrison and Taylor, 1976) suggested that there, too, the early attrition was the most severe and the deaths of the youngest patients were due to deaths in epilepsy. The later deaths came from more complex associations with the seizure disorder. In both instances projections of the manner and extent of late mortality from early mortality would have been quite wrong. The studies also show that close follow-up must be maintained and no satisfactory global projection can be made for people lost to follow-up. When all patients have been followed to their death, there will be two slopes on the attrition curve, of which only the first will relate directly to our understanding of the disorders giving rise to the epilepsy.

The strange experience of finding, in two long-term follow-up studies, that most of the deaths were concentrated near the beginning of the follow-up and the chances of dying grew less as the population grew older gave me reason for serious thought. Although at first it seems unlikely, it is actuarially correct that the older one is the better the chances of surviving to any given older age. It is also logically likely that the deaths among a group of people identified through serious illness will be maximal near the beginning of a follow-up. This is because those likely to die of their disorder do and the rest of the group live, only later on succumbing to random causes of death. This is also true for the natural population of newborns.

There is an issue that concerns those of us gathered under the rubric of Epilepsy. Granted almost any statement based on any given type of clinical experience, an inner (or another) voice asks: But is the population representative? And I want to address myself to that. Of what should the population under study be representative? Epidemiology was properly the study of epidemics. There has been no epidemic of epilepsy. What was intended for epidemiology was to show the spread of a contagion, or the late consequences of an event (such as exposure to asbestos), or the distribution or incidence of some durable state of affairs. Although one can reasonably ask the point prevalence of cholera, asbestosis, or muscular dystrophy by collecting all the cases known to exist in a given population today, such a study for a behavior such as epilepsy is logically absurd. Because it is and because we insist on doing it just the same, or imagining that we can, we continue to be jarred by the possibility of generalizing from almost any given clinical finding.

Suppose I collect from the population of Oxfordshire all of the people actually convulsing at this moment. First, the prevalence would be low; second, the mortality would be unusually high. Instead, we might collect all of the people who have had a fit during the last week. The prevalence would increase and relative mortality would decrease because those whose fit last week proved lethal would be nonresponders; similarly, if we defined as "epileptic" those having had a fit in the last year, or 2, or indeed 30 years. "Epilepsy" in some definitions really means identifying an expectation; the expectation that another fit will occur. I know of no parallel to this.

The only way I can see of achieving a representative population is to collect and follow all those people in a given population who experience their first fit. At least that would give doctors the same view of the prognosis of epilepsy as is held in the group experience of the people we serve. Otherwise we necessarily fail to comprehend epilepsy since the people we know with epilepsy spend vastly variable lengths of time in that condition and are either caught up or not in the nets of our epidemiology depending entirely on the size we choose to make the holes. Does any clinical practice, for example, really feel in touch with all the available patients who have had a fit in the last, say, 5 years—keeping in mind, of course, the patients who have died? Probably not. What represents epilepsy to the physician is that experience drawn from whatever segment of the population served by their clinic, who are presently in active treatment for their disorder as defined by the length of time between fits which the doctor deems sufficient to warrant supervision and who are not precluded from his clinic on behavioral grounds.

Small wonder that our experiences differ, that we regard those different experiences as arcane, other people's findings unsound bases for generalizations, and the implications of suffering epilepsy as relatively slight.

The alternative strategy more often preferred is to work on populations defined through seizure type. Despite excellent work in this area it seems to me that the more we learn on this basis the more unsound seizure types become as bases for prognosis. Consider the variety incorporated in "neonatal seizures," "infantile spasms," or "temporal lobe epilepsy." Another device that is clinically sound but scientifically useless is to incorporate prognosis in the definition, as has been done in the case of febrile convulsions in some instances and in benign focal epilepsy of childhood (Lerman and Kivity, 1975). (Presumably any case that proved not to be benign would cease to be an instance.)

The virtue of follow-up studies is that what constitutes an instance to be followed up, if soundly and comprehensively defined at the beginning so as to be intelligible to others, cannot cease to be an instance because we do not like the way it is turning out. Those who die are not lost to us, neither are those who improve to the point of no longer suffering, and those whose chronic burden moves them to insalubrious places like mental hospitals or other institutions. Through follow-up studies we might derive what we really need to know: the factors that significantly alter the outlook for any given individual seeking our help and advice.

ACKNOWLEDGMENTS

The study was supported by the Clinical Medicine Board of the University of Oxford. Mr. Peter Schurr kindly permitted continuation of our study. Dr. C. Bruton and Dr. J. A. N. Corsellis provided neuropathological evidence. Dr. A. Barr gave statistical assistance. Dr. J. Lindsay and Dr. C. Ounsted helpfully commented on the manuscript.

REFERENCES

Ferguson, S. M., and Rayport, M. (1965): The adjustment to living without epilepsy. *J. Nerv. Ment. Dis.,* 140:26–37.
Flor Henry, P. (1974): Pyschosis, neurosis and epilepsy. *Br. J. Psychiatry,* 124:144–150.
Harrison, R. M., and Taylor, D. C. (1976): Childhood seizures: a 25-year follow-up. *Lancet,* 1:948–951.
Hill, J. D., Pond, D. A., Mitchell, W., and Falconer, M. A. (1957): Personality changes following temporal lobectomy for epilepsy. *J. Ment. Sci.,* 103:18–27.
Lerman, P., and Kivity, S. (1975): Benign focal epilepsy of childhood. *Arch. Neurol.,* 32:261–264.
Taylor, D. C., and Falconer, M. A. (1968): Clinical, socio-economic and psychological changes after temporal lobectomy for epilepsy. *Br. J. Psychiatry,* 114:1247–1261.

Epilepsy, The Eighth International Symposium,
edited by J. K. Penry. Raven Press, New York
© 1977.

Experience in the Long-Term Use of Carbamazepine (Tegretol®) in the Treatment of Epilepsy

M. N. Hassan and M. J. Parsonage

Neurological Department, General Infirmary at Leeds and the Neuropsychiatric Unit (Special Centre for Epilepsy), Bootham Park Hospital, York, England

The reported results of the treatment of epilepsy with carbamazepine have, in general, been consistently favorable. Furthermore, the drug's relative freedom from serious adverse effects has often been emphasized, although reports about its psychotropic effect have been conflicting.

Of late there have been two further trends in the history of the use of carbamazepine. First, the number of published controlled trials with pharmacological data has increased (Rodin et al., 1974; Cereghino et al., 1974; Simonsen et al., 1975). Second, more information about its long-term effects has become available (Bonduelle, 1973).

In this chapter we report our experience in the long-term use of carbamazepine in the treatment of generalized and partial epilepsies in 254 adults.

PATIENTS AND METHODS

Classification of the epilepsies in all cases was based on a combination of clinical and EEG findings. There were 186 patients (88 males and 98 females) with partial epilepsies. Of these, 53 had seizures with simple symptomatology that was associated with secondary generalization in 42, and 122 had seizures with complex symptomatology associated with secondary generalization in 82 cases. In the remaining 11 patients, the EEG revealed sources of seizure discharge in one or both temporal lobes, the seizures being clinically generalized from the onset.

Epilepsies were generalized in 68 patients (37 males and 31 females). These epilepsies were primary in 17 and of the secondary variety in 45 cases; in the remaining 6 the epilepsies were unclassifiable because of insufficient data (Table 1).

Figure 1 shows the age ranges when treatment with carbamazepine was started. Of the 129 women, 110 were of childbearing age.

The majority of the patients had severe epilepsies of long standing. Thus, in 160 the length of the epileptic history ranged from 10 to 30 years. A total of 60

TABLE 1. *Patients treated with carbamazepine, 1964–1976*

Type of epilepsy	Male	Female	Total
Partial epilepsies			
Simple symptomatology	25	28	53
Complex symptomatology	57	65	122
Partial seizures, secondarily			
generalized	6	5	11
Total	88	98	186
Generalized epilepsies			
Primary	11	6	17
Secondary	23	22	45
Unclassifiable	3	3	6
Total	37	31	68
Grand total	125	129	254

patients were mentally retarded, 30 with generalized epilepsies (chiefly secondary generalized) and 30 with partial epilepsies (chiefly with complex symptomatology).

Before treatment with carbamazepine, 75 patients were having an average of three seizures daily, 65 about three a week, 60 about four a month, and 54 about two a month (Table 2). We found that 60 patients were being treated with a combination of three or four of the commonly used antiepileptic drugs, 114 were on a combination of two drugs, and 75 on a single drug; only 5 patients were not receiving any antiepileptic therapy.

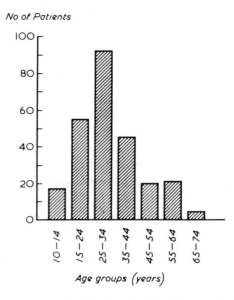

FIG. 1. Age at commencement of treatment with carbamazepine (254 patients).

TABLE 2. *Frequency of seizures before*
treatment with carbamazepine

No. of patients	No. of seizures
75	3/day
65	3/week
60	4/month
54	2/month

The duration of treatment with carbamazepine ranged from 1 to 12 years. In our series 86 patients were treated with carbamazepine for periods ranging from 1 year to just under 2 years, 127 for 2 to 5 years, 35 for 6 to 9 years, and 6 for 10 to 12 years. The initial dose of carbamazepine was 200 mg daily, and this was added to existing medication in all but five cases. The dosage was gradually increased to an average of 1,000 mg daily, and in 10 patients the maximum daily dosage ranged from 2,000 to 2,400 mg.

In addition to clinical and EEG assessment, each patient was subjected to full hematological and biochemical screening before starting treatment with carbamazepine, and in most cases this was repeated at intervals thereafter. Plasma concentrations of carbamazepine were determined on several occasions in most of the patients.

All patients (or a relative) kept a record of the occurrence of all seizures. Most of them had already been doing so for some time and the frequency of seizures during the 6-month period prior to starting treatment with carbamazepine was taken as the base line for assessment.

RESULTS

The results of treatment by the addition of carbamazepine were divided into six categories based on the number of seizures recorded (see Tables 3 and 4).

Partial Epilepsies

The results of treatment with carbamazepine in the partial epilepsies are shown in Table 3. Of the patients with partial epilepsies with simple symptomatology, 11% had no further seizures and 70% had a greater than 50% reduction in seizure frequency. In those with partial epilepsies with complex symptomatology, the corresponding figures were 13% and 54%, respectively. Of the 11 patients with partial seizures secondarily generalized from the onset, 3 had no further seizures and 4 others had more than a 50% reduction in seizure frequency.

Generalized Epilepsies

The response of the generalized epilepsies to carbamazepine is shown in Table 4. Of the patients with primary generalized epilepsy, 12% had no further seizures

TABLE 3. *Results of treatment with carbamazepine: partial epilepsies*

	No. of patients	Reduction in seizures			
		100%	>50%	25–50%	Unchanged or worse
Simple symptomatology					
Aphasic	5	—	3	—	2
Versive	3	1	—	—	2
Motor	18	1	14	—	3
Special sensory/somatosensory	11	—	9	1	1
Autonomic	13	3	4	2	4
Compound	3	1	1		1
Total	53	6	31	3	13
Percentage	100	11	59	6	24
Complex symptomatology					
Impaired consciousness	17	2	5	3	7
Cognitive	7	1	3	—	3
Affective	6	—	6	—	—
Psychosensory	12	2	4	2	4
Psychomotor	34	5	13	6	10
Compound	46	6	19	8	13
Total	122	16	50	19	37
Percentage	100	13	41	16	30
Partial seizures (secondarily generalized)	11	3	4	2	2

TABLE 4. *Results of treatment with carbamazepine: generalized epilepsies*

	No. of patients	Reduction in seizures			
		100%	>50%	25–50%	Unchanged or worse
Primary					
Absences	2	—	1	—	1
Tonic-clonic	6	1	4	—	1
Tonic-clonic + absences	9	1	3	—	5
Total	17	2	8	—	7
Percentage	100	12	47	—	41
Secondary					
Absences	5	—	3	1	1
Tonic-clonic	11	1	2	1	7
Tonic-clonic + absences	16	—	9	1	6
Tonic-clonic + absences + atonic	13	—	5	3	5
Total	45	1	19	6	19
Percentage	100	2	42	13	42
Unclassifiable	6	1	3	—	2

and 59% had a greater than 50% reduction in seizure frequency. Of those with secondary generalized epilepsies, the corresponding figures were 2% and 44%, respectively. Of the 6 patients with generalized epilepsies with inconclusive EEG findings, a single patient had no further seizures and 3 others had a greater than 50% reduction in seizure frequency.

Drug Combinations

Of the 134 patients with partial epilepsies who showed an improvement, 4 received carbamazepine as the first and only antiepileptic agent. In 46 patients, treatment with carbamazepine was more effective and completely replaced previous therapy (three drugs in combination in 9, two drugs in combination in 21, and a single drug in 16 cases). Of the remaining 84 patients in this group, all of whom were on combinations of drugs, two drugs were dispensed with in 10 and one drug in 29 cases. The remaining 45 patients continued with their previous medication in addition to carbamazepine.

Of the 40 patients with generalized epilepsies who showed an improvement, carbamazepine completely replaced previous medication in 16 cases (three drugs in combination in 3, two drugs in combination in 8, and a single drug in 5 cases). In 6 further cases, two drugs in combination and in 7 single drugs were withdrawn. In the remaining 11 the previous medication was continued in addition to carbamazepine.

Duration of Seizure Control

The 110 patients with partial epilepsies who had either no further seizures or a reduction of seizure frequency by over 50% remained in good control for the following lengths of time: 38 patients for 1 to 2 years, 54 for 2 to 4 years, 15 for 5 to 8 years, and 3 for 9 to 12 years (Table 5).

The seizures of the 34 patients with generalized epilepsies who also benefited remained in good control as follows: 4 patients for 1 to 2 years, 16 for 2 to 4 years, 12 for 5 to 8 years, and 2 for 9 to 12 years (Table 5).

It is noteworthy that of the 52 patients with partial epilepsies who at the final

TABLE 5. *Duration of seizure control*

Time (years)	Partial epilepsies[a]	Generalized epilepsies[a]
1–2	38	4
2–4	54	16
5–8	15	12
9–12	3	2
Total	110	34

[a] Patients with 100%, > 50%, or 25–50% reduction in seizures.

assessment had shown no improvement or had become worse, 11 had shown an initial improvement for periods ranging from 6 months to 2 years (average, 1 year). Similarly, of the 28 patients with generalized epilepsies who had not benefited at the final assessment, 6 had shown an initial improvement for periods ranging from 6 to 12 months (average, 9 months).

Plasma Levels

Plasma levels of carbamazepine ranged from 5.0 to 12.5 mg/liter (oral dosage range, 10 to 30 mg/kg).

Additional Effects

Twenty patients reported an improvement in mood or mental function, but all had had some or all of their previous medication withdrawn. The drugs withdrawn most commonly were phenytoin, phenobarbital, and primidone.

Adverse Effects

Of the 254 patients included in this study, 230 of them had had regular blood tests over the years. These revealed no evidence of either hepatotoxic or nephrotoxic effects. In 15 cases, a slight transient fall in white cell counts was observed, but these returned to normal within 2 to 4 months. Of the 110 women of childbearing age, 6 had children while on treatment with carbamazepine, there being no evidence of teratogenicity.

Adverse effects were recorded in 25 cases, as shown in Fig. 2 and Table 6. A low serum folate level was noted in 54 patients; 28 of these were on carbamazepine alone and 26 were on a combination of carbamazepine with other antiepileptic drugs, most commonly phenytoin, phenobarbital, and primidone.

The administration of carbamazepine was discontinued in 27 cases (Table 7). In six of these the drug was withdrawn within a month because of such adverse reactions as a skin rash (three cases), dizziness (two cases), and drowsiness (one case). The remaining 21 cases either showed no improvement or became worse,

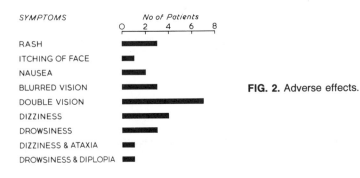

FIG. 2. Adverse effects.

TABLE 6. Adverse effects with dosages

Symptoms	No. of patients	Antiepileptic therapy (daily dose in mg)						
		Carba-mazepine	Etho-suximide	Pheno-barbital	Primidone	Phenytoin	Sulthiame	Sodium valproate
Rash	3	800, 1,200, 200						
Itching of face	1	600		60	750	300		
Nausea	2	200, 800				300		
Blurred vision	3	1,000, 1,200, 1,200	500					
Double vision	7	1,600, 2,400, 1,600, 1,600, 800, 1,000, 2,000		90	750	300		1,200
Dizziness	4	400, 1,200, 1,400, 800		90		350	600	400
Drowsiness	3	400, 1,200, 400			1,000, 500, 1,000	400		
Dizziness and ataxia	1	800				150		
Drowsiness and diplopia	1	1,400			750			

TABLE 7. *Reasons for withdrawal of carbamazepine*

Type of epilepsy	No. of patients	Clinical response	Other reasons for withdrawal
Generalized			
Primary	3	Not assessable	Rash (2); dizziness (1)
	5	Not improved	Drowsiness (1); diplopia (1)
Secondary	2	Not improved	
	2	Worse	Nausea (1)
Partial			
Simple symptomatology	4	Not improved	Dizziness and ataxia (1); drowsiness (1)
Complex symptomatology	3	Not assessable	Dizziness (1); drowsiness (1)
	7	Not improved	Diplopia (1)
	1	Worse	

and 6 of these had also experienced adverse effects (usually drowsiness, dizziness, and blurred or double vision).

DISCUSSION

The recently published controlled trials of the antiepileptic action of carbamazepine have indicated that it is as effective as phenobarbital and phenytoin in controlling psychomotor and convulsive seizures. There is also evidence that it may be effective when used in combination with these drugs (Cereghino et al., 1975), perhaps because plasma concentration of its epoxide derivative may be increased in these circumstances (Dam et al., 1975).

Information about the long-term effects of carbamazepine is also important. There are now a number of reports attesting to its long-term value in maintaining seizure control, to its safety, and to its psychotropic effect. Our own findings in this context do not add anything new; indeed, they are essentially confirmatory of those already reported. We would, however, like to comment on them briefly.

Just over half (57%) of our total series of previously drug-resistant cases have had reasonable control of seizures for periods lasting as long as 12 years in some instances. Of the remainder of our patients, less than a third of them showed either no improvement or a worsening in the control of their seizures, and just over a tenth of them experienced only marginal change for the better.

Such psychotropic effects as were observed could not, in our view, be ascribed with certainty to a direct action of carbamazepine. Indeed, it seemed equally likely that they could be the outcome of better control of seizures or of the withdrawal of other medication, or perhaps even of both factors. Reports in the literature are contradictory about the alleged psychotropic effect of carbamazepine. Those claiming a positive effect seem to be based mainly on clinical impression, whereas attempts at making controlled observations have tended to produce negative results (Rennick et al., 1975). Clearly, there must be reasons for these contradictions and perhaps more account should be taken of the types of patients treated, considering both personality and the type and cause of the epilepsy.

The incidence of adverse effects has been low in our patients. Such minor effects as drowsiness, double vision, and ataxia have generally been dose dependent and reversible or perhaps due to the effects of other drugs. In only six cases was it necessary to withdraw carbamazepine because of unacceptable side effects. Low serum folate levels were sometimes observed in patients on carbamazepine alone, but we have yet to encounter a serious blood dyscrasia. According to Troupin (1976), only 14 reported cases of aplastic anemia are attributable to carbamazepine therapy, and these have mostly occurred in elderly subjects being treated for trigeminal neuralgia. Most commonly, in our experience, the reasons for discontinuation of treatment with carbamazepine have been failure to improve or worsening of the control of seizures.

In conclusion, we would emphasize that our evaluations are based on uncontrolled clinical observations and we realize that our patients might have responded just as well, or as badly, if we had treated them differently. All we can say is that some benefit has accrued to some of them where previously it was lacking and that such benefit has sometimes been long continued. A few of our patients were temporarily incommoded by treatment, but none of them has been harmed seriously.

SUMMARY

A total of 254 patients have been treated with carbamazepine for periods ranging from 1 to 12 years. All but five had intractable epilepsies that were unresponsive to treatment with other antiepileptic agents. There were 186 patients with partial epilepsies, which were associated with secondary generalization of seizures in 135, and 68 patients had generalized epilepsies.

Seizure frequency was reduced by more than 50% in 62% of the patients with partial epilepsies and in 56% of those with generalized epilepsies. Good control of seizures has been maintained in a number of patients for as long as 12 years.

There were no serious adverse reactions. A few minor adverse effects were encountered in 25 patients, but in only 6 was it necessary to withdraw carbamazepine. In a further 21 cases the drug was withdrawn, either because of lack of improvement or because of a worsening of the clinical state. Twenty patients reported an improvement in either mood or mental function.

It is concluded from these observations that carbamazepine can be an effective agent in the treatment of intractable epilepsies of both the partial and the generalized types. Furthermore, control of seizures can be maintained with safety for long periods of time.

ACKNOWLEDGMENTS

We are grateful to Ciba-Geigy, Ltd., for financial help, to our colleagues for clinical assistance, and to Mrs. Jennifer Bedford for secretarial assistance.

REFERENCES

Bonduelle, M. (1973): My study of Tegretol in the treatment of epilepsy. In: *Tegretol in Epilepsy.* Report of an International Symposium, edited by C. A. S. Wink, pp. 80–88. C. Nicholls, Manchester.

Cereghino, J. J., Brock, J. T., Van Meter, J. C., Penry, J. K., Smith, L. D., and White, B. G. (1974): Carbamazepine for epilepsy. *Neurology (Minneap.),* 24:401–410.

Cereghino, J. J., Brock, J. T., Van Meter, J. C., Penry, J. K., Smith, L. D., and White B. G. (1975): The efficacy of carbamazepine combinations in epilepsy. *Clin. Pharmacol. Ther.,* 18:733–741.

Dam, M., Jensen, A., and Christiansen, J. (1975): Plasma level and effect of carbamazepine in grand mal and psychomotor epilepsy. *Acta Neurol. Scand.* [*Suppl.* 60], 52:33–38.

Rennick, P., Keiser, T., Rodin, E., Rim, C., Clifford, C., and Lennox, K. (1975): Carbamazepine (Tegretol): Behavioral side-effects in temporal lobe epilepsy during a short-term comparison with placebo. *Epilepsia,* 16:198.

Rodin, E. A., Rim, C. S., and Rennick, P. M. (1974): The effects of carbamazepine on patients with psychomotor epilepsy: Results of a double-blind study. *Epilepsia,* 15:547–561.

Simonsen, N., Olsen, P. Z., Kuhl, V., Lund, M., and Wendelboe, J. (1975): A double-blind study of carbamazepine and diphenylhydantoin in temporal lobe epilepsy. *Acta Neurol. Scand.* [*Suppl.* 52], 60:39–42.

Troupin, A. (1976): The choice of anticonvulsants—a logical approach to sequential changes—a comment from an American neurologist. In: *Textbook of Epilepsy,* edited by J. Laidlaw and A. Richens, pp. 248–271. Longman, New York.

Epilepsy, The Eighth International Symposium,
edited by J. K. Penry. Raven Press, New York
© 1977.

A Comprehensive Interdisciplinary Approach to the Care of the Institutionalized Person with Epilepsy

Brian P. O'Neill, Barbara Ladon, Linda M. Harris, Harold L. Riley, III, and Fritz E. Dreifuss

Department of Neurology, University of Virginia, Charlottesville, Virginia 22904

Two years ago, the Lynchburg Training School, in conjunction with the Department of Neurology at the University of Virginia Medical Center, instituted a program to upgrade the care of institutionalized patients with epilepsy. Of 3,000 residents in the institution, 892 were identified as suffering from epilepsy. During the second year of the program, the Division of Health Services Research instituted an evaluation of demographic and health-related data on these patients.

The treatment program relied primarily on the use of a nurse specialist in epilepsy who coordinated the care of patients, developed in-service education programs for the staff, and conducted a ward survey of the residents diagnosed as epileptic, that is, approximately one-third of the total institutional population. The epileptic patients were classified as controlled if they had had no seizures for 1 year, partially controlled if they had had at least one seizure but less than four seizures in any one quarter, and uncontrolled if four or more seizures had occurred in any one quarter. Initially, there were 92 patients in the uncontrolled group. It was predicted that as seizure identification improved, this group would enlarge; this hypothesis was fulfilled. However, the uncontrolled group rapidly shrank with the institution of particular attention to its problems. All patients with seizure problems received careful medical evaluations and were seen in weekly seizure clinics staffed by a neurologist. An important part of the service aspect of the program was the provision of diagnostic services and follow-up using GLC blood anticonvulsant level capability, which was developed at the Lynchburg Training School. At the same time, a systematic evaluation program was taking place, and this led to recommendations for future studies based on the experience of the model.

There was no statistical difference in age, race, sex, length of hospitalization, or severity of mental retardation between patients in the controlled and uncontrolled groups. Further analysis by specific medical diagnosis of underlying disorders is proceeding.

In the course of 1 year of study, 39% of uncontrolled patients became seizure-free and a further 21% became partially controlled. Of those identified as partially controlled or controlled, 90% remained within this subgroup. Those patients who were classified in a downward direction subsequently were brought under control within one quarter, and it is believed that the transient increase in the number of patients classified as uncontrolled was the result of increased recognition ability on the part of the hospital staff.

During the program, episodes of status epilepticus numbered 47, whereas in the 2 years prior to the study, this condition occurred in 91 patients. Moreover, in the preceding 2 years 7 patients died of seizure-related causes in a total of 22 deaths, and in the subsequent 2 years only 1 death of a total of 34 was seizure-related. Anticonvulsant drug toxicity was reduced and a number of patients who suffered with uncontrolled seizures during toxicity became controlled with relief of this condition. The overall information level of the nonphysician staff toward epilepsy was raised, referrals to the clinic increased, and accurate categorization of seizure types was instituted. The improvement of clinical state of the residents has provided visible evidence that such an approach can be productive. Many recommendations for translation of such a program to other institutions have been developed for improving the care of the institutionalized epileptic and for providing follow-up evaluation for deinstitutionalized patients.

ACKNOWLEDGMENTS

Funded by the Department of Health, Education, and Welfare, Office of Human Development, Developmental Disabilities Office, Region III. Administered by the University Affiliated Facility, Johns Hopkins University and The John F. Kennedy Institute. Implemented by the Department of Neurology, University of Virginia, Charlottesville, Virginia, with the Lynchburg Training School and also by NINCDS Comprehensive Epilepsy Center Contract NO1-NS-5–2329.

Epilepsy, The Eighth International Symposium,
edited by J. K. Penry. Raven Press, New York
© 1977.

Anticonvulsive and Psychotropic Effects of Carbamazepine in Hospitalized Epileptic Patients: A Long-Term Study

*Amarendra Narayan Singh, *Bishan M. Saxena, and
**Marcel Germain

*Hamilton Psychiatric Hospital, Hamilton, Ontario, Canada and **Ciba Geigy,
Quebec, Canada*

Carbamazepine (Tegretol®) is a derivative of dibenzazepine, namely, 5-carbamoyl-5H-dibenz[b,f]azepine, with the structural formula shown in Fig. 1. The empirical formula is $C_{15}H_{12}N_2O$, which structurally is closer to the tricyclic antidepressants but also resembles to a lesser extent the phenothiazines. Carbamazepine was first introduced by the laboratories of J. R. Geigy, S.A., in 1953, and was first marketed in the United Kingdom in October, 1963. Since then, numerous clinical studies (more than 7,500 published case reports) have confirmed that carbamazepine is an effective and well-tolerated antiepileptic drug that has been found to be particularly efficacious in the treatment and management of grand mal epilepsy, temporal lobe or psychomotor epilepsy, post-traumatic epilepsy, and for the symptomatic relief of pain associated with trigeminal neuralgia, other cranial nerve pain, and atypical headaches. It was established during the early clinical studies that the therapeutic efficacy of this compound was not restricted to epileptic seizures but also extended to the behavioral and personality disorders commonly associated with epilepsy (Lorgé, 1963; Burner et al., 1965; Donner and Frisk, 1965; Martinez-Lage et al., 1965; Schneider et al., 1965; Simpson et al., 1965; Rajotte et al., 1967; Bratto and Greppi, 1968; Burner, 1968; Lehmann and Ban, 1968; Marjerrison et al., 1968; Schwartz, 1968;

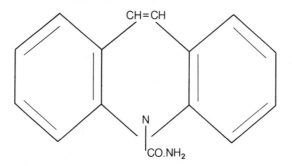

FIG. 1. Structural formula of carbamazepine.

Singh et al., 1976). Clinical trials conducted in Canada and elsewhere demonstrated the psychotropic properties of carbamazepine, as shown by beneficial effects of the drug on the behavior often occurring with epilepsy.

Bonduelle and colleagues (1962) were among the first clinical investigators reporting on the psychotropic efficacy of carbamazepine in treating behavioral disorders, especially for the symptoms of aggressivity and lack of interest which are often associated with epilepsy. According to these workers, slightly over one-third showed great improvement and a similar proportion showed a perceptible improvement, whereas the remaining less than one-third showed no improvement. Furthermore, therapeutic exhaustion of psychotropic effect was not seen in spite of a 9-year follow-up study.

This open study was planned to assess the long-term psychotropic, anticonvulsant, and therapeutic safety of carbamazepine when used as an adjuvant medication in a population of chronic institutionalized epileptic patients with pronounced behavior disorders.

PATIENTS AND METHODS

We studied 20 patients (9 males and 11 females) with the primary diagnosis of epilepsy complicated by behavior disorders. The patients ranged in age from 20 to 63 years (mean 48 years). Selection criteria were an age of between 20 and 65 years, a minimum of 2 years' hospitalization, and seizure control maintained by at least two anticonvulsant drugs, one of which was phenobarbital. Each patient had a history of seizures observed while he was in the hospital. In 15 cases the epilepsy was accompanied by personality disorder, and in 5 cases by psychosis (paranoid schizophrenia). Patients with a history of sensitivity to tricyclic antidepressants or presently on tricyclic antidepressants, were excluded from the study. In addition, patients with hepatic disease, blood dyscrasia, cardiovascular disease, or pregnancy were excluded from the study.

All patients were stabilized on phenobarbital and carbamazepine. The initial mean dosage of phenobarbital was 180 mg/day. Carbamazepine was added to the regular dosage of phenobarbital and was individually adjusted for each patient, depending on the clinical response. The daily dosage of carbamazepine ranged from 600 to 1,000 mg (mean 800 mg).

The psychotropic activities of the compounds were evaluated by the use of Rajotte's Scale and rated by senior investigators at four weekly intervals. Detailed reports were recorded by the ward nurses who observed the behavioral adjustment on the ward and the frequency of seizures. Simultaneously, the Brief Psychiatric Rating Scale was also completed by the psychiatrist to evaluate alteration of psychopathological parameters.

Both before and after the clinical trial, each patient underwent a detailed physicial examination. Detailed laboratory blood and urine tests were completed prior to the trial and at 12-week intervals thereafter.

Each time period was evaluated statistically by the analysis of variance test, that is, at 8, 16, 24, 32, 48, 60, 72, 80, and 96 weeks of treatment.

Two patients who developed leukopenia did not complete the clinical trial.

RESULTS

Seizures

The number of seizures occurring in each month was recorded for each patient for a 24-month follow-up period, as well as in the month prior to administration of trial drugs. The mean number of seizures during each month is summarized in Fig. 2.

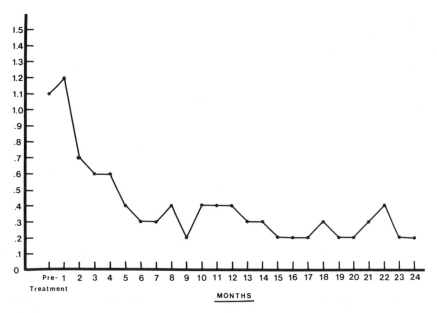

FIG. 2. Mean number of seizures in the month before treatment with carbamazepine and in the 24-month follow-up period.

There was a gradual reduction in the mean number of seizures over the first 3 or 4 months from about 1/month at the beginning of the study to approximately 0.4/month. A statistically significant result from carbamazepine was obtained in controlling seizures, thereby confirming its anticonvulsant activity.

Behavior Characteristics

Changes in behavior characteristics of the patients were assessed using Rajotte's Scale and the Brief Psychiatric Rating Scale. These were analyzed separately.

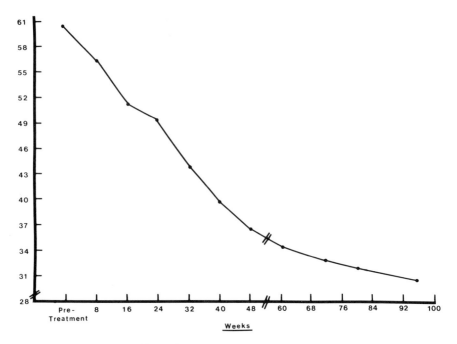

FIG. 3. Mean scores on Rajotte's Scale.

Rajotte's Scale includes 16 characteristics, each of which is rated on a seven-point scale, where a score of one denotes absence and a score of seven indicates a frequent occurrence and maximum severity.

The total score was analyzed and an assessment then made of changes over time in specific characteristics. Assessments were made before treatment and at 8, 16, 24, 32, 40, 48, 60, 72, 80, and 96 weeks after the start of therapy with carbamazepine.

The mean total score for the treatment group is shown in Fig. 3 and the mean reduction in total scores is shown in Fig. 4. The mean pretreatment score was 60.4, and the addition of carbamazepine produced a statistically significant ($p < 0.01$), gradual, and consistent reduction of pathological behavior characteristics, as illustrated by a reduction in the mean score from 60.4 to 30.2 by the 96th week of the study.

Item analysis of Rajotte's Scale revealed that carbamazepine addition improved the following 12 items: clastic, abusive, angry, quarrelsome, touchy, rude, fault-finder, domineering, restive, obstinate, suspicious, and noisy. Figure 5 shows the gradual reduction after adding carbamazepine. A reduction of at least two points in the item scores was seen, e.g., 6 to 4, or 5 to 2, during analysis, which confirms the statistically significant result obtained during this study. In 12 of 18 patients on carbamazepine, a significant improvement occurred in all charac-

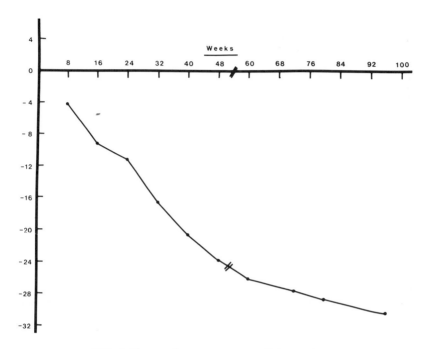

FIG. 4. Changes in mean scores on Rajotte's Scale.

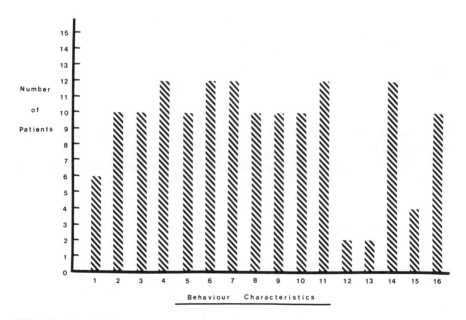

FIG. 5. Number of patients showing significant improvement in specific behavior characteristics.

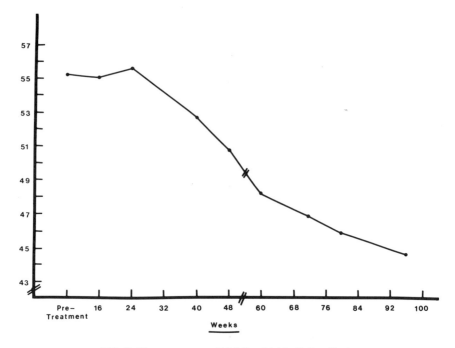

FIG. 6. Mean scores on Brief Psychiatric Rating Scale.

teristics except items 1, 12, 13, and 15, which were invariably absent or manifested only minimally in the patients.

The Brief Psychiatric Rating Scale covers 18 symptoms which are assessed on a seven-point scale, from not present to extremely severe. Item analysis and cluster analysis were done on all patients. Cluster analysis was done in four groups (1 to 5, 6 to 10, 11 to 13, and 14 to 18). Although assessment was done monthly, analysis was restricted to assessment before treatment and at 16, 24, 40, 48, 60, 72, 80, and 96 weeks, since these would be adequate to determine whatever benefits there might be.

The mean total scores and the mean score for four clusters are summarized in Fig. 6. A statistically significant reduction in total scores and the mean scores for four clusters was observed during the 96 weeks of study.

Item analysis revealed that the carbamazepine group showed improvement in the symptoms of irritability, hostility, uncooperativeness, and excitement.

Nurses' Clinical Observations

The nurses' clinical observations showed an improvement in the general ward behavior of the patients, mainly in elevation of mood and increased interest in ward activities.

Laboratory Examinations

Two patients developed leukopenia, one in the 13th month of treatment, with a leukocyte count of 3,100 and another in the 15th month, with a leukocyte count of 3,400. The dosage of carbamazepine was 800 mg/day for both patients. They were dropped from the study immediately and were put on ethosuximide, along with phenobarbital. Their leukocyte counts became normal within 6 weeks of withdrawing carbamazepine. Otherwise, there was no evidence of any other abnormalities in all other laboratory tests.

Detailed physical examinations before and after the study and at 12 weeks showed no abnormality. The ophthalmic examination was also within normal limits.

Adverse Reactions

Adverse reactions were evaluated on the Treatment Emergent Symptoms Scale, and all were of a mild nature. Table 1 summarizes the adverse reactions seen during the 96 weeks of the trial period.

TABLE 1. *Side effects in 20 patients during treatment with carbamazepine*

Adverse reactions	No. of patients
Dry mouth	4
Mild headache	3
Weight gain	2
Tremor	1
Nausea	1
Leukopenia	2 (dropped from study)

DISCUSSION

With more than 7,500 published case reports, carbamazepine has established itself as a potent anticonvulsant drug in the present armamentarium of antiepileptic agents. Findings from numerous controlled studies, including ours, indicate that its anticonvulsive properties resemble and are equal to those of other antiepileptic drugs.

In addition, carbamazepine has been found to possess significant psychotropic properties, all of which have an added advantage for the treatment of epileptic patients who in the majority of cases show behavior disorders or psychoses, and sometimes both. The improvement in behavior disorders, psychoses, or both, without the use of a neuroleptic, which often lowers the convulsive threshold, is an important advance in the treatment of the epileptic patient.

The third most important aspect of the treatment of epilepsy is sustenance of long-term efficacy and safety, and the present study, like many previous studies, shows that in the therapeutic range of dosage, carbamazepine is a safe and potent drug that has only mild adverse reactions.

The reduction in seizure activity to a statistically significant level confirms that carbamazepine possesses adequate anticonvulsive properties, at best when administered in conjunction with another anticonvulsive agent.

From the present study, however, no definite conclusion can be drawn about the anticonvulsive properties of carbamazepine when administered alone. Nevertheless, in epileptics requiring major anticonvulsant drugs, it is not a usual practice to rely heavily on any single compound.

Drug-related EEG changes were observed, and the overall disorganization of the EEGs may be attributed to the drug's tricyclic structure.

The presence of significant psychotropic properties was demonstrated by the analysis of Rajotte's Scale and the nurses' observations of ward behavior. The addition of carbamazepine improved agitation, as well as retardation in verbal and motor behaviors, and a significant improvement was seen in the patients' cooperation on the ward. Our clinical observations are in agreement with previously published reports that carbamazepine elevates the patient's mood, thus increasing activities and interest.

To achieve reasonable control of seizures and symptoms of hostility and excitement, it is usually necessary to administer heavy sedative doses of anticonvulsants in the majority of the chronic epileptic population, but with the addition of carbamazepine, our findings suggest that relative control of seizures and symptoms of behavioral disturbance can be maintained without producing a significant degree of sedation.

The therapeutic efficacy of carbamazepine in controlling seizure activity, and its significant psychotropic properties, lower frequency of side effects, and better tolerance make carbamazepine a drug of choice in the treatment and management of chronic hospitalized epileptic patients with predominant symptoms of behavior disturbance.

CONCLUSION

This open study confirms the potent anticonvulsant properties, the psychotropic properties, the long-term therapeutic safety, and better tolerance of carbamazepine in chronic institutionalized epileptic patients with behavior disorders.

The conjunction of psychotropic, anticonvulsant, and antipsychomotor epileptic properties in a drug resembling the tricyclic antidepressants to a major extent, and the phenothiazines to a lesser extent, makes carbamazepine an attractive and useful drug in the armamentarium of anticonvulsants. Carbamazepine also becomes a drug of choice when predominant symptoms of behavior disturbances are present in chronic epileptics and mood enhancement is needed.

There was no obvious incompatibility between carbamazepine and other anticonvulsants. Adverse reactions with carbamazepine were minimal and of a transitory nature. Except for two cases of leukopenia, no other abnormalities were seen in laboratory tests.

The psychotropic effect of carbamazepine was particularly useful in obtaining a change in the general behavior of these epileptic patients without the use of neuroleptics, which often lower the convulsive threshold.

SUMMARY

The long-term anticonvulsive and psychotropic properties of carbamazepine were evaluated in 20 chronic hospitalized epileptic patients with pronounced behavior disorders. All patients were taking at least two anticonvulsant drugs, and carbamazepine replaced one of these. It was administered in a flexible dosage schedule between 200 and 1,000 mg/day. The dosage was individually adjusted for each patient, depending on the clinical response. Carbamazepine significantly reduced the severity of behavior disorders and the frequency of seizures. The psychotropic effect of carbamazepine was particularly useful in obtaining a change in the general behavior without the use of a neuroleptic, which often lowers the convulsive threshold. Carbamazepine was well tolerated and was associated with only minimal and transitory side effects. There was no obvious incompatibility between carbamazepine and other anticonvulsants. Electroencephalograms showed no marked changes.

REFERENCES

Bonduelle, M., Bouygues, P., Sallou, C., and Chemaly, R. (1962): A review of clinical trials conducted with the anti-epileptic G 32 883: Results obtained with 89 cases. Proc. C.I.N.P. Congress, Munich, 1962, pp. 312–315.

Bratto, M., and Greppi, G. (1968): The success of carbamazepine in the treatment of severe epilepsy and its associated character disturbances. *Riv. Sper. Freniat.*, 92:1217.

Burner, M. (1968): The treatment of character disturbances: Results obtained with Tegretol. Proceedings of the Fourth World Congress of Psychiatry, Madrid, 1966, pp. 2240–2243. Excerpta Medica International Congress Series No. 150, Amsterdam.

Burner, M., Haynal, A., de Quervain, P. F., Zurn, A., and Pagani, J. P. (1965): Antiepileptic and psychotropic effects of Tegretol in outpatient practice. C. R. Congr. Psychiatr. Neurol. Langue Franc., Lausanne, pp. 675–683.

Donner, M., and Frisk, M. (1965): Carbamazepine treatment of epileptic and psychic symptoms in children and adolescents. *Ann. Paediatr. Fenn.*, 11:91–97.

Lehmann, H. E., and Ban, T. A. (1968): Studies with new drugs in the treatment of convulsive disorders. *Int. J. Clin. Pharmacol.*, 1:230–234.

Lorgé, M. (1963): Clinical experiences with Tegretol (G-32 883) a new antiepileptic with a special influence on epileptic character changes. *Schweiz. Med. Wochenschr.*, 93:1042–1047.

Marjerrison, G., Jedlicki, S. M., Keogh, R. P., Hrychuk, W., and Poulakakis, G. M. (1968): Carbamazepine: Behavioral, anticonvulsant and EEG effects in chronically-hospitalized epileptics. *Dis. Nerv. Syst.*, 29:133–136.

Martinez-Lage, F. M., Molina, P., Madox, P., and Villanueva, F. A. (1965): Clinical evaluation of the psychotropic and antiepileptic effects of Tegretol. *Rev. Med. Univ. Navarra*, 10:195–205.

Rajotte, P., Jilek, W., Jilek, L., Perales, A., Giard, N., Bordeleau, J.-M., and Tetreault, L. (1967): Antiepileptic and psychotropic properties of carbamazepine (Tegretol). *Union Med. Can.*, 96: 1200–1206.

Schneider, P. B., Burner, M., and Pagani, J. P. (1965): Initial results of antiepileptic and psychotropic effects of Tegretol obtained in a study based on outpatients. *Encephale,* 54:433–439.

Schwartz, J. F. (1968): Recent advances in treating epileptic children. *Postgrad. Med.,* 44:107–111.

Simpson, G. M., Kunz, E., and Watts, T. P. S. (1965): Behavioral and anti-epileptic effects of an iminostilbene derivative. Proceedings of the Fourth International Congress of Neuropsychopharmacology, Birmingham, 1964, pp. 442–448. Elsevier, Amsterdam.

Singh, A. N., Saxena, B. M., and Gent, M. (1976): Carbamazepine and diphenylhydantoin in the treatment of grand mal epilepsy: A comparative clinical trial. In: *Total Care in Severe Epilepsy,* edited by M. J. Parsonage, pp. 87–91. International Bureau for Epilepsy, London.

Epilepsy, The Eighth International Symposium,
edited by J. K. Penry. Raven Press, New York
© 1977.

Long-Term Treatment in Severe Epilepsy (Institutionalized Patients): II. Retrospective Evaluation of Carbamazepine

H. Schneider

Leiter der Neurophysiologischen Abteilung der Gesellschaft für Epilepsieforschung E.V. Bethel, Maraweg 13, D-4800 Bielefeld 13, and Section on Epilepsy, Institution "Eckhardtsheim," v. Bodelschwingh Institutions, Federal Republic of Germany

Carbamazepine (Tegretol®, 5-carbamyl-5H-dibenz[b,f]azepine) was introduced as an antiepileptic drug in Germany in 1964. Since then, numerous reports on its clinical efficacy have been published, but only a few have dealt with long-term treatment with carbamazepine and its evaluation.

Dreyer (1965) studied 120 adult inpatients with mixed forms of epilepsy under continuous treatment of 400 to 2,400 mg (average 1,166 mg) carbamazepine daily over a mean period of 21 months. In Dreyer's study 4 patients received carbamazepine only, and 116 were on mixed medication. The best effect was reported in sole grand mal and grand mal combined with psychomotor seizures, 33 patients being seizure-free within the observation period. However, it was mentioned that five patients after some months of treatment with carbamazepine resumed their previous seizure frequency. A discrepancy between clinical effect and EEG was found in 15 patients. Side effects such as dizziness and loss of appetite were minor. A rash was reported in five patients. A slight decrease in hemoglobin and leukocytes was also reported and attributed to the mixed medication rather than to carbamazepine alone.

Vasconcelos (1967) studied the efficacy of carbamazepine in 125 outpatients being treated for 1 to 36 months (most for less than 1 year) with 600 to 2,000 mg/day. The results were very favorable in isolated grand mal and less favorable in psychomotor epilepsies. A decreasing effect with time could not be established. Eight patients had short-lasting side effects (four with skin rashes, two with dizziness, one with gastric and intestinal complaints, and one with leukopenia with burning mouth syndrome). In another four patients, the treatment had to be stopped for continuous side effects: two patients with reversible leukopenia, one with fever and vomiting, and one with dizziness, diplopia, and walking difficulties.

Krüger (1972) reported the results obtained in 59 outpatients treated with carbamazepine. Minimum daily dosages were 400 mg and maximum 2,400 mg (mean 1,000 mg); co-medication was not mentioned. Most of these patients (61%)

had only one type of seizure, the others combined forms of grand mal with focal, psychomotor, or pyknoleptic seizures. The results were favorable in the single-type epilepsies and less favorable in combined forms; no increase in seizure frequency was noted after years of treatment. The "borderline dose" toward recurrence of seizures was reported as 300 to 400 mg daily. No relation was found between the clinical effect and the EEG; in particular, the EEG could still be altered or even worsened although the patient was clinically improved. Regular blood cell counts every 3 to 6 months revealed no changes due to toxicity.

PATIENTS AND METHODS

This study included 70 adult patients from two homes of the institution "Eckardtsheim." There were 31 women aged 19.7 to 80.8 years (mean 44.1 years) who had been under continuous observation in our institution for 0.7 to 51.6 years (mean 18.9 years). Diagnosis of epilepsy was given as genuine in 11, symptomatic in 15, and not clear in 5 patients. Carbamazepine was given in daily dosages of 200 to 1,200 mg for an average of 5 years (range 0.4 to 13.8 years). The 39 male patients, aged 19.5 to 60.9 years (mean 36.9 years), had been under long-term observation for 0.3 to 48.9 years (mean 19.2 years). Diagnosis of epilepsy was given as genuine in 12 patients and symptomatic in 27 patients. Carbamazepine was taken in daily dosages of 200 to 1,800 mg over an average of 6.9 years (0.2 to 13.1 years).

Only 1 patient was on sole carbamazepine treatment; 69 received a combined medication with phenytoin, phenobarbital, primidone, and/or other drugs. The effect of carbamazepine was assessed by comparing the seizure frequency in the years and months before and after the addition or exchange of carbamazepine. Although all patients had other types of seizures as well, only clinically defined psychomotor and grand mal attacks were evaluated. Sixty-three patients had combined psychomotor, grand mal, and other types of seizures; five had combined psychomotor and other seizures without grand mal; and two had other types of seizures. This means that our group consisted of patients previously reported to benefit least from treatment with carbamazepine. Routine blood cell counts and EEG controls, usually obtained at least once a year, were also included in the evaluation.

RESULTS AND DISCUSSION

Psychomotor Attacks

Complete control of psychomotor seizures was achieved in three patients (4%) with dosages of 1,000 to 1,600 mg daily. Further, 15 patients (22%) showed a reduction in seizures of more than 50% with daily dosages of 600 to 1,200 mg, whereas up to 50% seizure control was achieved in 21 patients (31%), mainly with dosages of 600 mg/day. Uncertain results were seen in 16 patients (24%), and an increase in psychomotor attacks was seen in 13 patients (19%), mainly due to concomitant changes of co-medication. Some of these patients were part of a study performed earlier (Schneider, 1975), which revealed a good correlation between seizure control and mean serum concentrations of carbamazepine: 4.6 ± 1.3 μg/ml in the first group with complete control, 3.7 ± 1.9 μg/ml in the second group with seizure control in excess of 50%, and 2.3 ± 1.4 μg/ml in the last group (up to 50% seizure control).

In general, dosages of up to 400 mg/day produced uncertain, slight, or no effects, and dosages of 600 mg/day reduced seizures up to 50% in most cases. Also, sometimes noted was an increase in seizures when carbamazepine was exchanged against phenytoin or phenobarbitol, as well as a reduction in seizures in excess of 50% when the drug was added to preexisting therapy. Dosages of 800 to 1,000 mg/day were mainly followed by a 50 to 99% control of seizures, and only 1,000 to 1,600 mg/day of carbamazepine was able to control psychomotor attacks over long periods.

Grand Mal Seizures

In four patients (6%) complete control of grand mal seizures was achieved by the addition of carbamazepine, and another five (8%) showed an improvement of 50 to 99% in seizure frequency. Further, 18 (29%) had a slight improvement in their grand mal attacks, whereas 4 (6%) had completely unfavorable results and 32 (51%) were questionable, again mainly due to changes in concomitant phenytoin, phenobarbital, and/or primidone treatment. Dosages of 400 mg daily and less showed only slight, uncertain, and even unfavorable results, whereas 600 to 1,000/per day reduced grand mal attacks, mainly up to 50%. Complete control of grand mal attacks by the addition of carbamazepine was achieved by 900 to 1,600 mg/day, with one patient's attacks being completely controlled with 600 mg/day.

In general, with both types of seizures and in the patients involved, the absence of seizure control or the minor degree of seizure control achieved seemed to be solely or mainly the result of low dosages of carbamazepine of up to 400 or 600 mg daily. Occasionally, seizure frequency even worsened through concomitant withdrawal of major antiepileptic drugs in sometimes higher dosages. The expectation from this study that carbamazepine is effective to a greater extent also in our group of patients with severe epilepsies (mixed forms) has to be investigated in a controlled prospective study.

Increase in Seizure Frequency

An increase of psychomotor attacks was seen in four patients after treatment with carbamazepine for 2 to 3 years. The failure to give long-term antiepileptic protection in these cases may be attributed *in part* to the epilepsy itself, as adjustment and even alteration of the medication in two patients did not result in lasting seizure control. On the other hand, the compliance of patients by blood-level controls was not studied at that time.

An increase in grand mal attacks was seen in one patient under long-term additional treatment with carbamazepine. In this patient, too, an alteration in medication could not produce a lasting antiepileptic effect.

Discontinuation of Carbamazepine Treatment

In 25 patients carbamazepine treatment was terminated after periods of 0.3 to 11.2 years.

In 12 patients an increase of seizures (4 patients) or drug adjustment due to lack of efficacy (8 patients) was the reason stated. Another patient showed behavioral disturbances, two patients had skin disorders (rash; one with a preexisting rash and generalized edema), and two experienced drowsiness. In one patient polyneuropathy was suspected. In six patients no clear-cut cause was documented. The dosages involved in these patients were 200 to 1,200 mg daily; no specific CNS side effects such as diplopia or ataxia were noted. The side effects mentioned were fully reversible after termination of carbamazepine.

Electroencephalogram

EEG recordings showed no consistent changes under carbamazepine treatment as compared to controls obtained before the initiation of carbamazepine. In 21 patients there was no alteration of preexisting EEG activities and in another 12 only minor changes were observed. Moreover, 10 patients showed an increase and 14 an improvement in common cerebral activity. Focal activity increased in three patients, whereas focal signs improved in seven patients. Specific epileptic activity worsened in 11 patients and improved in 8 patients. Thus, background activity and focal symptoms improved only slightly, if at all, whereas specific ictal activities may have even increased. It must be stated, however, that slight alterations of the preexisting co-medication may also have contributed to this effect.

Laboratory Data

Findings from the routine blood evaluations performed at least once yearly before and after initiation of carbamazepine treatment were compiled for the 45 patients still under carbamazepine treatment (Fig. 1).

Female Patients

A slight increase in erythrocyte count from 4.2 to 4.28 mill./mm^3 and a corresponding increase in hemoglobin from 12.5 to 12.9 g% was seen in 22 patients, whereas the hemoglobin per erythrocyte (Hb$_E$) decreased from 32.7 to 29.3 $\gamma\gamma$ (14 patients). Leukocyte counts were slightly higher, on the average

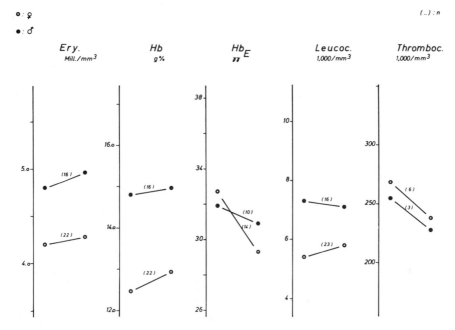

FIG. 1. Averaged blood count data before *(left)* and after *(right)* the initiation of carbamazepine. Ery., erythrocytes; Leucoc., leukocytes; Thromboc., thrombocytes.

5,800, as compared with 5,400/mm³ before carbamazepine treatment. Thrombocyte counts before and after initiation of carbamazepine treatment could be evaluated in only six patients and showed a decrease from 268,500 to 238,-000/mm³.

Male Patients

There was also a slight increase in erythrocytes from 4.8 to 4.95 mill./mm³ and a corresponding slight increase in hemoglobin from 14.8 to 14.9 g% in 16 patients, whereas the Hb_E again showed a decrease from 31.9 to 30.9 $\gamma\gamma$ (10 patients). Leukocytes decreased slightly from 7,300 to 7,100/mm³ (16 patients); there was also a decrease in the thrombocytes in 3 patients from 254,700 to 227,900/mm³.

In general, routine blood cell counts showed statistically a slight increase in erythrocytes and hemoglobin, whereas thrombocytes and Hb_E decreased slightly; leukocytes on the average (male and female) showed no significant change. The decrease in thrombocytes (and also Hb_E) is in agreement with the findings of the above-mentioned authors and others (see also review by Pisciotta, 1975), whereas the slight increase in erythrocytes and hemoglobin and the unchanged leukocyte counts would not corroborate statistically the hypothesis of a drug-induced bone marrow insufficiency. As Pisciotta (1975) has pointed out, however, this may not be detected by routine blood cell counts. On the other hand, some other cause may underlie these changes noted in routine blood cell counts and may only be speculated on at present. Furthermore, before attributing these effects to the carbamazepine treatment, one has to bear in mind that preexisting co-medication was also changed quite often in the course of time. After other antiepileptic drugs, in particular phenytoin, were withdrawn, a normalization of previously low figures of these parameters, especially erythrocytes, hemoglobin, and leukocytes, could be observed not infrequently.

SUMMARY

In 70 patients (39 men, 31 women) from two homes of the institution "Eckardts-heim" the beneficial therapeutic effect of carbamazepine on psychomotor and grand mal seizures could be demonstrated with daily dosages of at least 600 mg for treatment periods up to 13.8 years; dosages of 400 mg or less showed only slight or no effects and must therefore be regarded as subtherapeutic in our patients. In four patients an increase in psychomotor seizures and in one patient an increase in grand mal attacks were observed after 2 to 3 years of carbamazepine treatment, but these increases are thought to be partly due to the epilepsy itself. Side effects leading to termination of treatment were slight and fully reversible. No striking EEG alterations could be observed, with occasional discrepancies between clinical control and EEG abnormalities. Routine blood cell counts revealed only a slight decrease in thrombocytes as well as Hb_E, whereas on the average erythrocytes, hemoglobin, and leukocytes remained the same or showed a slight improvement. These changes are briefly discussed.

ACKNOWLEDGMENTS

This study would not have been possible without the permission of Dr. med. J. Berenguer and Dr. med. H. Stegmann, head of the institution "Eckardtsheim," to study their patients and patients' files, which is thankfully acknowledged. The assistance of Fr. B. Kleine in the evaluations is greatly appreciated.

REFERENCES

Dreyer, R. (1965): Erfahrungen mit Tegretal®. *Nervenarzt,* 36:442–445.
Krüger, H. J. (1972): Katamnestische Erhebungen über einen Zeitraum von 9 Jahren zur Therapie der Epilepsie mit Carbamazepin. *Med. Welt.,* 23:896–898.
Pisciotta, A. V. (1975): Hematologic toxicity of carbamazepine. In: *Complex Partial Seizures and Their Treatment, Advances in Neurology, Vol. 11,* edited by J. K. Penry and D. D. Daly. Raven Press, New York.
Schneider, H. (1975): Carbamazepine: An attempt to correlate serum levels with anti-epileptic and side-effects. In: *Clinical Pharmacology of Anti-Epileptic Drugs,* edited by H. Schneider, D. Janz, C. Gardner-Thorpe, H. Meinardi, and A. L. Sherwin. Springer-Verlag, Berlin.
Vasconcelos, D. (1967): Die Behandlung der Epilepsie mit Tegretal®. *Nervenarzt,* 38:506–509.

Epilepsy, The Eighth International Symposium,
edited by J. K. Penry. Raven Press, New York
© 1977.

Therapy-Resistant Epilepsies with Long-Term History—Slow Spike-and-Wave Syndrome

T. Osawa, M. Seino, M. Miyokoshi, K. Yamamoto, N. Kakegawa, K. Yagi, T. Hirata, T. Morikawa, and T. Wada

National Institute of Epilepsy-Shizuoka, 886 Higashi, Shizuoka, Shizuoka, Japan

The Lennox-Gastaut syndrome has been regarded as one of the typical clinical entities among secondary generalized epilepsies in the sense of the International Classification of the Epilepsies (Gastaut, 1970) and the terminology described in the *Dictionary of Epilepsy* (Gastaut, 1973). This syndrome has also been taken into account as one of the epilepsies most resistant to every kind of antiepileptic drug.

Since the syndrome occurs most often in infancy and childhood, and rarely in preadolescence, it has been largely accepted that the age dependency and therefore state of brain immaturation were important etiological factors. According to our study, the clinical manifestations similar to those of the Lennox-Gastaut syndrome were not infrequently observable in the older ages.

In the present chapter, first, we disclose the existence of the Lennox-Gastaut syndrome in adulthood based on the strictly defined diagnostic criteria for this syndrome and confirm the approximate upper limit of the age; and, second, we clarify the difference in clinical and electroencephalographic symptomatology between the Lennox-Gastaut syndrome and other types of secondary generalized epilepsy, commonly with slow spike-wave discharges in the interictal tracing.

SUBJECTS

The distribution of epilepsy in 1,200 subjects, based on the International Classification of Epilepsy, was as follows:

Generalized epilepsies	577 (48.1%)
Primary	276 (23.0%)
Secondary	282 (23.5%)
Undetermined	19 (1.6%)
Partial epilepsies	576 (48.0%)
Unclassifiable epilepsies	47 (3.9%)
Total	1,200

Approximately 25%, an unexpectedly large percentage, of these subjects were in the category of secondary generalized epilepsies. This is partly because our Institute was opened as a sole special center for epilepsy in Japan.

The subjects of this study were 116 patients, all with diffuse bursts of spike-wave discharges slower than 3/sec in the interictal recording, who were selected from the 282 patients with secondary generalized epilepsy. Of the 116 patients, 72 were below the age of 15 years and 44 were above the age of 16 years.

RESULTS

For the purpose of confirming the unusual presence of the Lennox-Gastaut syndrome in elder subjects, we carefully reconsidered each of the diagnostic criteria previously proposed by other authors and adopted the following three criteria:

1. Evidence of diffuse bursts of slow spike-wave discharges in the interictal electroencephalogram, especially with pseudorhythmicity.
2. Presence of a combination of two or more types of epileptic seizures in a certain stage throughout the chronology of epilepsy.
3. Presence of definite neurological and/or psychiatric deficits indicative of underlying brain pathology, such as signs of retarded psychomotor development.

Provided that all three criteria were completely satisfied in a patient, the diagnosis of Lennox-Gastaut syndrome was given.

Lennox-Gastaut Syndrome in Older Patients

Number of Patients with the Lennox-Gastaut Syndrome

The Lennox-Gastaut syndrome, carefully diagnosed by the above-mentioned criteria, was found in 91 (7.6%) of the 1,200 subjects—62 of 442 subjects below the age of 15 years, and 29 of 758 subjects above the age of 16 years. This included 17 patients above the age of 20 years, of which the oldest was a man of 38 years.

Although patients younger than 15 were found about four times as often as patients above 16, the considerable number of adult patients with this syndrome should be mentioned, along with the existence of the oldest case at 38 years.

Presumable Age at Onset of the Lennox-Gastaut Syndrome

The presumable age at onset of this syndrome was studied by either reviewing the old electroencephalograms recorded in other clinics or confirming the alternating point in chronology at the time when multifold epileptic seizures took place and/or definite signs of neuropsychiatric deficits became manifest. We found that 67 cases had their onset below 19 years of age and 7 cases above 20 years.

Types of Seizures

The types of seizures occurring throughout the history of 91 cases with this syndrome were atypical absences, tonic and tonic-clonic seizures, which were most common, followed by myoclonic seizures, epileptic drop attacks, and atonic seizures in decreasing order. There was no difference in the ictal symptomatology between the group below 15 and the group above 16.

Other Cases with Slow Spike-Wave Discharges in the Interictal EEG

If the interictal electroencephalogram revealed a run of diffuse slow spike-wave discharges but the clinical and electroencephalographic manifestations did not completely satisfy the three criteria, the patient was not included in the Lennox-Gastaut syndrome but tentatively was categorized into two syndromes, that is, multi-ictal and uni-ictal slow spike-wave syndromes, depending on the presence or absence of multifold combinations of seizures and neuropsychiatric deficits. For example, when two criteria, pseudorhythmicity in the paroxysmal discharges and multifold combination of seizures, were satisfied, but there was only the slightest evidence of neuropsychiatric deficits, the epilepsy was denominated as the multi-ictal slow spike-wave syndrome. With a single type of seizure, e.g., atypical absence, a pseudorhythmic paroxysmal pattern, and a positive sign of mental deterioration, the epilepsy was denominated as the uni-ictal slow spike-wave syndrome.

Difference in Types of Seizures Among the Three Syndromes

In the Lennox-Gastaut syndrome as well as the so-called multi-ictal slow spike-wave syndrome, atypical absences and tonic and tonic-clonic seizures were most common; whereas in the uni-ictal slow spike-wave syndrome, myoclonic seizures, epileptic drop attacks, and atonic seizures were not found. These findings are our logical basis for proposing that the multi-ictal slow spike-wave syndrome can be oriented as a syndrome immediately adjacent but not identical to the Lennox-Gastaut syndrome, and the uni-ictal slow spike-wave syndrome as the one less immediately adjacent.

Effectiveness of Antiepileptic Drugs on the Three Syndromes

The effectiveness of antiepileptic drugs on the three syndromes appears to be remarkably different. For example, one-third of the patients with the Lennox-Gastaut syndrome showed more than a 75% reduction in seizure frequency, whereas three-fourths of those with the multi-ictal slow spike-wave syndrome and all of those with uni-ictal slow spike-wave syndrome experienced this reduction in seizure frequency (Fig. 1).

Antiepileptic drugs such as sodium valproate, clonazepam, ethosuximide, and barbiturates were mostly used in polypharmacy.

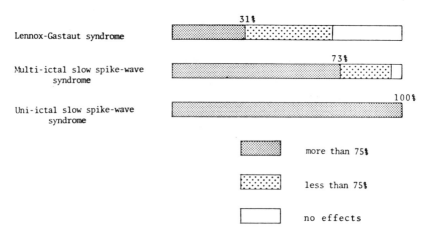

FIG. 1. Effect of antiepileptic drugs on the Lennox-Gastaut syndrome and on the multi-ictal and uni-ictal slow spike-wave syndromes.

DISCUSSION

We reported 29 patients with the Lennox-Gastaut syndrome in post-adolescence, of which 17 patients were older than 20 years, and the oldest was a man of 38 years. The clinical symptomatology of the Lennox-Gastaut syndrome in adulthood was identical with that in childhood.

Gastaut et al. (1975) recently reported that they found patients with the Lennox-Gastaut syndrome in 0.6% of 2,430 patients with epilepsy above the age of 15 years. This figure appears to be low compared to the 3.8% of our result above the age of 16 years. Gastaut et al. (1975) reported a patient of 34 years as the oldest, and Niedermeyer (1972) reported a case at 31 years. According to these reports, there is no doubt that the Lennox-Gastaut syndrome might be observed in adulthood, as well as in childhood, and the upper limit of the age might be around 30 years. Taking into account that this syndrome is not infrequently found among adult patients and that it may possibly begin in adolescence and adults with an identical clinical symptomatology, the question may be posed whether the age dependency and therefore state of immaturation of the central nervous system in affected children can be crucial etiological factors. Our data indicating the presence of the Lennox-Gastaut syndrome in adulthood, in spite of the rather rigidly defined criteria for diagnosis, suggest such a plausibility that the age dependency does not bear an inevitable part in its pathogenesis, but a suitable set of brain lesional conditions, in terms of anatomy as well as physiology, may yield a particular epileptogenicity even in adult's brain, although the underlying pathology appears to be unspecific.

Although there is no substantial evidence as to the origin of the Lennox-Gastaut syndrome, the role of mesodiencephalon (Gastaut et al., 1966) and frontal lobe cortices, for example, has been emphasized. Niedermeyer (1972) reported that diffuse slow spike-wave discharges were demonstrated in patients with frontal lobe lesions caused by trauma. It might be reasonable to consider that the anatomical substrates concerning the pathophysiology of the Lennox-Gastaut syndrome in both infancy and adulthood remain uncertain until the neuropathological anatomy will reveal the nature of these questions.

In order to ascertain the presence of the Lennox-Gastaut syndrome in adulthood, it is of immediate necessity to make the diagnostic criterion as rigid as possible. We gave preference for the presence of pseudorhythmicity in slow spike-wave discharges as one of the crucial factors. Gastaut et al. (1966) have emphasized that the absence of rhythmicity in the interictal paroxysmal discharges is one of the important factors for diagnosis of this syndrome, although he gave no details in his original paper. The difference between orthorhythmic and pseudorhythmic spike-wave discharges might reflect the fact that the pace-making mechanism responsible for production of this type of paroxysm is not identical. Namely, the cerebral pathophysiology, rather specific to the Lennox-Gastaut syndrome, might be of significance for the formation of pseudorhythmicity as well as the multi-ictal symptomatology, to a certain extent.

The Lennox-Gastaut syndrome is demarcated as a rather well-defined clinical entity characterized by the above-mentioned criteria in the realm of secondary generalized epilepsies with slow spike-wave discharges. In addition, we found two other categories of secondary generalized epilepsies, which by the criteria failed to be classified as the Lennox-Gastaut syndrome. That is, the Lennox-Gastaut syndrome is in its own right a more typical entity and the two other syndromes of symptom complexes are less typical entities in the secondary generalized epilepsies, which were characterized by the presence of slow spike-wave discharges in the interictal recordings.

An attempt to propose such categories among secondary generalized epilepsies is not for theoretical interest but is of practical usefulness. The effectiveness of antiepileptic drugs on the three syndromes appears to be remarkably different. In terms of therapy resistance, the Lennox-Gastaut syndrome was most refractory, and it can be regarded as a nuclear entity among the secondary generalized epilepsies.

In short, it would be reasonable to arrange in the following order the three types of secondary generalized epilepsies with slow spike-wave discharges as syndromes or symptom complexes: (1) Lennox-Gastaut syndrome, (2) multi-ictal slow spike-wave syndrome, and (3) uni-ictal slow spike-wave syndrome. This kind of clinical categorization may be worthwhile for exploring the possibility of disclosing some new clinical and, consequently, nosological entities to be extracted among the secondary generalized epilepsies.

SUMMARY

Reconsidering the diagnostic criteria for the Lennox-Gastaut syndrome, we found the presence of pseudorhythmicity in diffuse slow spike-wave discharges and of multifold clinical seizures to be of fundamental significance. According to the criteria, we found 91 cases to satisfy these norms out of 116 patients belonging to secondary generalized epilepsy.

The results are summarized as follows:

1. Notwithstanding the rather rigid diagnostic criteria, the Lennox-Gastaut syndrome was evidently found in adulthood. Of patients 16 years of age or older, 29 (3.8%) had Lennox-Gastaut syndrome; 17 (2.7%) of these patients were older than 20 years. The oldest was a man of 38 years with presumed onset at about 17 years of age. There was no difference in symptomatology of the Lennox-Gastaut syndrome between childhood and adulthood.

2. In the secondary generalized epilepsies, which were characterized by the presence of slow spike-wave discharges in the interictal EEG, the Lennox-Gastaut syndrome was demarcated as the more typical entity, with two other syndromes or symptom complexes as less typical.

3. The drug therapy resistance was not identical among these three syndromes, and the Lennox-Gastaut syndrome was most refractory. This allowed us to presume that the presence of pseudorhythmic slow spike-wave discharges might be a token of malignancy if the discharges coexist with multifold combinations of epileptic seizures.

4. All above-mentioned clinical characteristics may justify our diagnostic criteria tentatively established for the Lennox-Gastaut syndrome.

REFERENCES

Gastaut, H. (1970): Clinical and electroencephalographical classification of epileptic seizures. *Epilepsia,* 11:102–113.

Gastaut, H. (1973): *Dictionary of Epilepsy. Part 1: Definitions.* World Health Organization, Geneva.

Gastaut, H., Gastaut, J. L., Goncalves e Silva, G. E., and Fernandez Sanchez, G. R. (1975): Relative frequency of different types of epilepsy: A study employing the classification by the International League Against Epilepsy. *Epilepsia,* 16:457–561.

Gastaut, H., Roger, J., Soulayrol, R., Tassinari, C. A., Regis, H., Dravet, C., Bernard, R., Pinsard, N., and Saint-Jean, M. (1966): Childhood epileptic encephalopathy with diffuse slow spike-waves (otherwise known as "petit mal varient") or Lennox syndrome. *Epilepsia,* 7:139–179.

Niedermeyer, E. (1972): *The Generalized Epilepsies. A Clinical and Electroencephalographic Study.* Charles C Thomas, Springfield, Ill.

Epilepsy, The Eighth International Symposium,
edited by J. K. Penry. Raven Press, New York
© 1977.

Clinical, Therapeutic, and Social Status of Epileptic Patients Without Seizures for More than Five Years

*L. Oller-Daurella, **L. Oller F-V, and †R. Pamies

*Centro de Lucha Antiepileptica; **Instituto Neurologico Municipal and Centro de
PENEPA; and †Centro de PENEPA, Barcelona, Spain*

At the Seventh International Symposium on Epilepsy, which was held in Berlin in 1975, we presented a paper based on the study of 356 epileptics who were seizure-free for more than 5 years, and of these, 138 in whom medication had been suppressed (Oller-Daurella et al., 1976). A review of our present casuistic permits us to restate the problem of a much more important casuistic composed of 522 epileptics among whom 241 have had medication completely suppressed.

The existing bibliography on the suppression of treatment among epileptics was reviewed in our previous study. Let us point out the works published by Juul-Jensen (1964, 1968), which show a 29% relapse rate upon suppression of medication (after 2 years without crises) in the first year without treatment, and of 15%, 3%, 6%, and 3% in the subsequent years. Our results seem to be more optimistic, perhaps because we have not suppressed medication until arriving at a minimum period of 5 seizure-free years. To the bibliography cited in the previous paper, we should add the interesting works published by Loiseau (1972) and Loiseau et al. (1972), based on 250 patients in whom medication had been suppressed after a variable period and in whom a 50% relapse rate was observed.

PATIENTS

Our study population consisted of 568 patients who have been seizure-free for more than 5 years. Following the criterion that only those patients who have suffered recurrent crises can be considered epileptics, we have excluded 46 cases in which the patient had only a single crisis or episode.

Of the 522 authentic epileptics who have been seizure-free for more than 5 years, 241 are presently without treatment, while 281 are going through the phase of diminished treatment. Of the 241 epileptics in whom treatment has been suppressed, 82 relapses (34%) have occurred, and 159 patients (66%) continue to be seizure-free. Of the 281 patients in whom medication is being reduced progressively, 49 relapses (17.4%) have occurred, while 232 patients (82.6%) continue to be seizure-free. It should be noted that the average observation period since the time of control of seizures is 10.1 years, extending to 30 years in one case.

Total Suppression of Treatment: 241 Epileptics

Of the total number of relapses, 35 (42.7%) occurred during the first year. In the following 9 years, the percentage of relapses was much lower, but an important number of cases showed a relapse extremely late, even after 24 to 25 years without an attack.

In Table 1, we have analyzed the clinical seizure types of 228 epileptics who have been seizure-free for more than 5 years and in whom medication has been suppressed *progressively*. This is the same group of 241 patients mentioned earlier in which we have excluded 13 patients who abruptly suppressed treatment on their own initiative, without following our guidelines.

In these 228 epileptics, 69 relapses (30.3%) have occurred, a percentage somewhat higher than the one in our previous study, possibly due to the longer period of observation.

TABLE 1. *Suppression of medication in 228 patients: types of epilepsy and evolution*

	No. of patients	No. and % of relapses
Epileptics seizure-free for more than 5 years who have suppressed medication (not included are 13 patients who because of abrupt suppression of medication had 13 relapses)	228	69 (30.3)
Primary generalized epilepsy	57	9 (15.8)
Absences	22	1 (4.6)
Absences + myoclonias	1	1 (100.0)
Grand mal	17	5 (29.4)
Myoclonias	4	1 (25.0)
Absences + grand mal	3	0
Grand mal + myoclonias	7	0
Grand mal + absences + myoclonias	1	0
Other primary generalized epilepsies	2	1
Secondary generalized epilepsy	24	6 (25.0)
West syndrome	7	2 (28.6)
Lennox-Gastaut syndrome	7	3 (42.9)
Tonic crises	5	1
Other secondary generalized epilepsies	5	0
Partial epilepsy	78	29 (37.1)
Partial elementary	13	3 (23.1)
Partial complex	9	3 (33.3)
Secondary generalized	16	8 (50.0)
Elementary + secondary generalized	17	4 (23.5)
Complex + secondary generalized	23	11 (47.8)
Unilateral epilepsy	34	15 (44.1)
Unilateral	30	11 (36.7)
Unilateral + partial	4	4 (100.0)
Unclassified epilepsy	35	10 (28.6)

Primary generalized epilepsy shows the minimum number of relapses (15.8%), undoubtedly because typical absences that have only a 4.6% relapse rate are included. The unilateral and partial epilepsies have the highest percentage of relapses, 44.1% and 37.1%, respectively. For partial epilepsy, the incidence of relapses is greater when there is secondary generalization of crises (41.1%) than when there are partial complex or elementary crises without secondary generalization (27.3%), and even among the latter the isolated partial elementary crises show a relapse rate of 23.1%.

We have purposely left for the end our comments on relapses in secondary generalized epilepsy, in which only 25% of the cases have relapses, even though it is considered to be the most serious of all the epilepsies. Nevertheless, the conditions of our study, 5 previous years seizure-free under medication, caused us to exclude the majority of the serious forms of this type of epilepsy.

Progressive Diminution of Treatment Before Reaching Complete Suppression: 281 Epileptics

Table 2 shows that 49 relapses occurred among the 281 patients (17.4%). This percentage is perceptibly lower than that of the previous groups in which treat-

TABLE 2. *Reduction of medication in 281 patients: types of epilepsy and evolution*

	No. of patients	No. and % of relapses
Epileptics seizure-free for more than 5 years who have progressively diminished treatment	281	49 (17.4)
Primary generalized epilepsy	69	10 (14.5)
Absences	13	1 (7.7)
Absences + myoclonias	0	0
Grand mal	28	2 (7.1)
Myoclonias	0	0
Absences + grand mal	15	4 (6.7)
Grand mal + myoclonias	7	0
Grand mal + absences + myoclonias	4	1 (25.0)
Other primary generalized epilepsies	2	2
Secondary generalized epilepsy	20	3 (15.0)
West syndrome	5	1 (20.0)
Lennox-Gastaut syndrome	6	2 (33.0)
Tonic crises	3	0
Other secondary generalized epilepsies	6	0
Partial epilepsy	132	27 (20.5)
Partial elementary	11	3 (27.3)
Partial complex	13	3 (23.1)
Secondary generalized	41	8 (19.5)
Elementary + secondary generalized	26	6 (23.1)
Complex + secondary generalized	38	6 (15.9)
Elementary + complex	2	1
Elementary + complex + secondary generalized	1	0
Unilateral epilepsy	31	7 (22.6)
Unclassified epilepsy	29	2 (6.9)

ment was completely suppressed, which seems logical because these patients continued treating themselves even though at very low doses.

It is interesting to observe how the percentages of relapses, according to the different clinical forms of seizures, maintain a certain relation to those obtained in the previous series of total suppression of treatment. In the primary generalized epilepsies there is less difference (15.8% in the previous series, against 14.5% in the present series). The principal difference to note is that the total number of patients with grand mal crises or grand mal crises and myoclonic jerks only shows a 5.7% relapse rate during the diminution of treatment, although this group experiences a 20% relapse rate when medication is totally suppressed.

In this series, the unilateral epilepsies continue to show a higher percentage of relapses (22.6%), followed closely by the partial epilepsies (20.5%).

PROGRESSIVE SUPPRESSION OF TREATMENT

The norms that have been followed for the progressive suppression of treatment are the following:

1. Only patients who have been seizure-free for a minimum of 5 years have been used.
2. The reduction of medication has been realized during a minimum period of 1 year, passing from eventual polytherapy to monotherapy, ending in a daily dose of medication in the final phase.
3. Final monotherapy has always been phenobarbital when convulsive crises existed, even if they were generalized initially or secondarily. We have chosen this drug because it has the longest "half-life." In the remaining types of crises, the most recently used drugs have varied according to the types of seizures and the previously administered medication.
4. It is not necessary to say that the diminution of medication has been interrupted if an extremely small crisis has occurred.
5. Periodic EEG controls have been executed, which on occasion have made it advisable not to continue the reduction of medication.
6. Especially during the monotherapy phase, a great number of cases have had the serum level of medication controlled, to which we shall refer later.
7. Special social and work-related circumstances have made it advisable in some cases not to reach complete suppression of medication.
8. In the great majority of cases, these general guidelines have been followed, with the exception of several patients who abruptly suppressed the medication, which resulted in an immediate relapse in most cases.

SOCIAL CIRCUMSTANCES

This review of the social circumstances will consider epileptics who are seizure-free for more than 5 years and in whom medication has been suppressed progressively. It has not been possible among all of the patients, but it has been realized in 281 of them: 89 of school age and 192 of work age.

It is extremely exceptional that the rare crises of these patients (only two cases) have created either school- or work-related problems. In effect, the relapses that have occurred have consisted almost entirely of a single crisis that has not recurred from the moment that treatment was reestablished. Among the majority of the patients in this group who are not working, the problems are, with rare exception, due to concomitant psychic problems, in general, an oligophrenia due to a perinatal encephalopathy (30 cases). The cases of deterioration practically do not exist in our casuistic (only one doubtful case), and dysthymias and behavioral problems are exceptional (eight cases). In some patients (six cases), the cause of their inability to work consisted of permanent neurological problems, such as tetraplegia and hemiplegia, and was even due to nonneurological causes (two cases).

The most important social problem that the suppression of treatment has created has been to realize suppression in those individuals who, because they had been seizure-free for many years, possessed a driver's license. Although we have not followed a strict rule in each case, our advice has been that the patient not drive any motor vehicle for a certain number of weeks following each progressive diminution of the treatment. Following this guideline, we have had not a single failure to date.

The patients in whom we have progressively suppressed medication have professions that would not be dangerous given an eventual crisis, a fact which has facilitated our work in this aspect. Among the patients in this casuistic, a great number have university professions (19 patients), are university students (11 patients), or have administrative positions of great responsibility (9 patients).

BLOOD SERUM LEVELS IN PROGRESSIVE SUPPRESSION OF MEDICATION

In a large number of our patients in whom we have progressively suppressed medication, we have periodically evaluated the blood serum level of medication.

In order to conserve homogeneity in this casuistic, we have included in this series only those patients affected by initially or secondarily generalized convulsive crises, excluding those patients affected by absences and by partial nongeneralized crises or unilateral crises. We have also limited this review to the serum level of phenobarbital, as the majority of patients in the final phase of monotherapy are using this drug.

The 34 patients who continue to be seizure-free presently have an average level of phenobarbital of 18.3 μg/ml, the amount varying between quite ample limits in relation to the dosage administered previous to the experiment and also in relation to the phase of suppression of medication.

Of the 10 patients with relapses, the crises reappeared when the level of phenobarbital in the blood serum varied between 18.4 μg/ml, in the case in which its concentration in the blood was highest, and an almost imperceptible level in two cases. The average level of serum concentration at which relapses occurred was 9.9 μg/ml.

It is curious to note that the levels at which the relapses occur are quite variable, which leads us once again to believe that one cannot speak of a therapeutic serum level of phenobarbital, as this varies in each particular case with the seriousness of the epilepsy. However, it seems interesting to us to note once again that a relapse has never occurred in these forms of epilepsy above 18 μg/ml, which seems to imply that upon reducing medication, one should take special precautions when going below this level.

DISCUSSION

All of the previously disclosed data and all of the information provided in the literature establish a series of problems that we think should be discussed briefly:

1. Can antiepileptic medication be suppressed in a patient who has been seizure-free for several years? We believe that in the majority of cases the intention of suppressing medication can be realized with the patient's prior agreement, explaining to him or her the risks involved in the suppression of medication. The possibility of a relapse in 30% of the cases, according to our data, should be taken into account. But one should also appraise the risk represented by indefinitely maintaining medication, because if with time the patient succumbs to the temptation of trying to suppress the medication without medical supervision, the risks are much greater.

2. How should one arrive at the suppression of medication? There is no doubt that medication should be suppressed with maximum precautions and, in our opinion, during a very prolonged period of time, taking as a minimum period 1 or 2 years. The steps to be taken from polytherapy and the manner of realizing the progressive diminution of medication have been explained above.

3. When should the progressive reduction of medication be initiated? We believe that this point is essential for the successful suppression of treatment. At the International Colloquium on Epilepsy that we organize annually in Barcelona, we were able to see the disparity of criteria that exist in this respect. Our personal experience was initiated among patients who had been seizure-free for 10 years. Subsequently, we began to suppress treatment in all patients who had been free of all types of crises for 5 years. The results have been practically identical. A larger reduction of time seems dangerous to us, as the statistics based on patients who have been seizure-free for only 2 years seem to show a percentage of relapses higher than that of our patients.

On the other hand, it is difficult to appraise the results without a prolonged follow-up after the period of suppression. Look at the relapses that we have recorded after 24 or 25 years without a crisis. However, we do not believe that medication is justified because of the possibility that the patient may suffer a crisis 25 years later.

REFERENCES

Juul-Jensen, P. (1964): Frequency of recurrence after discontinuance of anticonvulsant therapy in patients with epileptic seizures. *Epilepsia,* 5:352–363.

Juul-Jensen, P. (1968): Frequency of recurrence after discontinuance of anticonvulsant therapy in patients with epileptic seizures. *Epilepsia,* 9:11–16

Loiseau, P. (1972): Quand faut-il arrêter un traitement antiépileptic? *Nouv. Presse Med.,* 1:47–49.

Loiseau, P., Henry, P., and Prissard, A. (1972): Considerations sur l'arrêt des traitement antiepileptiques. *Bourdeaux Med.,* 19:2631-2640.

Oller-Daurella, L., Pamies, R., and Oller F-V, L. (1976): Reduction or discontinuance of antiepileptic drugs in patients seizure-free for more than 5 years. In: *Epileptology,* Proceedings of the Seventh International Symposium on Epilepsy, Berlin (West), June 1975, edited by D. Janz, pp. 218–227. Thieme/PSG, Stuttgart.

Epilepsy, The Eighth International Symposium,
edited by J. K. Penry. Raven Press, New York
© 1977.

Long-Term Combination Therapy with Phenytoin and Phenobarbital— Evaluation of Serum Levels

F. O. Müller, H. K. L. Hundt, A. K. Aucamp, L. Olivier, W. Wessels, and J. M. Steyn

University of the Orange Free State Medical School, Bloemfontein 9301, Republic of South Africa

A long-term clinical study over a period of 103 days with phenytoin-phenobarbital combination therapy is reported. The study was undertaken in an effort to resolve the controversy still surrounding the results obtained in previous combination therapy studies (Buchthal and Svensmark, 1971; Kutt and Louis, 1972).

PATIENTS AND METHODS

Fifteen adult institutionalized patients suffering from generalized tonic-clonic epilepsy and who had been under good control for at least 3 months prior to the study on a combination tablet (Garoin®, containing 90 mg diphenylhydantoin and 45 mg phenobarbital) were selected. The group included ten black and five white patients.

The flow chart for the trial was elaborated as follows:

1. On day 0 combination therapy was stopped and phenytoin (Epanutin®) substituted at 2.3 mg/kg/day. This relatively low dosage scheme was chosen in the light of findings of Morselli et al. (1971) that discontinuation of phenobarbital may be associated with a significant rise in phenytoin levels.
2. At day 15 the phenytoin dosage was doubled to 4.6 mg/kg/day and 14 days allowed for steady-state levels of phenytoin to be reached.
3. At day 30 phenobarbital at a dose of 2 mg/kg/day was added to the existing regimen.
4. At day 80 the patients were switched back to the combination tablet (Garoin®) in equivalent dosage.
5. Day 103 was the end of the trial period.

Laboratory investigations done at the start of the trial revealed a slight elevation of alkaline phosphatase levels in four patients and neutropenia in six patients.

Serum levels of phenytoin and phenobarbital were monitored simultaneously by means of gas chromatography during the entire trial period.

Statistical analysis was undertaken to determine if significant differences could be shown in mean serum levels at the start of the trial, when maximum levels were reached, and at the end of the trial.

RESULTS

Evaluating phenytoin serum levels at the end of the trial, it was concluded that:

1. Serum phenytoin levels did not increase significantly in this group of patients when phenobarbital was stopped.
2. Doubling the dosage of phenytoin after 14 days led to a significant increase in serum phenytoin levels.
3. Adding phenobarbital to the dosage regimen evoked a further increase of serum phenytoin levels, probably as a result of competitive metabolism.
4. Maximum levels of phenytoin were reached with widely varying intervals of time, the average delay being 34.9 days (range 14 to 49 days). This maximum was reached when phenobarbital levels had already stabilized.
5. No significant difference was found between end values of serum phenytoin and those values ruling before phenobarbital was added to the regimen, i.e., serum phenytoin levels reverted to more or less prephenobarbital levels. The average delay in time to reach prephenobarbital levels was 18 days (range 7 to 33 days). Again a wide interindividual variation was noted.

Table 1 shows the results of serum phenytoin levels monitored during the trial period.

TABLE 1. *Effect of the addition of phenobarbital (2 mg/kg/day) on mean phenytoin serum levels during chronic administration of phenytoin (4.6 mg/kg/day)*

Patient group	Phenytoin serum levels after 2 weeks monotherapy (dosage: 4.6 mg/kg/day)	Max. phenytoin serum levels reached during 11 weeks of combination therapy	Phenytoin serum levels at the end of 11 weeks of combination therapy
	A	B	C
Blacks	12.37	18.20	11.52
($N = 10$)	(SE ± 2.12)	(SE ± 2.38)	(SE ± 1.80)
Whites	11.22	20.24	15.10
($N = 5$)	(SE ± 3.31)	(SE ± 4.70)	(SE ± 5.17
Blacks			
+	11.98	18.88	12.71
whites	(SE ± 3.09)	(SE ± 2.14)	(SE ± 2.03)
($N = 15$)			

The values in column A differ significantly ($p < 0.01$) from those in column B except for the white group where N was too small for any valid statistical conclusions. The values in column B do not differ significantly from those in column C. The values in column A do not differ significantly from those in column C.

DISCUSSION

Long-term combination therapy with phenobarbital and phenytoin in epileptic patients yielded results that are of some importance in the clinical situation. It became clear that the time needed to reach maximum serum levels of phenytoin shows a very wide individual variation.

Secondly, one finds that, after an initial rise and reaching of a maximal value, serum phenytoin levels eventually revert to more or less the same levels that were found before phenobarbital was added to the regimen. Again, wide individual variations were found.

Thirdly, it is necessary to monitor serum levels of phenytoin closely for an extended period of time after introducing phenobarbital to the dosage regimen in order to avoid overenthusiastic adjustments in phenytoin dosage during the critical period of approximately 60 days during which phenytoin levels constantly change.

REFERENCES

Buchthal, F., and Svensmark, O. (1971): Serum concentrations of diphenylhydantoin (phenytoin) and phenobarbital and their relation to therapeutic and toxic effects. *Psychiatr. Neurol. Neurochir.,* 74:117–136.

Kutt, H., and Louis, S. (1972): Anticonvulsant drugs. *Drugs,* 4:227–255.

Morselli, P. L., Rizzo, M., and Garattini, S. (1971): Interaction between phenobarbital and diphenylhydantoin in animals and in epileptic patients. *Ann. N.Y. Acad. Sci.,* 179:88–107.

Epilepsy, The Eighth International Symposium,
edited by J. K. Penry. Raven Press, New York
© 1977.

The Middle Age of Epilepsy

A. Earl Walker

*Department of Surgery (Neurosurgery), University of New Mexico School of Medicine,
Albuquerque, New Mexico 87131*

Epilepsy has usually become manifested by the time a person reaches the early twenties. A great deal has been written about its course in the next few years and its effect on the lives of those who suffer attacks. However, after some years, the epileptic person seems to be forgotten and little is written about the middle-aged person who had seizures in youth. What happens to these individuals? Do they merge into and become lost in the general population? Do they die off? Or do they continue to be plagued by their affliction in business, life, home, and play? Moreover, with the present interest in pollution, perhaps it is time that we began to look at the long-term effects of some drugs that we have been giving our epileptic patients. Granted that in most cases no significant effects on the immediate well-being of the patient have been noted, do we know what the effect of such drugs will be over a period of 20 or 30 years? We have been loading our patients with diphenylhydantoin and other anticonvulsive drugs known to have such side effects as depression of bone marrow, hyperplasia of epithelial tissue, peripheral neuritis, and probably degeneration of the Purkinje cells of the cerebellum. Do patients under such chronic medication develop an aplastic anemia, neoplasms of the liver, or other disturbances that may shorten their life expectancy? No serious study of these questions has been reported as yet, but surely such a longitudinal epidemiological study is desirable. This dissertation is an attempt to answer some of these questions. Accordingly, several series of patients with epilepsy that the author has been intimately acquainted with will be discussed. The first is a series of 1,000 men head-injured in World War I, many with epilepsy, who were followed for more than 50 years (Walker et al., 1971). The second is a group of 240 men who developed epilepsy after head wounds in World War II and who have been followed for more than 25 years (Walker, 1972). The third is a group of 50 patients with intractable psychomotor epilepsy whose discharging temporal lobes the author removed 10 to 25 years ago. It is acknowledged that these series are not representative of epilepsy in the community for, in general, these patients have much more organic neurological pathology. However, the medical, social, and vocational problems are not too dissimilar, and in the absence of follow-up data of other epileptic individuals, these series should give an idea of the life of a middle-aged person who suffered seizures in young adult life.

SEIZURES

Although they are generally considered first, seizures are not the major problem of this population. It is frequently quoted that the epileptic attacks may be controlled at the present time in about two-thirds of cases. But these figures are based on short-term evaluations. Rodin (1968) could find only 10% of persons free from attacks for 10 years. Ghosh (1976) reported that of 600 patients followed 6 to 20 years, 230 were free of attacks for 4 or more years—and about half of them without medication. In the World War I series of 300 patients with posttraumatic epilepsy followed 45 years, 25% of the individuals had no attacks after the initial 3 to 4 years. In the 240 World War II epileptic veterans, approximately half of the original group were having no seizures 25 years later—irrespective of whether or not they were taking anticonvulsant medication. Approximately one-third of the temporal lobectomized group were also free of attacks, and this figure is similar to reports from other centers—Falconer (1972) in London and Rasmussen (1975) in Montreal. However, in all series it is noted that patients after 10 or 15 years of freedom from attacks may have a single or a cluster of seizures in a few days and then none for many years. In some cases these recurrences are related to inadvertent stopping of medication, in some to periods of severe physical or mental stress, in some instances to other neurological conditions involving the brain, and in a few to no known cause. However, these attacks that occur in 10 to 15% of seizure-free patients do not portend recurrent seizures. In fact, many patients with such recurrences have been free of attacks for the next 7 to 15 years. Whether or not a patient continues to take anticonvulsant medication over several decades in the absence of attacks is not so much a medical as a personal consideration. Irrespective of medical advice, about half of the patients stop all medication after a few months or years of freedom from attacks. Most of the remainder continue with token amounts, usually at bedtime, and a few take therapeutic doses even though they have had no attacks for 25 years and they must pay nearly $1,000 per year for their medications.

TABLE 1. *Initial and 15-year follow-up EEG findings*

Epilepsy Type and frequency	EEG abnormality– percentage of cases					
	None		General		Focal	
	Initial	15 year	Initial	15 year	Initial	15 year
Minor						
None (*N* = 33 & 42)	30.3	40.5	18.2	7.1	51.5	52.4
One + (*N* = 26 & 44)	23.1	34.1	15.4	6.8	61.6	59.1
Major						
None (*N* = 33 & 43)	27.3	46.5	15.2	4.7	57.6	48.8
One + (*N* = 27 & 43)	22.2	27.9	22.2	9.3	55.6	62.8
Major and minor						
None (*N* = 21 & 28)	28.6	53.6	14.3	3.6	57.1	46.4
One + (*N* = 26 & 58)	23.1	31.0	23.1	8.6	53.8	60.3

What about the patients who continue to have attacks? The follow-up data on such cases suggest that their attacks, with few exceptions, tend to become fewer and less severe as they grow older. Some seem to cease having attacks with the menopause. In general, those unfortunate ones with continuing major seizures constituted only about 10% of the entire epileptic population 25 years previously.

The electroencephalograms of the older persons tend to have fewer abnormalities and may even be normal in spite of occasional clinical seizures. The improvement is mainly in the greater number of normal records and the fewer records with generalized abnormalities (Table 1). The focal abnormalities remain approximately the same, at least percentage-wise.

SOCIAL ADJUSTMENT

A rough index of the adjustment of an individual to his epilepsy may be obtained by noting his domicile (Table 2). The fact that approximately 25% of

TABLE 2. *Domicilary status 25 years after posttraumatic epilepsy*

Status	No. of patients
Home with wife	92
Home with family	12
Living alone	34
Living in hospital	2
Unknown	6
Total	146

this group are unmarried and living alone distinguishes them from the normal population of a similar sex and age in which less than 10% are single. To some extent the bachelors represent the more severely injured men having seizures, but this is not the whole story, for many loners have no neurological deficit or seizures. However, if their story is correct, most of the men in both groups are living a contented life, although happiness prevails slightly more in the married group (90% as compared with 84% in the single men).

Those men who were married were not only happy but content with their lot, for only 11% sought divorce—as compared with 25% among U.S. men in general. This marital stability probably is based on the fidelity of both partners for, as will be shown later, the wives of these men seem to have a devoted feeling for their spouse to a degree rarely seen in a family of normal people.

Other indices of social adjustment include community activities and motor car driving, which is now a social symbol. The patients with epilepsy seemed to have a good relationship to community life irrespective of their epileptic status. Sixty percent of the patients drive a car and, relative to highway accidents and traffic violations, are better than the average driver if their records are reliable (Table 3).

TABLE 3. *Driving records (10-year period)*

Traffic violations	No.
None	65[a]
One or more	25
Traffic accidents	
None	43[a]
One or more	55

[a] The frequency of such occurrences among all drivers is difficult to ascertain because of nonreported or multiple occurrences. The unofficial data suggest that the figures for this series are better than those for the general population by a factor of 100 to 200%.

LIFE EXPECTANCY

Data on death rates and life expectancy are based on males because adequate series of women with epilepsy have not been reported. Men with posttraumatic epilepsy have a higher death rate at all ages and a shortened life expectancy (Walker et al., 1971). The role that the convulsions play in shortening the life span is not clear. It may be that brain damage is the important determining factor. If such is the case, it would seem that the compensations for the injured brain fail when stresses of aging become severe. Whether these are related to vascular changes or to primary neuronal deficiencies is not evident from the available data. Possibly, subtle functional changes induced by the various cerebral impairments resulting from the head injury render the general defense mechanisms of the body more vulnerable to the stresses of aging.

PHYSICAL OR MENTAL DETERIORATION

There has been the suspicion that after years of epileptic attacks, a certain mental deterioration develops. However, some writers have denied this conclusion; Lennox and Lennox (1960; p. 699) wrote, "The natural tendency for the seizure state and brain waves to improve may extend to the mental state. Although adequate longitudinal studies are lacking . . . the I.Q.'s of many patients will increase."

Data on this point are available from the posttraumatic epilepsy group of World War II (Walker, 1972). After 25 years, approximately 25% of the men and a few more of their wives admitted that there had been some deterioration, either physically or mentally. This mental failing took the form of emotional instability, failing memory, easy fatiguability, and hypersomnia—changes common in persons of 70 to 80 years of age—but these patients were in their late forties. These changes seem to be related to many factors. Illnesses during the last 10 years of the period of observation were more common in individuals showing signs of aging than in those who did not. Perhaps a corollary to the aging process, a certain tendency to accident proneness, was apparent. Whether the chronic ingestion of anticonvulsant medication had an effect on aging is difficult to judge, but there was no doubt that those showing aging were much more likely to be taking medications than those who did not. However, these are trends and do not prove to have statistical significance. Similarly, the definite preponderance of aged individuals in the unemployed group of men may or may not be the result of the aging process. However, the rate of aging did not seem to correlate with the continuing occurrence of minor, major, or any type of fit. Hence, the deterioration may result more from organic brain damage than from the seizures.

SUMMARY

With the onset of middle age, the person who had seizures in childhood is likely to become free of attacks. However, stresses, either physical or mental, may precipitate an isolated seizure or cluster of seizures followed by an indefinite free period.

The social and economic adjustment of these middle-aged persons is good, and few serious deviations from the characteristics of the general population are detectable. However, as a class, these individuals have a higher death rate and lower life expectancy than controls. This early demise is not the result of any specific vulnerability, for the causes of death are similar to those in the general population. Mental deterioration, which occurs in about 25% of the cases, is probably related more to brain damage or medication than to recurrent seizures.

REFERENCES

Falconer, M. A. (1972): The surgical treatment of temporal lobe epilepsy. *Neurochirurgia (Stuttg.)*, 8:161–172.

Ghosh, T. K. (1976): Long-term follow-up in convulsive seizures. *Proceedings of the National Seminar on Epilepsy,* Bangalore, India, 6(5):146–149.

Lennox, W. G., and Lennox, M. A. (1960): *Epilepsy and Related Disorders, Vols. 1 and 2.* Little, Brown and Co., Boston.

Rasmussen, T. (1975): Cortical resection in the treatment of focal epilepsy. *Adv. Neurol.,* 8:139–154.

Rodin, E. A. (1968) *Prognosis of Patients with Epilepsy.* Charles C Thomas, Springfield, Ill.

Walker, A. E. (1972): Long term evaluation of the social and family adjustment to head injuries. *Scand. J. Rehabil. Med.,* 4:5–8.

Walker, A. E., Leuchs, H. K., Lechtape-Grüter, H., Caveness, W. F., and Kretschman, C. (1971): Life expectancy of head injured men with and without epilepsy. *Arch. Neurol.,* 24:95–100.

Epilepsy, The Eighth International Symposium,
edited by J. K. Penry. Raven Press, New York
© 1977.

Chromosomal Damage in Patients with Epilepsy: Possible Mutagenic Properties of Long-Term Antiepileptic Drug Treatment

*Jan Herha and †Günter Obe

*Psychiatrische Klinik and †Institut fuer Genetik der Freien Universitaet Berlin,
Berlin, West Germany*

The long-term drug treatment of patients, in our case, epileptics, raises the question of teratogenic, carcinogenic, and mutagenic side effects of the drugs taken over many years. These three effects are suspected to be induced by anticonvulsive drugs in man (Annegers et al., 1974; Janz, 1975; Neubert et al., 1975). In 1974 the Arzneimittelkommission der Deutschen Aerzteschaft reported that 11 retrospective studies with 1,461 mothers using antiepileptics revealed a rate of malformed children of 6% as compared with 2.5% in controls.

Analyses of leukocyte chromosomes in epileptics have not been conclusive up to now because they are undertaken with patients on therapy with different drugs and with inadequate methods (Grosse et al., 1972; Bartsch, 1975). In our analysis, we investigated the leukocyte chromosomes of epileptics on monotherapy with carbamazepine (CBZ) and with diphenylhydantoin (DPH) and found a significant elevation of exchange-type aberrations of the chromosome type (dicentric and ring chromosomes) and of the chromatid type (chromatid interchanges) as compared with a control sample (Herha and Obe, 1976). Data concerning sex, age, duration of therapy, drug intake, blood levels of the drugs, and the chromosomal findings can be seen in Table 1.

PATIENTS AND METHODS

In this chapter we report on results of a further analysis with 10 probands on therapy with CBZ and DPH, and with 6 probands on therapy with CBZ and primidone (PRIM). As in our previous study we used whole blood cultures incubated for 48 hr with exclusively first *in vitro* mitoses coming into appearance (Dudin et al., 1974; Obe et al., 1976*a*). The data concerning sex, age, drug intake, blood levels of the drugs, duration of therapy, and chromosomal findings can be seen in Table 2 for CBZ + DPH and in Table 3 for CBZ + PRIM.

TABLE 1. Epileptics on monotherapy with carbamazepine and diphenylhydantoin and a control sample

Drug	No. of probands	Sex	Age in years (range)	Duration of therapy in years (range)	Drug intake in grams (range)	Blood level µg/ml (range)	Mitoses analyzed per proband (total)	Exchange-type aberrations	
								Chromatid type	Chromosome type
CBZ	10	6 M, 4 F	38.1 (16–61)	4.5 (1–8)	1,526 (109–3,557)	8 (3–12)	200 (2,000)	7	2
DPH	14	8 M, 6 F	34.4 (18–54)	6.1 (2–10)	830 (220–1,626)	15 (7–22)	200 (2,800)	—	9
Controls	20	10 M, 10 F	30.8 (22–54)	—	—	—	200 83 in 1 case (3,883)	3	—

Sex, average age, average duration of therapy, average values of drug intake, average blood level of drugs, mitoses analyzed, and exchange-type aberrations (data from Herha and Obe, 1976). The blood levels (from blood gained in the morning) of CBZ were determined after the method of B. Herrmann (see Riedel, 1975; Diehl et al., 1976). The blood levels of DPH were determined after the method of Svensmark and Kristensen (1963).

TABLE 2. *Epileptics on therapy with carbamazepine and diphenylhydantoin*

Drug	Proband	Sex	Age in years	Duration of therapy in years		Drug intake in grams		Blood level in $\mu g/ml$		Mitoses analyzed	Exchange-type aberrations
				CBZ	DPH	CBZ	DPH	CBZ	DPH		
CBZ + DPH	1	M	34	10	16	5,402	3,066	11	7	200	1 dicentric chromosome
CBZ + DPH	2	F	34	6	2	5,256	146	11	14	200	—
CBZ + DPH	3	F	25	6	10	4,818	1,460	8	7	200	—
CBZ + DPH	4	M	27	8	12	4,480	1,060	8	12	200	—
CBZ + DPH	5	M	49	6	16	2,628	1,206	7	11	200	—
CBZ + DPH	6	M	36	4	8	2,518	1,096	9	12	200	2 dicentric chromosomes
CBZ + DPH	7	M	40	6	3	2,190	329	9	11	200	1 dicentric chromosome
CBZ + DPH	8	M	46	5	23	1,095	2,049	7	14	200	2 dicentric chromosomes
CBZ + DPH	9	F	18	2	2	876	292	5	13	200	2 dicentric chromosomes
CBZ + DPH	10	M	24	2	4	438	515	5	19	200	1 dicentric chromosome

Sex, age, duration of therapy, drug intake calculated for the whole time of therapy, average blood level of drugs, mitoses analyzed, and exchange-type aberrations. The blood levels were determined during the last 2 years of therapy after the method of B. Herrmann (see Riedel, 1975; Diehl et al., 1976) concerning CBZ, and after the method of Svensmark and Kristensen (1963) concerning DPH.

TABLE 3. *Epileptics on therapy with carbamazepine and primidone*

Drug	Proband	Sex	Age in years	Duration of therapy in years		Drug intake in grams		Blood level in µg/ml		Mitoses analyzed	Exchange-type aberrations
				CBZ	PRIM	CBZ	PRIM	CBZ	PRIM		
CBZ + PRIM	1	M	27	6	8	3,139	2,097	8	12	200	1 dicentric chromosome
CBZ + PRIM	2	M	36	9	14	2,044	4,597	5	9	200	2 chromatid translocation
CBZ + PRIM	3	M	71	9	16	2,044	3,196	6	28	200	2 dicentric chromosomes[a]
CBZ + PRIM	4	F	34	7	10	1,956	3,580	9	13	200	—
CBZ + PRIM	5	F	35	6	12	1,798	3,178	8	10	200	—
CBZ + PRIM	6	M	44	3	6	1,314	3,223	5	30	200	1 acentric ring

[a] In 1 mitosis.

Sex, age, duration of therapy, drug intake calculated for the whole time of therapy, average blood levels of drugs, mitoses analyzed, and exchange-type aberrations. The blood levels were determined during the last 2 years of therapy after the method of B. Herrmann (see Riedel, 1975; Diehl et al., 1976) concerning CBZ, and after the method of Bush and Helman (1965) concerning primidone.

RESULTS

In the CBZ + DPH group we found exclusively dicentric chromosomes, all associated with fragments. In two probands (CBZ + DPH 7 and CBZ + DPH 9) we found two dicentrics, in the other probands we found only one (CBZ + DPH 2, 8, 10). This result is similar to our findings with patients on monotherapy with DPH where also only dicentric chromosomes have been found (see Table 1 and Herha and Obe, 1976). In the DPH series we found nine dicentrics in 2,800 mitoses, or 0.0032 per mitosis, and in the CBZ + DPH series seven in 2,000 mitoses, or 0.0035 per mitosis. In the control series analyzed in our previous investigation (Herha and Obe, 1976) we found no dicentric chromosomes. In control material compiled from the literature and from our own data we have found 11 dicentric chromosomes in 52,007 mitoses from 463 probands or 0.0002 per mitosis (Obe et al., 1976b), a frequency around 17 times lower than that found in patients treated with DPH.

In the CBZ + PRIM group (Table 3) we found two chromatid translocations in one proband (CBZ + PRIM 2), two dicentric chromosomes with one fragment each in one mitosis of one proband (CBZ + PRIM 3), one dicentric chromosome without fragment (CBZ + PRIM 1), and one acentric ring chromosome (CBZ + PRIM 6). Some of these aberrations can be seen in Figure 1. The finding of chromosome- and chromatid-type exchanges in this group resembles our previous findings in a group of probands on monotherapy with carbamazepine (see Table 1 and Herha and Obe, 1976) where also all these three exchange types were found. In the CBZ + PRIM group we found three dicentric chromosomes in 1,200 mitoses, i.e., 0.0025 per mitosis; this is 12.5 times higher than in the 463 control probands referred to above. We found two chromatid translocations in 1,200 mitoses in the CBZ + PRIM group, i.e., 0.0016 per mitosis. In our control series with 20 probands (Table 1 and Herha and Obe, 1976) we found three chromatid translocations in 3,883 mitoses, i.e., 0.0008 per mitosis, and this is two times lower than the frequency in the CBZ + PRIM group. In a control series with 647 probands and 35,296 mitoses compiled from the literature and from our own data (Obe et al., 1976b), we found 15 chromatid translocations or 0.0004 per mitosis; this is 4.25 times lower than the value found in the CBZ + PRIM group.

In our whole analysis with epileptic probands we found 25 dicentric chromosomes in 10^4 mitoses (20/8,000), as compared to 2.1 in 10^4 mitoses (11/52,007) found in the control sample with 463 probands (Obe et al., 1976b). Furthermore, we found 11.25 chromatid translocations in 10^4 mitoses (9/8,000), as compared with 4.25 in 10^4 mitoses (15/35,296) from the control sample with 647 probands (Obe et al., 1976b).

DISCUSSION

Our data indicate that long-term treatment with antiepileptic drugs leads to an elevation of exchange-type aberrations in the lymphocytes of the patients.

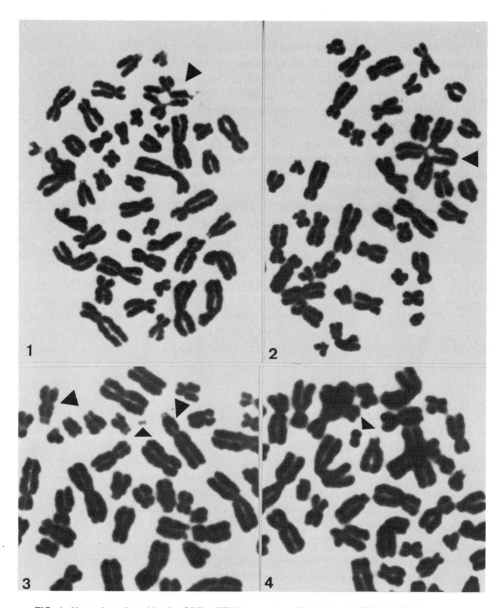

FIG. 1. Aberrations found in the CBZ + PRIM group (see Table 3). **1:** CBZ + PRIM 2, symmetric chromatid translocation *(arrow)* between two homologous chromosomes of the C-group. **2:** CBZ + PRIM 2, asymmetric chromatid translocation *(arrow)* between two A1-chromosomes. **3:** CBZ + PRIM 3, two dicentric chromosomes *(large arrows)* and a double fragment *(small arrow)*. The fragments which belong to the dicentric chromosomes are not shown. **4:** CBZ + PRIM 6, acentric ring chromosome *(arrow)*.

Chromosomal aberrations induced in somatic cells such as lymphocytes indicate that similar aberrations may also have been induced in germ cells. Chromosomal aberrations in germ cells are normally eliminated and so they are mostly without genetic consequences. However, chromosomal aberrations indicate that point mutations may also be present which cannot be detected by our cytogenetic method. Point mutations are carried to the progeny and will eventually lead to severe genetic consequences.

SUMMARY

We analyzed the leukocyte chromosomes of: (a) 10 epileptic probands on therapy with carbamazepine and diphenylhydantoin and (b) 6 epileptics on therapy with carbamazepine and primidone. We compared the results with control material compiled from the literature and from our own data. The finding of chromosome- and chromatid-type exchanges resembles our previous findings in epileptic patients on monotherapy with CBZ and DPH. Our data indicate that long-term treatment with antiepileptic drugs leads to an elevation of exchange-type aberrations in the lymphocytes of the patients.

ACKNOWLEDGMENTS

We thank Prof. Dr. Mueller-Oerlinghausen and his staff from the Psychiatrische Klinik der Freien Universitaet Berlin for the determination of the blood levels (supported by the Deutsche Forschungsgemeinschaft, He 916/1). We thank Mrs. R. Jonas and Mrs. A. Hille from the Institut fuer Genetik der Freien Universitaet Berlin for technical assistance.

REFERENCES

Annegers, J. F., Elveback, L. R., Hauser, W. A., and Kurland, L. T. (1974): Do anticonvulsants have a teratogenic effect? *Arch. Neurol.,* 31:364–373.

Arzneimittelkommission der Deutschen Aerzteschaft (1974): Antiepileptika und Missbildungen. *Dtsch. Aerzteblatt.,* 71:2230.

Bartsch, H. D. (1975): Cytogenetic testing of antiepileptic drugs in human patients. *Mutat. Res.,* 29:279.

Bush, M. T., and Helman, E. (1965): Quantitative determination of primidone. *Life Sci.,* 4:1403–1404.

Diehl, L. W., Mueller-Oerlinghausen, B., and Riedel, E. (1976): The importance of individual pharmacokinetic data for treatment of epilepsy with carbamazepine. *Int. J. Clin. Pharmacol. (in press).*

Dudin, G., Beek, B., and Obe, G. (1974): The human leukocyte test system. I. DNA synthesis and mitoses in PHA-stimulated 2-day cultures. *Mutat. Res.,* 23:279–281.

Grosse, K.-P., Schwanitz, G., Rott, H.-D., and Wissmueller, H. F. (1972): Chromosomenuntersuchungen bei Behandlung mit Anticonvulsiva. *Hum. Genet.,* 16:209–216.

Herha, J., and Obe, G. (1976): Chromosomal damage in epileptics on monotherpay with carbamazepine and diphenylhydantoin. *Hum. Genet.,* 34:1–9.

Janz, D. (1975): Teratologische Wirkungen von Antiepileptika. Antiepileptische Langzeitmedikation, Pharmakokinetik—Klinische Begleitwirkungen *Bibl. Psychiatr.,* 151:86–98.

Neubert, D., Helge, H., and Roehnelt, M. (1975): Zum Problem praenataler Schaedigungen bei antiepileptischer Therapie. Antiepileptische Langzeitmedikation, Pharmakokinetik—Klinische Begleitwirkungen. *Bibl. Psychiatr.,* 151:99–113.

Obe, G., Beek, B., and Slacik-Erben, R. (1976*a*): The use of human leukocyte test system for the evaluation of potential mutagens. *Excerpta Medica International Congress Series,* 376:118–126.

Obe, G., Ristow, H.-J., and Herha, J. (1976*b*): Chromosomal damage by alcohol in vitro and in vivo. Alcohol intoxication and withdrawal: experimental studies, III. *Adv. Exp. Med. Biol. (in press).*

Riedel, E. (1975): Methoden des Nachweises von Antiepileptika. Antiepileptische Langzeitmedikation, Pharmakokinetik—Klinische Begleitwirkungen. *Bibl. Psychiatr.,* 151:1–14.

Svensmark, O., and Kristensen, P. (1963): Determination of diphenylhydantoin and phenobarbital in small amounts of serum. *J. Lab. Clin. Med.,* 61:501–507.

INTENSIVE MONITORING

Epilepsy, The Eighth International Symposium,
edited by J. K. Penry. Raven Press, New York
© 1977.

Intensive Monitoring of Patients with Intractable Seizures

J. Kiffin Penry and Roger J. Porter

*Epilepsy Branch, Neurological Disorders Program, National Institute of Neurological
and Communicative Disorders and Stroke, National Institutes of Health,
Bethesda, Maryland 20014*

Intensive monitoring means detailed, frequent, and accurate quantitative observations and determinations. Intensive monitoring of patients with epileptic seizures means detailed, frequent, and accurate recording of the clinical seizures, the electrical manifestations of these seizures, and the serum concentration of the antiepileptic drugs circulating in the blood to combat these seizures. Simultaneous monitoring of these three factors is essential.

Who needs to be intensively monitored? When a patient has suffered recurring seizures for many years, has failed to respond adequately to antiepileptic drugs, singly or in combination, and has failed to respond to the skills of one or more physicians through conventional outpatient treatment and one or more hospitalizations, it is time to admit the failure of conventional approaches. Those methods of treatment have often failed because the physician is unable to obtain accurate information. When the multiple events occurring in the patient cannot be accurately documented or temporally related to each other, the physician is unable to determine the cause of failure of therapeutic intervention. In addition, cumulative toxic side effects of the medications all too often complicate the therapeutic effort. When patients suffer from intractable seizures, the complexity of events, such as the frequency, duration, and magnitude of seizures—both clinically and electroencephalographically—and the efficacy and toxicity of multiple drugs and their metabolites make intensive monitoring a necessity if the physician hopes to bring order out of chaos.

Reasonably adequate techniques have evolved over the past 10 years so that intensive monitoring of patients with intractable seizures can be effectively and economically carried out (Penry and Dreifuss, 1969; Porter et al., 1971; Porter et al., 1976). Nevertheless, intensive monitoring is sufficiently expensive to preclude its use when conventional therapeutic management techniques will suffice. It is estimated that less than 5% of all epileptic patients should require intensive monitoring.

VIDEOTAPE RECORDING

Some clinical manifestations of epileptic seizures may be readily apparent through stiffening or jerking movements of some part of the body. These movements often occur in many different parts of the body. The patient or other observer rarely gives an adequate and detailed description of the seizures. Even the physician who witnesses such seizures often fails to observe some features of the movements (Penry, 1973). The clinical manifestations of seizures may be subjective and only reported by the patient, but objective events, such as slowing of movement, are often present. The dysfunction of mental performance as a clinical manifestation of seizures may be apparent but may need to be accurately defined and quantified (Penry et al., 1975). This usually requires some type of interaction with the patient, for example, testing the patient's ability to perform such high-level mental functions as arithmetic, memory, and speech.

Another important aspect of documenting the clinical manifestations of epilep-

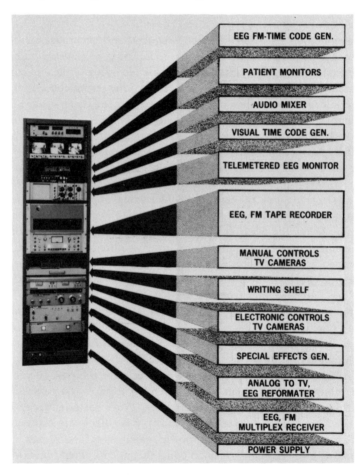

FIG. 1. Equipment used for intensive monitoring of epileptic patients studied in the Clinical Epilepsy Research Program of the NINCDS. Each component of the system is labeled. Components not shown are small EEG transmitter mounted on the patient's head, two television cameras in the patient's room, and two videotape recorders in the central television studio.

tic seizures is the variation of the seizures. The patient or the observer can remember only the major features and may consider several seizures to be the same. When these are studied in detail, however, there may be a central theme, often with significant variations on this theme (Penry et al., 1975). This can be documented only through study of the seizures by video recording.

The technical aspects of video recording have been developed over a period of 10 years and have recently been reviewed (Porter et al., 1976). Two cameras are necessary: one for the whole body and another to show the features of the face, especially the eyes. The whole-body view and the close-up view of the face are simultaneously displayed on a video screen, which also has space to include the electrical manifestations of the seizure. It is absolutely essential that a time code also be displayed so that the date and time of the attack are documented. It is true that the patient's activity is somewhat restricted because freedom of movement is limited to the range of the cameras. Nevertheless, activity can be near normal for a living room, dining room, and bedroom mode of living. This is far superior to being in the EEG laboratory, where the patient must be essentially immobilized. Figure 1 illustrates our monochromatic monitoring equipment.

TELEMETERED EEG

With improvement in techniques of intensive monitoring, the telemetered EEG has proved of vital importance in the evaluation of patients with seizures and the evaluation of the effects of drugs on these seizures. The telemetered EEG offers a reliable recording, although usually with a reduced number of electrodes, in which the effect of normal behavior on the seizure frequency may be taken into consideration. The telemetered EEG contains less artifact and offers an opportunity to record spontaneous seizures. These techniques have been reviewed by Porter and colleagues (1971, 1976). It is of vital importance that a time code for hour, minute, and second be recorded on the magnetic tape, so that events may be searched and written out for quantitative analysis or study of the EEG patterns. In intensive monitoring, the telemetered EEG may be displayed on the video screen with the face and whole-body views of the patient, so that the electrical and clinical manifestations of the abnormal neuronal discharge may be correlated. The sequence of these events is of vital importance.

EEG DIGITAL CASSETTE RECORDING SYSTEM

Although seizures usually occur less frequently when the patient is engaged in a full range of activity, seizures may occur only with specific activities or behavioral precipitants. Also, for prolonged recording of the EEG, patients are unable to stay within the range of the EEG telemetering transmitter and receiver. Techniques have been developed to have the patient wear an EEG amplifier and small tape recorder with an ordinary magnetic tape cassette for recording the

EEG continuously (Sato et al., 1976). This provides an opportunity to capture seizures that are less frequent or that have a tendency to occur in relation to a specific activity. A digital clock must be a part of the system, frequently encoding the hour, minute, and second on the tape, not only for the telemetered EEG but also for documentation of the continuity of recording.

SERUM ANTIEPILEPTIC DRUG CONCENTRATIONS

The usefulness of serum antiepileptic drug concentrations in the treatment of epilepsy has been rapidly increasing over the past 10 years (Rose et al., 1971; Woodbury et al., 1972; Kutt and Penry, 1974). Not only are these determinations extremely valuable in assessing toxic manifestations in the patient, but they are also of increasing value in improving control of epileptic seizures by the adjustment of blood levels of the drugs. Sherwin and colleagues (1973) have demonstrated the practical application of blood levels in the treatment of absence seizures. Antiepileptic drug determinations, however, have been of greatest value in detecting the lack of patient compliance, determining toxic levels, and defining effective levels, primarily in outpatients.

The use of antiepileptic drug concentrations in intensive monitoring requires frequent determinations of the drugs and, often, of their metabolites. Patients with intractable seizures require large amounts of medication, in which an effective drug level nearly always borders on a toxic level. The exact time of serum sampling in relation to drug intake becomes extremely important, as well as additional blood sampling to show the direction of a rise and fall of serum levels. For example, a 23-year-old epileptic man, having several complex partial seizures each week, had ineffective serum carbamazepine concentrations. With an increasing dosage, the carbamazepine levels were raised to an effective level at which seizures were under control, but the patient complained of diplopia each morning. The diplopia lasted approximately 20 min. Changing the administration of carbamazepine to after meals and delaying absorption eliminated the diplopia. Delaying absorption, of course, slightly reduced the peak blood level. In addition, patients with intractable seizures are always on multiple drugs, so that the problem of drug interaction must be taken into account. Intensive monitoring of serum antiepileptic drug concentrations is necessary to determine these interactions.

NECESSITY OF SIMULTANEOUS DATA COLLECTION

It is absolutely essential that all of the monitored factors be precisely identified by time. The multiple variables interacting among abnormal neuronal discharge, electrical manifestations, behavioral manifestations, and the kinetic activity of antiepileptic molecular agents in the body must be considered in order to understand the interrelationships. The essence of an epileptic seizure is the abnormal and excessive paroxysmal discharge of neurons. It is important to study all of the clinical and electrical manifestations. The recording of either manifestation alone is of limited value. For example, in order for one to evaluate brief episodes of strange behavior to determine if they are the manifestations of an epileptic seizure, the EEG must be recorded simultaneously. Likewise, it is essential to know the clinical manifestations when abnormal EEG patterns are recorded. Epileptic patients have been treated for more than 40 years from information obtained by a small sample of the interictal EEG recording. Although some meaningful correlations have been developed from such recordings, the data are all too frequently inadequate, and overextrapolations from such small samples of asynchronous data are all too often misleading. Consequently, there is no substitute for simultaneous recording of clinical events and the EEG—both ictally and interictally.

Simultaneous evaluation of blood samples is equally important. Although serum antiepileptic drug concentrations do not change as instantaneously as the EEG, it is important to determine rising and falling levels in relation to abnormal clinical and EEG events. Serial samples of blood are often necessary to detect rises and falls in serum drug concentrations. Assumptions should not be made from prescribed dosages or single isolated determinations.

OBJECTIVES OF INTENSIVE MONITORING

The purpose of intensively monitoring a patient with intractable seizures is twofold. First, the frequency, duration, and magnitude of seizures must be reliably determined, along with any toxic effects of the medication, and the serum concentration of all drugs. The dose : level ratios must be determined. When these data are studied in light of the history, neurologic examination, and ancillary studies, it becomes possible to plan a therapeutic intervention. Second, intensive monitoring must continue to evaluate the effects of intervention, whether the result of increasing or decreasing blood levels of antiepileptic drugs, minimizing fluctuations in blood levels, withdrawing some of the antiepileptic drugs, or substituting a new drug.

Patients with intractable seizures are nearly always severely handicapped. If the immediate objectives of intensive monitoring are controlling all seizures and removing all side effects of drugs, the long-range objective of intensive monitoring is improvement in the patient's social adjustment, resulting in successful rehabilitation of the individual. Success in rehabilitation extends beyond the benefit of antiepileptic drugs and includes the patient's improved ability to partake of educational, vocational, and recreational opportunities.

BENEFITS OF INTENSIVE MONITORING

Since epilepsy is a chronic paroxysmal disorder, assessing the benefits of intensive monitoring is difficult because any improvement must be maintained over a long period of time. Porter and colleagues (1977) have critically evaluated the benefit of intensive monitoring in 23 of 105 patients who suffered from intractable seizures. Ages ranged from 19 to 30 years in 19 patients and from 8 to 17 years in 4 patients. The average duration of attacks in the 21 older patients was 12 years. On discharge from the hospital, 14 patients had a reduced seizure frequency, and 9 remained unimproved. Of the improved patients, ten had complex partial seizures, three had absence attacks, and one had atonic-myoclonic attacks. Toxicity, mostly due to barbiturates, was eliminated in all but six patients during hospitalization, although the side effects were reduced to some degree in five of the six patients. Follow-up after discharge ranged from 3 to 15 months (mean, 8 months; median, 7 months). Of the 23 patients, 16 had improved seizure control and 19 had a reduction of medication side effects; 11 had a significant improvement in social adjustment when compared to preadmission status. Thus, it appeared that the immediate benefits of intensive monitoring were extremely valuable in a group of patients who were considered to have little or no hope for rehabilitation.

Although it is the purpose of this paper to define the benefits of intensive monitoring for the diagnosis and treatment of patients with intractable seizures, it should at least be mentioned that intensive monitoring provides an opportunity for enormous secondary benefits in both clinical research and medical education. When the clinical and electrical seizure manifestations are videotape recorded for a research protocol, it is possible to define seizure types specifically and to further define the pattern of electrical spread of the abnormal discharges within the brain. It is also possible to determine the effect of a specific drug upon a specific seizure type with adequate recording before and after the administration of the drug. Finally, video tapes of seizures become a valuable resource for teaching those who would otherwise never observe a seizure. Repeated viewing of the video tape is invaluable in teaching medical students about the various seizure types and members of the allied health disciplines about the patient with epilepsy. Furthermore, selected material is of value in the education of the patient, the family, and members of the general public. The school teacher who is aware of absence seizures, for example, is able to detect their occurrence and refer the students for appropriate treatment.

SUMMARY

Intensive monitoring means detailed, frequent, and accurate quantitative observations and determinations; it is indicated in patients who have intractable seizures. Effective and reliable technologies have evolved over the past 10 years. These include multicamera videotape recording of the clinical manifestations of seizures and simultaneous telemetering of the EEG. Blood samples are taken daily and sometimes serially for determination of serum antiepileptic drug concentrations. These data can then be used to plan a therapeutic intervention, with the effect of the intervention being evaluated by further monitoring. Preliminary results from intensively monitored patients with long-standing intractable seizures showed a significant improvement in the majority (61%) of these patients.

REFERENCES

Kutt, H., and Penry, J. K. (1974): Usefulness of blood levels of antiepileptic drugs. *Arch. Neurol.,* 31:283–288.

Penry, J. K. (1973): Behavioral correlates of generalized spike-wave discharge in the electroencephalogram. In: *Epilepsy: Its Phenomena in Man, Vol. 17,* UCLA Forum in Medical Sciences, edited by M. A. B. Brazier. Academic Press, New York.

Penry, J. K., and Dreifuss, F. E. (1969): Automatisms associated with the absence of petit mal epilepsy. *Arch. Neurol.,* 21:142–149.

Penry, J. K., Porter, R. J., and Dreifuss, F. E. (1975): Simultaneous recording of absence seizures with video tape and electroencephalography. A study of 374 seizures in 48 patients. *Brain,* 98: 427–440.

Porter, R. J., Penry, J. K., and Lacy, J. R. (1977): Diagnostic and therapeutic re-evaluation of patients with intractable epilepsy. *Neurology (Minneap.),* in press.

Porter, R. J., Penry, J. K., and Wolf, A. A., Jr. (1976): Simultaneous documentation of clinical and electroencephalographic manifestations of epileptic seizures. In: *Quantitative Analytic Studies in Epilepsy,* edited by P. Kellaway and I. Petersén, pp. 253–268. Raven Press, New York.

Porter, R. J., Wolf, A. A., Jr., and Penry, J. K. (1971): Human electroencephalographic telemetry: A review of systems and their applications and a new receiving system. *Am. J. EEG Technol.,* 11: 145–159.

Rose, S. W., Smith, L. D., and Penry, J. K. (1971): Blood level determinations of antiepileptic drugs. Clinical value and methods. National Institutes of Health, Bethesda.

Sato, S., Penry, J. K., and Dreifuss, F. E. (1976): Electroencephalographic monitoring of generalized spike-wave paroxysms in the hospital and at home. In: *Quantitative Analytic Studies in Epilepsy,* edited by P. Kellaway and I. Petersén, pp. 237–251. Raven Press, New York.

Sherwin, A. L., Robb, J. P., and Lechter, M. (1973): Improved control of epilepsy by monitoring plasma ethosuximide. *Arch. Neurol.,* 28:178–181.

Woodbury, D. M., Penry, J. K., and Schmidt, R. P. (Eds.) (1972): *Antiepileptic Drugs.* Raven Press, New York.

Epilepsy, The Eighth International Symposium,
edited by J. K. Penry. Raven Press, New York
© 1977.

Antiepileptic Drugs in Human Cerebral Cortex: Clinical Relevance of Cortex: Plasma Ratios

A. L. Sherwin,* C. D. Harvey,* and I. E. Leppik**

*Montreal Neurological Institute, 3801 University St., Montreal, Quebec, Canada
**Department of Neurology, University of Minnesota,
St. Paul—Ramsey Hospital, St. Paul, Minnesota 55101

The intensity and duration of the therapeutic action of antiepileptic drugs depend on maintenance of adequate concentrations of drug at hypothetical receptor sites, presumably in neuronal membranes. Indeed, anticonvulsant activity has been correlated with the concentration of a drug or its active metabolite in brain (Kupferberg and Yonekawa, 1974). Although most of the drug present in brain is bound nonspecifically by various tissue components, the total drug content of the tissue presumably reflects the concentration of freely diffusible drug in plasma water and indicates specific binding by putative specific receptor sites. Moreover, in the case of drugs with similar chemical structures such as phenytoin and phenobarbital, empirically determined therapeutic plasma levels may, in part, be a function of the relative distribution of these drugs in gray matter and plasma (cortex : plasma ratios). Correlations involving concentrations of drug in brain, especially in gray and white matter, may offer a quantitative refinement of the plasma concentration : response curve. At the least, the meaning of the plasma concentration in relation to drug in brain is given added perspective.

Previous studies of brain excised during neurosurgical therapy for focal epilepsy reveal good correlations between whole brain and plasma drug levels (Sherwin et al., 1973; Vajda et al., 1974; Houghton et al., 1975). The studies of Rapport et al. (1975) emphasize the importance of separating gray and white matter, as the phenytoin concentration of cerebral cortex is always lower than that of the underlying white matter. In the present study, the cortex : plasma ratios of phenobarbital and phenytoin were determined in patients undergoing neurosurgical therapy. The steady-state plasma levels of a second group of medically treated patients were then used to estimate the theoretical concentrations of phenobarbital and phenytoin present in cerebral cortex. The data show that the calculated molar concentrations of the two drugs in cerebral cortex were similar and that the total brain antiepileptic drug concentration was significantly greater in patients whose seizures were well controlled.

METHODS

Patients were selected from those undergoing neurosurgery for the treatment of focal epilepsy. All were at steady state having received fixed maintenance doses of various anticonvulsants for a period of at least five half-lives up to the time of operation. Cerebral tissues and plasma were assayed by gas chromatography as previously described (Sherwin et al., 1973).

A group of 187 patients with epilepsy (86 females, 101 males) were selected according to the following criteria: daily dose of at least 60 mg phenobarbital and 200 mg phenytoin, no other antiepileptic drugs, management by an experienced neurologist, evidence of compliance by regular plasma drug monitoring, no drug toxicity, and adequate information regarding seizures. Approximately half of the samples were obtained during periods of hospitalization. The average age of the patients was 37.1 ± 14.8 (SD) years and the average weight was 67.7 ± 13.9 kg. Partial seizures were found in 91 patients (simple, complex, and secondarily generalized), whereas 96 had generalized tonic-clonic seizures. Seizure frequency was classified as follows: one or more per month; less than one per month but more than one per year; and one per year or fewer. Steady-state plasma antiepileptic drug levels were used to calculate the theoretical gray matter concentrations using the cortex : plasma ratios of 1.44 for phenytoin and 0.74 for phenobarbital.

RESULTS

Phenobarbital

Phenobarbital was uniformly distributed between the gray matter of cerebral cortex and the underlying white matter (10 patients). The white : gray phenobarbital concentration ratios ranged from 0.83 to 1.34; mean 1.10 ± 0.04 (SE). Plasma levels ranged from 4.2 to 38.3 μg/ml (mean 14.8 μg/ml). There was a highly significant correlation between gray matter and plasma levels ($r = 0.97$, $p < 0.001$); mean cortex : plasma ratio, 0.74 ± 0.75.

Phenytoin

In contrast to the results with phenobarbital, there was a marked difference in the phenytoin concentrations in gray and white matter (5 patients). Phenytoin levels were 1.4-fold greater in the white matter. There was a good correlation between the drug concentrations in gray matter and plasma ($r = 0.86$). The cortex : plasma ratio was 1.44 ± 0.17, which is approximately twofold greater than that of phenobarbital.

Phenobarbital and Phenytoin Levels in Cerebral Cortex

The mean plasma levels in 187 patients were 17.8 ± 0.7 μg/ml (SE) for phenobarbital and 9.8 ± 0.5 μg/ml for phenytoin. However, when differences in the

TABLE 1. *Dose, plasma levels, and calculated brain concentrations of anticonvulsant drugs in 187 patients receiving combination therapy*

Drug	Daily dose (mg)	Daily dose (mg/kg)	Plasma level (μM/l)	Brain concentration (μM/kg)
Phenobarbital	100 ± 43[a]	1.5 ± 0.6[a]	76.7 ± 3.0[b]	56.8 ± 5.8[b,c]
Phenytoin	307 ± 74[a]	4.5 ± 1.1[a]	38.9 ± 1.9[b]	56.0 ± 9.8[b,d]

[a] ± SD.
[b] ± SEM.
[c] Cortex : plasma ratio 0.74 ± 0.05 [b]; molecular weight 232.
[d] Cortex: plasma ratio 1.44 ± 0.17[b]; molecular weight 252.

cortex : plasma ratios and molecular weights were taken into account, the estimated concentration of phenobarbital was 56.8 ± 5.8 μM/kg compared to 56.0 ± 9.8 μM/kg for phenytoin. Hence, although plasma drug levels differed widely, the concentrations of the two drugs in cerebral cortex were similar (Table 1).

Antiepileptic Drug Levels and Seizure Frequency

When patients with different seizure types and frequency were compared, phenobarbital plasma levels exceeded those of phenytoin in all groups studied. Table 2 shows the plasma antiepileptic drug concentrations observed in patients with partial epilepsy related to seizure frequency. There was a significantly higher estimated total brain antiepileptic drug concentration in those patients having one seizure per year or fewer as compared to those with more frequent attacks.

TABLE 2. *Drug concentrations in cerebral cortex in partial epilepsy related to seizure frequency*

	More than 1/month	Less than 1/month, more than 1/year	1/year or fewer
Plasma phenobarbital μg/ml	17.4 ± 1.2[a]	14.6 ± 2.4	26.7 ± 4.4
Plasma phenytoin μg/ml	9.3 ± 0.6	11.3 ± 2.5	13.1 ± 1.7
Total drug in cortex μM/kg	108.6 ± 5.4	111.2 ± 19.6	160.1 ± 20.4[b]
No. of patients	64	15	19

[a] SEM.
[b] $p < 0.01$ compared to groups with more frequent seizures.
   Cortex: plasma ratios—phenobarbital 0.74 ± 0.05[a], molecular weight 232; phenytoin 1.44 ± 0.17, molecular weight 252.

A similar trend was observed in patients with generalized epilepsy and tonic-clonic seizures.

DISCUSSION

Although there is no clear evidence of specific binding of antiepileptic drugs by receptors in brain, anticonvulsant activity does parallel brain concentration in the experimental animal (Baumel et al., 1973). We have recently demonstrated that similar molar concentrations of phenobarbital and phenytoin are required for protection in the maximal electroshock seizure test. When various combinations of phenobarbital and phenytoin were tested, the drugs acted in an additive fashion and seizure protection was dependent on the total concentration of antiepileptic drug present in the brain (Leppik and Sherwin, 1976).

The finding that phenobarbital was evenly distributed between gray and white matter with slightly less drug in brain than plasma agrees with the observations of Domek et al. (1960) and van der Kleijn et al. (1973) who studied the regional distribution of this drug in cat and monkey, respectively. The cortex : plasma ratio of phenobarbital in the present study (0.74) was lower than the whole brain : serum ratio of 1.1 reported by Houghton et al. (1975). Vajda et al. (1974) found the whole brain : plasma level to be 0.59 in seven patients. The cortex : plasma ratio of phenytoin of 1.44 observed in relatively nonaffected cortex from epileptic patients in our study is within the range observed by Rapport et al. (1975) in three nonepileptic patients. These investigators found a marked decrease in phenytoin binding in focal epileptogenic lesions characterized by fibrous astrogliosis.

Our review of the 187 carefully monitored patients treated with phenobarbital and phenytoin in combination revealed that the neurologists were using the individual drugs at the lower end of the therapeutic range. Effective seizure control was probably dependent on the synergistic action of the two agents. It is of interest that the widely differing plasma levels resulted in similar estimated drug concentrations in the cerebral cortex. Possibly careful titration of phenytoin dosage would achieve the same effects with a single drug (Reynolds, 1976). Similarly, the degree of seizure control attained in patients with partial epilepsy was directly related to the antiepileptic drug concentration estimated to be present in the cerebral cortex.

At present, perhaps the only value of the cortex : plasma ratio is to focus the clinician's attention on the fact that plasma levels do correlate with antiepileptic effects in brain. The ratios illustrate the relative ease by which an antiepileptic drug enters and binds to brain constituents. Goldberg and Todoroff (1976) have speculated that the binding of phenytoin to brain proteins enhanced by phospholipids may contribute to the action of this drug as a membrane stabilizer. In recent experimental studies in the rat we found the brain : plasma ratio of valproate to be in the order of 0.2, hence a plasma level of approximately 50 $\mu g/ml$ would result in a molar concentration in brain of the same magnitude as 20 μg/ml of phenobarbital or 10 μg/ml of phenytoin. Recently it has been possible to demonstrate stereospecific receptor binding of neuroleptic drugs in brain. Seeman (1974) has been able to correlate the relative clinical potencies of these drugs in treating schizophrenia with presynaptic blockade of dopamine release in electrically stimulated slices from rat caudate nucleus. In fact, this assay is now being used to screen potentially new neuroleptic drugs. It is most likely that specific receptors exist for antiepileptic drugs, especially for extremely potent agents such as clonazepam. Perhaps similar studies will aid our understanding of the mechanism of action of antiepileptic drugs as well as provide new insight into functional membrane abnormalities underlying the genesis of the epilepsies.

SUMMARY

Studies of cerebral tissue excised during neurosurgical therapy reveal that phenobarbital was equally distributed between gray and white matter and that the cortex : plasma ratio was 0.74 ± 0.05 (10 patients). In contrast, phenytoin concentrations averaged 1.4-fold greater in white matter and the cortex : plasma ratio was 1.44 ± 0.17 (4 patients). In 187 patients receiving these drugs as medical therapy, the mean plasma levels were phenobarbital 17.8 ± 0.7 μg/ml (SE), and phenytoin 9.8 ± 0.5 μg/ml. However, molar cortical concentrations calculated by using the cortex : plasma ratios were almost equal. In patients with partial seizures, the total brain antiepileptic drug concentration was significantly higher in those patients with one seizure or less per year.

ACKNOWLEDGMENTS

This work was supported by a grant from the Medical Research Council of Canada.

REFERENCES

Baumel, I. P., Gallagher, B. B., DiMicco, J., and Goico, H. (1973): Metabolism and anticonvulsant properties of primidone in the rat. *J. Pharmacol. Exp. Ther.,* 186:305–314.
Domek, N. S., Barlow, C. F., and Roth, L. J. (1960): An ontogenetic study of phenobarbital-C^{14} in cat brain. *J. Pharmacol. Exp. Ther.,* 130:285–293.
Goldberg, M. A., and Todoroff, T. (1976): Enhancement of diphenylhydantoin binding by lipid extraction. *J. Pharmacol. Exp. Ther.,* 196:579–585.
Houghton, G. W., Richens, A., Toseland, P. A., Davidson, S., and Falconer, M. A. (1975): Brain concentrations of phenytoin, phenobarbitone and primidone in epileptic patients. *Eur. J. Clin. Pharmacol.,* 9:73–78.
Kupferberg, H. J., and Yonekawa, W. (1975): The metabolism of 3-methyl-5-ethyl-5-phenylhydantoin (Mephenytoin) to 5-ethyl-5-phenylhydantoin (Nirvanol) in mice in relation to anticonvulsant activity. *Drug Metab. Dispos.,* 3:26–29.
Leppik, I. E., and Sherwin, A. L. (1976): Anticonvulsant activity of phenytoin in combination with phenobarbital. *J. Pharmacol. Exp. Ther. (in press).*
Rapport, R. L., Harris, A. B., Friel, P. N., and Ojemann, G. A. (1975): Human epileptic brain. *Arch. Neurol.,* 32:549–554.

Reynolds, E. H., Chadwick, D., and Galbraith, A. W. (1976): One drug (phenytoin) in the treatment of epilepsy. *Lancet,* 923–926.
Seeman, P. (1974): The actions of nervous system drugs on cell membranes. *Hosp. Prac.,* 9:93–101.
Sherwin, A. L., Eisen, A. A., and Sokolowski, C. D. (1973): Anticonvulsant drugs in human epileptogenic brain: correlation of phenobarbital and diphenylhydantoin levels with plasma. *Arch. Neurol.,* 29:73–77.
Vajda, F., Williams, F. M., Davidson, S., Falconer, M. A., and Breckenridge, A. (1974): Human brain, cerebrospinal fluid, and plasma concentrations of diphenylhydantoin and phenobarbital. *Clin. Pharmacol. Ther.,* 15:597–603.
van der Kleijn, E., Pijnappel, H., van Wijk, C., Guelen, P., and Rijntjes, N. (1973): Pharmacokinetic concepts for chronic treatment with anti-epileptic drugs. In: *Methods of Analysis of Anti-Epileptic Drugs,* edited by J. W. A. Meijer, H. Meinardi, C. Gardner-Thorpe, and E. van der Kleijn. American Elsevier Publishing Co., New York.

Epilepsy, The Eighth International Symposium,
edited by J. K. Penry. Raven Press, New York
© 1977.

Prolonged Monitoring of the EEG in Ambulatory Patients

J. F. Woods and J. R. Ives

Department of Neurology and Neurosurgery, McGill University and Montreal Neurological Institute, Montreal, Quebec H3A 2B4, Canada

Neurologists have long appreciated the importance of the EEG in the diagnosis of transient neurological symptoms. The concurrence of an epileptic discharge in the EEG with the patient's symptoms confirms the diagnosis while the absence of an epileptic discharge in the presence of symptoms is strong evidence against a diagnosis of epilepsy. The opportunity to record the EEG during an attack rarely presents itself in the EEG laboratory. Even if a patient does have an attack in the EEG laboratory, the chances that the attack will be recorded on the EEG are only about 50% in our experience. Specific paroxysmal discharges are seen in the interictal EEG of only 30 to 70% of patients depending on the type of epilepsy (Kooi, 1971).

On the other hand, epileptic changes in the interictal EEG do not prove that all of the patient's symptoms are due to epilepsy. For these and other reasons, it is often desirable to monitor a patient's EEG for a prolonged period in order to obtain a recording during an attack. Many systems have been devised for this purpose. Several laboratories are now using radiotelemetry for transmission of the EEG over short distances to a receiver that transfers the data to either a magnetic tape or an EEG machine or both. This eliminates the restriction of movement imposed by the wires used in routine EEG recordings, but the patient must still be confined within the radius of the range of the transmitter—usually no more than 50 feet from the receiver. This necessitates admission to hospital and close supervision by hospital personnel—either an EEG technician or nurses on the ward. It is useful for patients who must be confined to hospital for other reasons and provides recordings comparable in quality to those obtained by direct recording (Porter et al., 1971; Ives et al., 1973).

For prolonged recordings on outpatients, the only feasible system presently available is a cassette recorder. This has been developed for prolonged EKG recordings and can record continuously for 24 hr on a single standard cassette.

METHODS

The cassette recorder we use was designed by Oxford Instruments Co. in England for continuous EKG monitoring. It weighs under 400 g including batteries and cassette, and its dimensions are 10.6 × 8.6 × 3.6 cm. It will record for just over 24 hr on four channels using a standard C120 cassette.

Its major drawback is its noise level of about 50 μV. This is acceptable for EKG recording but clearly not for the EEG. In order to overcome this problem, we have devised a small preamplifier with a gain of 10 which in effect reduces the noise level to an acceptable 5 μV. This preamplifier is the key to the whole system.

Another disadvantage that applies to all analogue tape recording systems is their limited dynamic range of just over 30 db. The maximum signal which can be recorded without distortion is about 200 μV. Thus high-amplitude signals such as spike-and-wave complexes are distorted but still clearly recognizable.

Complete technical details have been reported elsewhere (Ives and Woods, 1975).

We use standard silver–silver chloride electrodes with electrode jelly injected through a hole using a blunt needle. The top of the electrode is insulated with epoxy to eliminate touch artifact. The electrode is connected to the preamplifier by a 28-gauge Teflon insulated wire; various colors are available to match the patient's hair. The electrodes are attached to the scalp in the standard manner using gauze and collodion glue. The subject takes home with him a syringe full of electrode jelly and a family member applies jelly to each electrode once a day. This system enables the electrodes to remain in place for up to 4 days. Some patients complain of scalp irrritation under the electrodes after 3 or 4 days, so we prefer not to leave the electrodes on for longer than 4 days as a rule. The patient also takes home with him three extra cassettes and one extra set of batteries. He is instructed to change the cassette every 24 hr and the batteries after 48 hr.

Female patients wear the cassette on a shoulder strap; males attach it to their belts.

If the purpose of the recording is to determine the nature of transient symptoms, the patient is asked to change the cassette 15 min after recovering from the symptoms. In this way, the exact epoch of EEG which correlates with the symptoms can be easily found and studied.

The recorded cassettes are played back on a high-speed playback unit. The EEG is written out by a mingograf ink-jet EEG machine that has an upper frequency response of 700 Hz as compared with 70 or 100 Hz for a machine using galvanometer ink pens. This permits the recording to be played back at 20 times the speed of recording, when the original band width of the recording, which is 0.5 to 35 Hz, becomes 10 to 700 Hz. The 24-hr recording can thus be written in just over 1 hr. With a paper speed of 30 cm/sec, the EEG printout is equivalent to 1.5 cm/sec real time.

It can also be written out at 60 times the recording speed so that 24 hr of data can be written out in 24 min. This reduces the upper frequency to 11 Hz but is adequate for identification of 3/sec spike-and-wave complexes.

RESULTS

Table 1 summarizes the results of our recording to date. We have made recordings on 38 patients. Some were recorded more than once giving a total of 54 recordings. The total time of the recordings was 3,458 hr with an average duration of 64 hr and a range of 24 to 120 hr.

The prerecording diagnosis is given in the left-hand column. Twenty-six patients had transient symptoms of unknown etiology. For these we normally record one channel of EKG and three of EEG. Nine patients were known to have epilepsy. These were recorded in order to determine the influence of various therapeutic measures on the frequency of their seizures. These had four channels of EEG recorded.

Two patients were suspected of having narcolepsy. These had two channels of EEG, one oculogram, and one of EMG in order to determine their circadian sleep pattern. One did have genuine brief sleep attacks, although these appeared to be of the non-REM type. The other had no excessive diurnal sleep during 3 days of recordings. It appeared that her so-called sleep attacks represented diurnal drowsiness secondary to nocturnal insomnia.

The one patient with torticollis had four channels of EMG recorded from her neck.

Of the 26 patients with transient attacks suspected to be epilepsy, 12 had attacks during the recordings. We select for recording those patients who have attacks once a week or more frequently. Occasionally, and especially when we started using the recorder, we did not apply this restriction rigidly and this accounts at least in part for our failure to obtain a recording during an attack in 14 patients. We prefer patients who have attacks daily, but patients are not often so cooperative. Indeed, occasional patients who have one or more attacks daily appear to derive considerable therapeutic benefit from wearing the recorder. This is not a lasting benefit, however, and in one patient the apparent effect wore off seconds after the recorder had been disconnected and the electrodes were being removed. This gave us our first opportunity to witness an attack and it appeared to be clearly hysterical. Patients seem to be much more aware of their symptoms

TABLE 1. *Prolonged EEG cassette recordings*

Diagnosis	No. of patients	No. of recordings	Total hr	Average duration (hr)	Range (hr)
Possible epilepsy	26	36	2,346	65.2	24–120
Known epilepsy	9	15	968	64.5	24–120
Narcolepsy	2	2	120	60	24–96
Torticollis	1	1	24	24	
Total	38	54	3,458	64	24–120

during the recording and sometimes give a much clearer description of their attacks after the recording than they had been able to give before. We ask them to write a description of their symptoms immediately following their attacks.

Two of the twelve patients had attacks accompanied by epileptic discharges in the EEG. Two others had cardiac irregularities during their attacks and were referred to a cardiologist for further investigation. Two had only muscle artifact during their attacks so that we could not interpret the EEG, but the description of the attacks and the concurrence of excessive muscle activity did not allow us to exclude epilepsy; therefore, they remained with a diagnosis of possible epilepsy. Three patients had attacks which were considered to be hysterical. In one of these, three attacks occurred during the recording. Each time, the recording ceased altogether a few minutes prior to the attack and resumed a few minutes after the attack. This could be explained only by the patient deliberately unplugging the electrodes from the recorder before the attack and replugging it afterward— strong evidence that the attacks were not true epilepsy.

Three patients whose symptoms consisted of recurrent brief episodes of dizziness had no changes in the EEG or EKG during the attacks, and they remained with a postrecording diagnosis of dizziness but with epilepsy and cardiac arrhythmia excluded as the cause.

Of the patients with known epilepsy, the efficacy of various forms of therapy in diminishing the frequency of seizure discharges were clearly demonstrated.

DISCUSSION

The cassette recorder, modified with the preamplifier, is a useful, practical instrument with a variety of clinical applications.

In patients with known epilepsy it can give us a clear picture of the influence of environmental and other factors on the frequency of seizure discharges. In patients with transient symptoms of unknown origin, it can sometimes be of great importance to exclude epilepsy or cardiac arrhythmia. It will not always provide the answer but we are dealing here with patients in whom all other methods of investigation including repeated EEGs both awake and asleep, EKGs, X-rays, CT scans, and often angiograms have failed to provide a diagnosis. If use of the cassette recorder can help even a small number of these patients, it represents a worthwhile advance. More experience in its use and improving technology will probably widen its applications and hopefully improve the percentage of positive results.

ACKNOWLEDGMENT

This work was supported by Canadian Medical Research Council Grant MA 4784 and a Killam Foundation Grant.

REFERENCES

Ives, J. R., Thompson, C. J., and Woods, J. F. (1973): Acquisition by telemetry and computer analysis of 4-channel, long term E.E.G. recordings from patients subject to "petit-mal" absence attacks. *Electroencephalogr. Clin. Neurophysiol.,* 34:665–668.

Ives, J. R., and Woods, J. F. (1975): 4-channel 24 hour cassette recorder or long-term E.E.G. monitoring of ambulatory patients. *Electroencephalogr. Clin. Neurophysiol.,* 39:88–92.

Kooi, K. A. (1971): *Fundamentals of Electroencephalography.* Harper and Row, New York.

Porter, R. J., Wolf, A. A., Jr., and Penry, J. K. (1971): Human electroencephalographic telemetry. *Am. J. EEG Technol., 11:145–159.*

Epilepsy, The Eighth International Symposium,
edited by J. K. Penry. Raven Press, New York
© 1977.

Evaluation of Reliability in Determination of Antiepileptic Drug Levels

Alan Richens

*Reader in Clinical Pharmacology, St. Bartholomew's Hospital,
London, EC1A 7BE, England*

Five years ago, my colleagues and I wished to set up methods for estimating the commonly used antiepileptic drugs, but as we had had little experience with gas chromatographic methods we were a little uncertain of the accuracy of our results. I decided, therefore, to send aliquots of a few specimens to five other laboratories in London who were offering a routine service for these estimations so that we could compare their results with ours. It was immediately obvious that there was no general agreement on the true concentrations of drugs in the specimens. In May, 1972, I called together a small group of clinical pharmacologists and clinical chemists to discuss the mechanism of setting up an informal quality control scheme, and following this meeting aliquots of pooled sera from epileptic patients were distributed at regular intervals. A great deal of interest was stimulated by this scheme, such that it was necessary to organize a larger meeting in October of the same year at which a number of workers from continental Europe were present. Since this time, the scheme has steadily grown and currently includes 123 participants working in laboratories in most European countries, as well as in South Africa, Malaysia, Canada, and the United States.

The results of 2 years' experience in organizing the scheme were presented at the Second Workshop on the Determination of Anti-Epileptic Drugs in Body Fluids (WODADIBOF II) in Bethel, West Germany, in 1974 (Richens, 1975). Among those present at the Workshop were Drs. Kiffin Penry and Charles Pippenger, and on their return to the United States they resolved to set up a similar scheme in their country. Their initial step was to mail to each laboratory which offered a service for drug estimations three pooled sera containing phenytoin, phenobarbital, primidone, and ethosuximide. By organizing distribution centers they were able to submit the specimens to the laboratories as if they had been taken from patients locally, and the samples were therefore run in the usual routine manner (unlike our specimens, which are always mailed out as quality control specimens). Their results deserve wide publicity because they highlight the urgent need for quality control of drug estimations (Pippenger et al., 1976). For each specimen the range of results reported was from zero to levels so high as to be compatible only with massive acute overdosage, and the coefficients of variation varied from 38 to 505%. Five laboratories who were known to have had a great deal of experience in estimating these drugs were chosen as reference laboratories, and they achieved coefficients of variation of 9 to 156%. Generally speaking, these reference laboratories obtained results that were acceptable for clinical purposes, although even their techniques left room for improvement. The results produced by many of the other laboratories, however, were entirely unacceptable and could often have led the clinician to adjust drug dosage in the wrong direction had the specimens come from real patients. Presumably, these results reflected the normal quality of drug estimations in these laboratories.

Our experience is, in general, a happier one, but there may be two reasons for this. First, as mentioned above, our specimens have always been sent out as quality control specimens and the results returned are often the mean of several separate estimations. Knowing that they are under test, laboratories naturally are anxious to return their best estimates (although anonymity is maintained when the results are published). Second, most European laboratories do not have a financial motive for offering a drug monitoring service, and therefore they are likely to do so only if they are scientifically motivated and this leads to a much higher standard of self-criticism. For instance, our quality control scheme has conclusively shown that spectrophotometric techniques for estimating phenytoin are very unreliable when used for analysis of samples from patients on multiple drug therapy (Table 1), and almost all of our participants have abandoned these methods in favor of gas chromatography or immunoassay. In contrast, an appreciable number of American laboratories still adhere to the older techniques.

In Table 1 it can be seen that gas chromatographic techniques involving methylation (usually flash methylation) give the most satisfactory results for phenytoin and phenobarbital, although nonderivative forming techniques appear to be superior for primidone. A number of laboratories are now using radio- or enzyme-immunoassay techniques, but insufficient results have yet accumulated to compare them with gas chromatography. Most research workers have a habit of making their own minor modifications to published methods for drug estimation, and therefore it is not possible from our results to conclude which specific method is the most satisfactory. With further experience it might be possible and this would obviously be useful to laboratories who are intending to set up assay methods.

Currently we send out two types of specimens: serum samples with weighed-in quantities of drugs (these have been prepared by Wellcomtrol, Biotrol, or members of the quality control scheme) or aliquots of serum pools to which a number (usually a large number) of patients receiving multiple-drug therapy have contributed. The latter specimens provide a much more severe test of an analytical method because they contain a variety of drugs in low dosage in addition to the drugs to be analyzed and, furthermore, they contain drug metabolites that can potentially cause interference in less specific assay methods. In general, the inter-laboratory coefficient of variation on these latter specimens is greater than for spiked standards. Quality control samples are provided for five drugs: phenytoin,

TABLE 1. Results of phenytoin, phenobarbital, and primidone estimations according to method used in the quality control scheme

Drug	Method	No. of labs	No. of specimens estimated	No. outside 95% confidence limits	Percentage outside 95% confidence limits
Phenytoin	GLC				
	No derivative	28	424	40	9
	Methylation[a]	35	480	23	5
	Spectrophotometric	4	41	22	54
	Modified				
	Wallace	5	78	14	18
	TLC	3	67	10	15
	HPLC	1	6	0	—[b]
	EMIT	4	13	0	—
	RIA	2	4	1	—
Phenobarbital	GLC				
	No derivative	25	442	47	11
	Methylation[a]	29	256	11	4
	TLC	3	65	3	5
	Spectrophotometric	3	17	3	—
	Modified				
	Wallace	1	4	0	—
	EMIT	4	14	1	—
Primidone	GLC				
	No derivative	19	200	10	5
	Methylation	17	128	14	11
	EMIT	3	6	0	—

[a] Occasionally ethylation.
[b] —indicates insufficient data for meaningful calculation.
The number of results which were outside the 95% confidence limits for each specimen has been calculated.

phenobarbitone, primidone, carbamazepine, and sodium valproate. The service has been provided free of charge, but as of January, 1977, a small charge will be made which will enable us to organize the scheme in a more professional manner. Negotiations with the Reference Bureau of the European Economic Community (EEC) have been initiated by a Steering Committee comprised of Professor Godfraind (Brussels), Professor Heusghem (Liege), Professor Siest (Nancy), and myself in order to set up a more formal quality control scheme covering all drugs being monitored for therapeutic purposes in all fields of medicine.

Clinical chemists have long accepted the need for quality control of analytical techniques, but in the drug monitoring field the concept is just being realized. This development is essential if the clinician is to be provided with reliable drug level estimations, and I would like to suggest that any European clinician who relies on the results of these assays should inquire as to whether his local laboratory takes part in the quality control scheme. If not, a tactful hint might be in order. Monitoring drug levels can greatly improve the management of epilepsy, but it is vital that a decision to alter a patient's treatment is based on an accurate result. Any laboratory wishing to join the scheme should write to me at the following address: Dr. A. Richens, Department of Clinical Pharmacology, St. Bartholomew's Hospital, London, EC1A 7BE, England.

REFERENCES

Pippenger, C. E., Penry, J. K., White, B. G., Daly, D. D., and Buddington, R. (1976): Interlaboratory variability in determination of plasma antiepileptic drug concentrations. *Arch. Neurol.,* 33:351–355.

Richens, A. (1975): Results of a phenytoin quality control scheme. In: *Clinical Pharmacology of Anti-Epileptic Drugs,* edited by H. Schneider, D. Janz, C. Gardner-Thorpe, H. Meinardi, and A. L. Sherwin. Springer-Verlag, Heidelberg.

Epilepsy, The Eighth International Symposium,
edited by J. K. Penry. Raven Press, New York
© 1977.

A Prospective Longitudinal Study of Serum Levels of Sulthiame and Phenytoin, Together with an Evaluation of Seizure Control

*N. Callaghan, *M. Feely, †M. O'Callaghan, and †B. Duggan

Departments of *Neurology and †Biochemisty, St. Finbarr's Hospital, Cork, Ireland

Sulthiame, a sulfonamide derivative with carbonic anhydrase–inhibiting properties, is used as an anticonvulsant for focal and generalized seizures. In most clinical trials, it has been given in combination with other anticonvulsants. Therefore, its effect as a single drug in the treatment of epilepsy has not been fully evaluated. Green et al. (1974) carried out a controlled trial using phenytoin as the control treatment. They concluded that sulthiame had little value as a primary anticonvulsant. However, it cannot be concluded from this study whether or not sulthiame is completely devoid of anticonvulsant properties, since phenytoin probably had a beneficial effect.

It has been suggested (Richens, 1976) that sulthiame is most effective when added to an established drug, the metabolism of which it inhibits, resulting in an increase in blood levels. It has been established (Hansen et al., 1968) that sulthiame is an inhibitor of phenytoin metabolism, resulting in increased levels of phenytoin when both drugs are used in combination. In view of the absence of comprehensive data on the effect of sulthiame when used as a single drug and in combination with phenytoin in seizure control, we set up a prospective longitudinal study in order to evaluate the anticonvulsant effect of this drug when used initially as a single anticonvulsant in epilepsy, and in combination with phenytoin, in patients in whom satisfactory control did not occur on sulthiame used as sole treatment. The purpose of this chapter is to report the preliminary results of this study.

PATIENTS AND METHODS

The patients were allocated sulthiame in a randomized fashion as part of a study set up to compare (1) the anticonvulsant effect of a group of anticonvulsant drugs, including sulthiame, and (2) blood levels with seizure control on a prospective longitudinal basis. Nine patients reported in this chapter were allocated sulthiame because of poor control on other drugs. One patient had had sulthiame initially but was included in the study, as the drug had been prescribed in a

TABLE 1. *Treatment before introduction of sulthiame*

Drugs	No. of patients
Phenytoin	3
Phenytoin + primidone	2
Phenytoin + phenobarbital	2
Phenytoin + sodium valproate	1
Carbamazepine + primidone	1
Sulthiame	1

subtherapeutic dose. The results in a total of ten patients are documented. The patients included six females and four males. The mean age of the male patients was 32.7 years (age range 18 to 70 years); the mean age of the female patients was 29.5 years (age range 14 to 75 years). The patients included six patients with grand mal epilepsy, one with temporal lobe absences, and three with a combination of grand mal seizures and temporal lobe attacks.

The anticonvulsant drugs the patients were receiving prior to the introduction of sulthiame are documented in Table 1. The anticonvulsant drugs which nine of the patients had been taking were discontinued, and sulthiame was introduced initially in a dosage of 3 mg/kg body weight. The dose was then increased at weekly intervals according to the patient's clinical requirements and tolerance to side effects. When phenytoin was used in combination with sulthiame, it was given in a dosage of 3 to 10 mg/kg. Blood was taken for the estimation of sulthiame and phenytoin levels 1 week following the start of treatment with each drug, and at intervals of 2 and 4 weeks thereafter, according to the progress of the patient. The serum levels of sulthiame and phenytoin were measured by gas-liquid chromatography. The method of Simons and Levy (1972) was used for the estimation of sulthiame, and the method of Roger et al. (1973) for the estimation of phenytoin. Before treatment with sulthiame was started, the serum levels of phenytoin were estimated for the eight patients to whom this drug was previously given as a single drug or in combination with other anticonvulsants. The levels were within the therapeutic range in four patients, in the toxic range in two patients, and at subtherapeutic level in two others.

RESULTS

The fit frequency per week prior to treatment with sulthiame was 7.8 ± SD 13.0. Sulthiame was given as a single drug over a mean period of 7 weeks, resulting in a reduction in fit frequency to 5.8 ± SD 5.3. The improvement was not significant. The dosage of sulthiame varied between 8 and 16.71 mg/kg with a mean dosage of 11.8 mg/kg. There was a wide range in the blood levels of sulthiame which varied between 2.50 and 18 μg/ml. A statistical test (Bartlett test X^2 (7) = 8.796, $p = 0.268$) showed that the variation of blood levels within each patient when on a fixed dose was the same for all patients and averaged 7.8, i.e., pooled within patient standard deviation = 2.8. A positive linear relationship between dose and blood level was established, using a regression analysis, whereby if the dose increased, the blood levels also increased.

When seizure control was not satisfactory on sulthiame, phenytoin was added to the regimen. This combination was used over a mean period of 15.3 weeks. The dose of sulthiame mostly remained the same and averaged 12.1 mg/kg during this period. The dosage of phenytoin varied between 3.33 and 7.50 mg/kg, and the serum levels varied between 13.36 and 43.00 μg/ml with a mean level of 25.18 μg/ml. In four patients, the serum levels of phenytoin were consistently elevated above 20 μg/ml, in two patients the levels fluctuated intermittently above and below 20 μg/ml, and in four patients the serum levels remained within the therapeutic range but were consistently below 20 μg/ml. The mean dosage of phenytoin in patients with consistently high levels was 7.5 mg/kg and 5.5 mg/kg in patients with fluctuating levels. In patients with levels consistently below 20 μg/ml the dosage was 3.5 mg/kg. The mean serum level of sulthiame when used in combination with phenytoin was 8.76 μg/ml $\pm$ SD 3.08. When sulthiame and phenytoin were used in combination, the fit frequency was reduced to 1.9 $\pm$ SD 2.9 per week. This improvement was significant ($p < 0.05$) when compared with the fit frequency on sulthiame used as a single drug.

SIDE EFFECTS

On sulthiame as a single drug, paresthesia occurred in three patients and hyperventilation in three others. Six patients developed headaches, two weight loss, and two others personality changes. When phenytoin was added to the sulthiame, four patients developed ataxia, and the personality changes that occurred initially in two patients on sulthiame alone progressed further, resulting in frank psychosis. The psychosis subsided when sulthiame was discontinued, and the ataxia improved in all patients when the dosage of phenytoin was reduced.

DISCUSSION

We have shown that sulthiame, when used as a single drug, is of no further benefit in a group of patients with frequent seizures who failed to respond to a variety of other drugs. It must be stressed, however, that the patients reported in this preliminary communication were patients with severe epilepsy who had failed to respond to other anticonvulsants, and our findings therefore would not exclude the possibility that sulthiame may be of benefit in patients with the less severe varieties of seizures. As part of our overall prospective longitudinal study of sulthiame, we are also investigating the less serious varieties of epilepsy, and based on our clinical observations, there is some evidence that this drug is of some benefit to patients who have had more than one seizure but whose attacks were occurring at infrequent intervals *(unpublished observations)*.

When phenytoin was added to sulthiame, a significant improvement in seizure control occurred, probably as a result of the inhibitory effect of sulthiame on phenytoin metabolism, resulting in serum levels of phenytoin which were adequate to improve seizure control. The improvement in seizure control could not be related to any additional benefit from sulthiame used in combination with phenytoin, as there was no significant change in serum sulthiame levels. The variation in the serum levels of phenytoin is of particular interest. This appeared to be dose related, as the patients with the toxic levels received the highest dose of 7.5 mg/kg, and the patients whose levels either fluctuated above and below the toxic level or were consistently below the toxic level had dosages that varied between 3.5 and 5.5 mg/kg. On the basis of this observation, we suggest that when phenytoin is used in combination with sulthiame, the initial dose should be 3.5 mg/kg and any increase in dosage should be based on careful and frequent monitoring of serum phenytoin levels. The improvement in seizure control in patients who previously had taken phenytoin as a single drug or in combination with other drugs was associated with an increase in serum levels in all patients. It is of interest that in the four patients whose levels were initially in the therapeutic range, further improvement in seizure control was associated with further increase in blood levels within the therapeutic range in two patients, and levels which were within the toxic range in two others. Two patients whose levels fluctuated above and below the toxic level previously had subtherapeutic levels of phenytoin, despite an adequate dose of that drug. Although the dosages in this study in both of these groups were different, the difference was not significant. This observation would suggest that serum levels of phenytoin when used in combination with sulthiame are subject to individual variation, depending on variations of phenytoin metabolism in different subjects.

There was a high incidence of side effects when sulthiame was used as a single drug. The personality changes in two patients on single-drug treatment were exacerbated when phenytoin was added. Although a definite relationship occurred between serum levels of phenytoin and ataxia, no definite correlation could be established between serum sulthiame levels and side effects because of the individual variation in sulthiame levels between different patients. Although no definite correlation could be obtained between serum levels and side effects, there appeared to be a relationship between dosage and certain side effects, such as hyperventilation, paresthesia, and headache, which improved with reduction in the dosage of the drug. It is possible that the variation in the psychiatric symptoms which occurred with high phenytoin levels was, in part, related to the high levels because this side effect subsided when sulthiame was discontinued with an associated reduction in phenytoin levels.

In conclusion, sulthiame did not appear to be of benefit to patients with severe and frequent seizures unless it was used in combination with another drug, such as phenytoin. The improvement was related to an increase in serum phenytoin levels even in some patients whose seizures were previously uncontrolled with this drug, and even with serum levels within the suggested therapeutic range. Therefore, this combination may be of further benefit to such patients by virtue of a further increase in phenytoin levels and to patients who show subtherapeutic levels of phenytoin despite an adequate therapeutic dose of the drug. It was not possible to establish any therapeutic range for sulthiame levels on the basis of this study.

ACKNOWLEDGMENTS

This work was supported by research grants from Bayer and Ciba-Geigy Laboratories. The statistical analysis was carried out by J. Seldrup and P. H. Poole, Mathematical Analysis Section, Ciba-Geigy, Simonsway, Manchester.

REFERENCES

Green, J. R., Troupin, A. S., Halpern, L. M., Friel, P., and Kanarek, P. (1974): Sulthiame: Evaluation as an anticonvulsant. *Epilepsia,* 15: 329–359.
Hansen, J. M., Kristensen, M., and Skovsted, L. (1968): Sulthiame (Ospolot) as an inhibitor of diphenylhydantoin metabolism. *Epilepsia,* 9:17–22.
Richens, A. (1976): *Drug Treatment of Epilepsy. Monographs in Controlled Medicine,* pp. 70–71. London, Henry Kimpton, Publishers.
Roger, J. C., Rodgers, G., Jr., and Soo, A. (1973): Simultaneous determination of carbamazepine (Tegretol) and other anticonvulsants in human plasma by gas liquid chromatography. *Clin. Chem.,* 19:590–592.
Simons, K. J., and Levy, R. H. (1972): GLC determination of sulthiame in plasma. *J. Pharm. Sci.,* 61:1252–1256.

Epilepsy, The Eighth International Symposium,
edited by J. K. Penry. Raven Press, New York
© 1977.

Long-Term Intensive Monitoring of Epileptic Patients

M. J. O'Kane and R. Sauter

Swiss Institute for Epilepsy, 8008 Zurich, Switzerland

The long-term registration of the EEG has become an accepted and well-documented procedure in the study of epilepsy. At the Swiss Institute for Epilepsy we have combined a 16-channel telemetry and video system to enable the documentation of the long-term registration and video recording from epileptic patients. This chapter aims to give a technical description of the complete system, which is shown as a block diagram in Fig. 1.

The transmitted composite signal of 16 channels of EEG is demodulated by the FM receiver. The receiver delivers three paralleled 16-channel outputs. The first series goes to PCM record electronics and is then relayed to an instrumentation tape recorder–reproducer. Integrated with this is a time-code generator synchronized by a video pulse. The generator displays days, hours, minutes, and seconds. The instrumentation tape recorder has an extended tape path resulting in a 30-sec delay between record and reproduce at a speed of 15/16 ips.

The 1-V RMS outputs from the reproduce side are delivered to an attenuator network in the EEG machine, thus allowing full use of the preamplifier stages. The timing is visually displayed and a slow BCD time code is written out on the timing channel of the EEG machine once every 10 sec.

The second series of outputs is relayed via a switch to a bandpass filter and amplitude trigger. An oscilloscope is used for identification. The trigger levels are then integrated and displayed on counters. The appropriate trigger is then selected for the driving of the EEG machine. A solid-state relay was fitted to the paper drive and conventional reed relays to the blocking control. These relays are activated from the writeout selector via a period generator and a 3-sec delay-width module. This arrangement allows the EEG machine to automatically start and stop for a length of time depending on the setting of the period generator. The amplifiers unblock 3 sec after the paper drive is activated and block 3 sec before the paper drive stops. A manual push-button control is also available to the neurophysiologist viewing the on-line monitor. With this method not only can we save an enormous amount of paper, but also, because of the 30-sec delay, we can obtain documentation of preictal, ictal, and postictal activity.

The third series of outputs goes via a switching unit to an on-line 16-channel monitor. The screen is large, measuring 50 × 40 cm, and a long decay P7 phos-

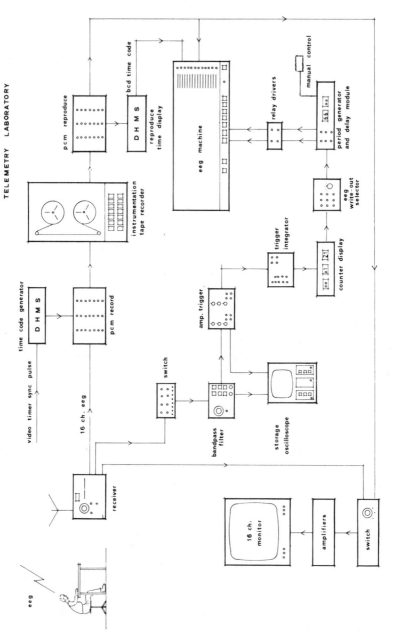

FIG. 1. Block diagram of EEG telemetry system.

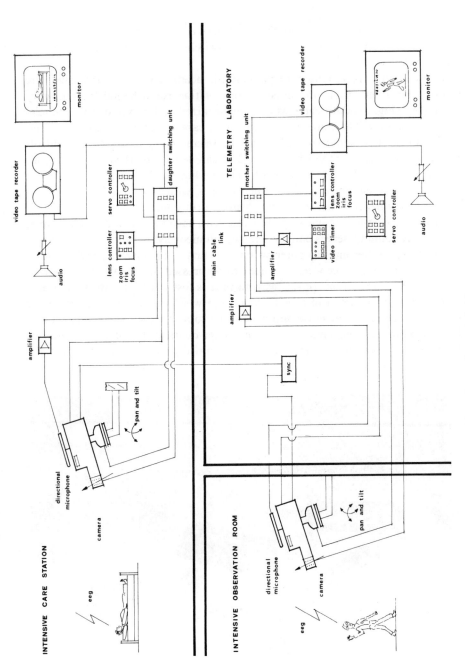

FIG. 2. Block diagram of video system.

phore in conjunction with a variable time base assures ample time for viewing the EEG. A timing graticule can also be switched on. Replay facility is also incorporated via this monitor.

Two cameras are mounted on pan-and-tilt heads, one in the intensive care station, the other one in the intensive observation room beside the telemetry laboratory (Fig. 2). Both cameras are synchronized and powered from the telemetry laboratory. The camera in the intensive care station serves two purposes: (1) it can be used simultaneously with the telemetry system with all controls switched downstairs to the laboratory; (2) it can be used by the nurses to record attacks which can later be reviewed by the medical staff.

Both cameras employ directional microphones, with motorized lens, zoom, iris and focus controls, as well as a servo pan-and-tilt control.

Video recorder and monitor are separate with each system and a video timer, continually running, serves both systems simultaneously. Because of the arrangement of the mother and daughter switching units, the "forward" and "motor" controls of the video recorder just need to be pressed to activate the system in the intensive care station. In this way no time is lost in documenting an attack.

The senders are worn in a belt around the waist and connections from the electrodes are via a low-noise antistatic cable to a montage selector panel also located in the belt. The senders consist of voltage-controlled oscillators, frequency modulated by mating amplifiers that are summed and then modulate the RF

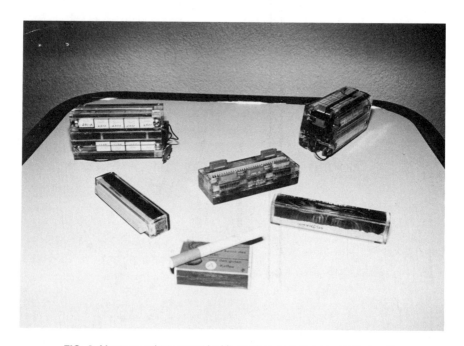

FIG. 3. Montage selector panel with senders and plug-in montage units.

carrier transmitter module. A specially made montage selector panel was constructed using plug-in montage modules. Its size is demonstrated against a cigarette in Fig. 3.

The intensive observation room has been furnished to accommodate different circumstances of recording, such as sleep, occupational therapy, school, or play.

The system took 1.5 years to install and has been running satisfactorily for a number of months.

In the video system we decided not to use a video mixer because resolution for combined 16 channels EEG and television was too poor. At present we are reviewing the possibility of splitting a TV projector. Automatic analysis is also being considered.

Epilepsy, The Eighth International Symposium,
edited by J. K. Penry. Raven Press, New York
© 1977.

Long-Term Monitoring of Antiepileptic Drugs in Patients with the Lennox-Gastaut Syndrome

*F. Viani, **G. Avanzini, A. Baruzzi, B. Bordo, L. Bossi,
†R. Canger, G. Porro, *A. Riboldi, M. E. Soffientini,
P. Zagnoni, and ‡P. L. Morselli

Milan Collaborative Group for Studies on Epilepsy

*Ospedale Provinciale di Neuropsichiatria Infantile "G. Corberi," Milan, Italy;
** Istituto Neurologico "C. Besta," Milan, Italy; Istituto di Ricerche Farmacologiche
"Mario Negri," 20157 Milan, Italy; †Centro per l'Epilessia dell'Università, Guardia II,
Policlinico, Milan, Italy; and ‡Département de Recherche Clinique,
LERS-Synthelabo, 75261 Paris, France*

The Lennox-Gastaut syndrome (LGS) is, by experience, defined as resistant to drug therapy (Lennox and Davis, 1950; Viani et al., 1975b); its clinical course involves wide variations in seizure frequency and type (Gastaut et al., 1966, 1973), and none of the drugs available up to now seems to be specific and efficacious in the long term.

Trying to cope with the difficult problem of managing patients with this particular type of epilepsy, clinicians often adopt frequent changes of therapeutic schedules and prescribe a large number of drugs, with a tendency toward high dosages, especially of the barbiturates (Viani et al., 1975a, 1975b; Beaumanoir, 1976).

This practice, although quite understandable from a psychological point of view, appears to have little rational basis; it may, in fact, worsen the patient's clinical situation, and it certainly makes it difficult to evaluate any correlations between drug therapy and clinical picture.

The present chapter summarizes the steps taken by the Milan Collaborative Group for Studies on Epilepsy, as an attempt toward a more rational therapeutic approach.

These were:

1. to obtain a preliminary picture of antiepileptic drug concentrations in a group of poorly controlled patients with the LGS, treated with several drug associations at dosages established on the basis of clinical experience;
2. to modify the therapeutic schedule in individual patients in order to achieve drug plasma levels which could be considered satisfactory on the

basis of data in the literature and our own experience (Woodbury et al., 1972; Morselli, 1973, 1977; Hvidberg and Dam, 1976);

3. after having chosen for each individual patient a drug combination promising clinical efficacy, to evaluate in the long term any changes in clinical symptoms during constant administration of the selected antiepileptic drugs at "therapeutic" plasma levels;
4. to evaluate, when possible, the effects of single drugs (or drug combinations) used.

PATIENTS AND METHODS

Nine patients with the LGS were followed for more than 21 months in a routine antiepileptic drug monitoring program. At the beginning of the observation their ages ranged from 5 to 15 years (mean 10 years). The mean duration of epilepsy was 8.3 years, with a range of 2 to 13 years; the mean duration of the LGS was 6 years, with a range of 1 to 12 years. All patients had been previously treated with phenobarbital (PB), diphenylhydantoin (DPH), carbamazepine (CBZ), ethosuximide (ETS), diazepam (DZ), and nitrazepam (NZ) in different combinations.

All patients had a high frequency of seizures, with a mean of 77/month and a range from 3/month to 14/day.

All patients had moderate to severe mental retardation. The EEG showed in all cases a diffuse pattern of "slow spikes and waves," except in one patient, who could be classified in a subgroup of the Lennox-Gastaut syndrome (Gastaut et al., 1973); this patient showed the specific seizures of the syndrome, but with an EEG pattern characterized by slow basal activity with rare discharges of slow spikes and waves.

Six of the patients were kept in hospital during the whole observation period, whereas three were outpatients.

Drug plasma levels were assayed and clinical and EEG examinations were made at regular monthly intervals. Blood samples for the determination of antiepileptic drugs were taken at 8 A.M. (before the morning drug administration) and 4 to 6 hr later. Gas chromatographic analysis was run according to McGee (1970) for PB and DPH, Morselli et al. (1973a) for CBZ, Gerna and Morselli (1976) for clonazepam (CNP), Morselli et al. (1973b) for DZ and desmethyldiazepam (NDZ), and Gerna et al. (1977) for dipropylacetate (DPA). Primidone (PRI) was determined as PB.

Clinical assessment was by the same physician for all patients during the whole study. The seizure frequency and type were observed by the nurses or parents.

RESULTS AND DISCUSSION

Initial Picture

Table 1 lists the therapy (doses and plasma concentrations) at the beginning of monitoring, resulting from several years of empirical treatment. The adminis-

TABLE 1. Daily drug doses (mg/kg), plasma concentrations (μg/ml) at 8 A.M. and 1 P.M., and total frequency of all seizure types per month in 9 patients with LGS

Case	Beginning of monitoring	After adjustment	End of constant therapy	Current picture
No. 1, M; 11 yr	PB 4.7 / 48–43 CBZ 18.7 / 5.4–9.2 DZ 0.62 / 0.400–0.560 NDZ— / 1.335–1.250	PB 2.8 / 32–35 CBZ 20.2 / 10.5–8.7 DZ 0.57 / 0.444–0.566 NDZ— / 1.116–1.465	PB 2.4 / 29–33 CBZ 17.0 / 6.4–7.1 DZ 0.60 / 0.800–n.p. NDZ— / 0.950–n.p.	PB 2.3 / 33–32 CBZ 20.6 / 7.4–7.5 DZ 0.57 / 0.500–n.p. NDZ— / 0.800–n.p.
seizures/month	400	600	120	145
No. 2, M; 10 yr	PB 6.4 / 52–58 DZ 1.6 / 0.605–0.710 NDZ— / 0.900–1.030	PB 2.9 / 29–31 CBZ 15.7 / 5.4–4.8 CNP 0.08 / 64–48	PB 2.7 / 30–27.3 CBZ 14.5 / 5.3–6.3 CNP 0.08 / 40–92	PB 2.7 / 31–29 CBZ 18 / 10.1–9.4
seizures/month	115	45	150	105
No. 3, M; 8 yr	PB 14.2 / 40–60 DZ 0.95 / 0.130–n.p. NDZ— / 0.780–n.p.	PB 9 / 43–40 DZ 1.4 / 0.200–0.800 NDZ— / 1.520–1.130	PB 8 / 39–44 DZ 0.8 / 0.200–0.361 NDZ— / 1.070–1.164	PB 6.8 / 35–36 CBZ 46.1 / 5.8–9.2
seizures/month	3	2	35	33
No. 4, M; 9 yr	PB 4.7 / 43–52 CBZ 28.6 / 4.0–6.2 DZ 0.71 / 0.590–0.260 NDZ— / 0.590–0.530 DPA 8 / 30–51	PB 3.4 / 30–n.p. CBZ 32 / 10–8 DZ 0.81 / 0.580–0.270 NDZ— / 0.485–0.635 DPA 16 / 120–110	PB 2.7 / 24–21 CBZ 26 / 5–7.4 DZ 0.65 / 0.207–0.441 0.777–0.806 DPA 13 / 98–131	PB 2.7 / 23–21 CBZ 34.8 / 5.5–7.2
seizures/month	10	0	11	0
No. 5, M; 13 yr	PB 6.2 / 60–74 DPH 3.3 / 2–1.3 CBZ 13 / 1.6–2.4 CNP 0.26 / n.p.–n.p.	PB 4.7 / 26–35 CBZ 26 / 5.1–6.3	PB 3.2 / 25–33 CBZ 26 / 5.8–6.5	PB 3.9 / 23–30 CBZ 21.6 / 6.7–9.1 CNP 0.094 / 18–21

TABLE 1. (cont'd)

Case	Beginning of monitoring	After adjustment	End of constant therapy	Current picture
seizures/month	13	33	36	5
No. 6, F; 15 yr	PB 5 (39–41) DPH 3.4 (1.9–3.5) DZ 0.6 (0.200–0.300) NDZ— (0.510–0.690)	PB 2.5 (22.7–26) DZ 0.8 (0.360–0.600) NDZ— (0.806–0.924)	PB 3.0 (23.5–23) DZ 0.73 (0.314–0.444) NDZ— (0.720–0.665)	PB 3.1 (33–36) CBZ 25 (7.6–9.3)
seizures/month	7	9	25	15
No. 7, M; 7 yr	PB 7.5 (53–71) CBZ 15 (3.5–5.7) DZ 0.87 (0.105–0.196) NDZ— (0.440–0.680)	PB 3.3 (42–36) CBZ 17 (2.6–3.9) DZ 0.76 (0.080–0.400) NDZ— (0.292–0.329)	PB 3.1 (24–25) CBZ 13 (3.6–2.9) DZ 0.79 (0.261–0.866) NDZ— (0.941–1.441)	PB 3.1 (29–29) CBZ 20.1 (5.9–7.4) DZ 0.72 (0.283–n.p.) NDZ— (0.715–n.p.)
seizures/month	35	31	30	6
No. 8, F; 14 yr	PB 7.9 (63–n.p.) DPH 4.9 (2.6–n.p.) DZ 1.5 (1.160–n.p.) NDZ— (2.240–n.p.)	PB 3.6 (40–33) CBZ 24 (8.2–8.0) DZ 1.1 (0.250–0.410) NDZ— (0.780–1.000)	PB 2.7 (33–34) CBZ 24 (4.8–8.3) DZ 1.1 (0.300–0.500) NDZ— (1.150–1.280)	PB 3.1 (32–32) CBZ 25 (5.6–7.0)
seizures/month	52	25	60	45
No. 9, M; 5 yr	PB 6 (40–54) DPH 8 (10–12) DZ 2 (0.250–0.290) NDZ— (0.265–0.360)	PRI 17.8 (20–20) DPA 50 (48–n.p.) DZ 0.71 (0.105–0.200) (0.540–0.530)	PRI 17.1 (24–24) DPA 44 (n.p.–53) DZ 0.62 (0.200–0.180) (0.240–0.235)	PRI 26.8 (42–38) CBZ 35.7 (4.4–6.4) 132

n.p., not performed.

tered drugs were PB (to all patients), DZ (to eight patients), CBZ (to four patients), DPH (to four patients), CNP (to one patient), and DPA (to one patient). Thus patients were all receiving fairly complex polytherapies, with a mean of three drugs each.

Interestingly enough, all patients had high phenobarbital plasma concentrations, with levels over 60 μg/ml in four patients, although plasma levels of the other drugs, particularly DPH, were low.

These data confirm the difficulty of establishing a satisfactory therapeutic schedule empirically, without assaying antiepileptic drug plasma levels.

Judging from these data, it might be assumed that the bad control of the epileptic symptomatology was related to overdosage of phenobarbital and underdosage of the associated drugs.

Therapeutic Adjustment

During a period of about 7 months, therapy was gradually adjusted according to plasma level data to attain satisfactory drug plasma concentrations. At the end of this period (Table 1), regimens were slightly simplified and the number of drugs was reduced to a mean of 2.7 for each patient: in particular, DPH was withdrawn from all patients.

During this period, improved behavior and a reduction in seizure frequency (> 50%) were observed in four patients (No. 2, 4, 7, and 9), possibly because they were no longer suffering from PB overdosage. However, the clinical picture of the other four patients showed no significant change, and in one patient (No. 5) seizure frequency significantly increased after withdrawal of DPH and CNP.

Period of Constant Therapy

As stated in the introduction, our aim was to evaluate any long-term correlations between clinical picture and "therapeutic" drug plasma levels. Drug plasma levels were therefore kept within the "therapeutic range" for 7 to 12 months, and throughout this period they remained fairly constant, the slight lowering found probably being due to weight gain (Table 1).

The clinical situation, however, did not follow this regular plasma level profile: The frequency of status epilepticus was low; four episodes of status epilepticus occurred in one patient (No. 1), and one in another (No. 2). In spite of satisfactory drug concentrations, the mean seizure frequency remained quite high: 60 seizures per month as opposed to 77 seizures per month at the beginning of monitoring. The most striking finding was the way seizures broadly varied over time, with a range of 0 to 600 seizures per month and variations within patients from 2- to 15-fold (mean, 7-fold). Alertness was judged to be satisfactory in four patients (No. 2, 4, 7, and 9) but remained low in five.

In short, in spite of constant and apparently satisfactory plasma concentrations of antiepileptic drugs, seizures remained frequent, unpredictable, and widely fluctuating, suggesting a poor correlation between drug therapy and clinical course.

Evaluation of Single Drugs and Drug Combinations Used

After this experience, we chose a different approach, trying to establish the effects of single drugs or drug combinations on seizure frequency and type.

We started with the association PB + CBZ, which was administered to all patients, at increasing CBZ dosages. The other drugs were gradually withdrawn. At the present time two patients are still taking DZ and one CNP (Table 1).

The mean number of drugs administered to each patient was therefore reduced to 2.33.

After 5 to 7 months (this phase is still in progress) we could make the following observations:

1. Drug plasma levels were all within the so-called therapeutic range.
2. The mean frequency of seizures in the last month of the study was slightly lower: 54 seizures per month (range 0 to 145), as opposed to the 77/month at the beginning of monitoring. In detail: seizures were more frequent ($> 50\%$) in three patients (No. 3, 6, and 9), unchanged in two (No. 2 and 8), less frequent ($> 50\%$) in three (No. 1, 5, and 7), and controlled in patient No. 4, who was classified according to this clinical feature and EEG features in a subgroup of the LGS.
3. Variations in seizure frequency were less broad in this last period of the study. In three patients (No. 1, 2, and 8), they varied very little, in four patients (No. 5, 6, 7, and 9) less than threefold, in patient No. 3 there was a tenfold variation, and in patient No. 4 seizures dropped from 11 to 0/month.
4. Eight patients showed marked behavioral improvement—alertness, communication skills, speech, motoricity, mood, and social awareness. In one patient (No. 1) alertness remained very low.
5. During this last period, which of course is quite short, no status epilepticus was observed.
6. As regards the effects of single drugs, we observed that withdrawal of diazepam (at concentrations from 180 to 500 ng/ml) was associated, in patients No. 3, 6, and 8, with a definite increase in seizure frequency, particularly of the myoclonic absence type. (In patients No. 4 and 9, however, the clinical picture showed no significant changes.)
7. Seizure frequency was reduced in three patients (No. 2, 4, and 7) out of four when the dose of CBZ was raised to 18 to 34.8 mg/kg (plasma levels 5.5 to 10.1 μg/ml). In other patients, however, the introduction of CBZ at similar dosages (and plasma levels) did not modify the clinical picture (No. 3, 6, and 9). In subjects who seemed to respond, CBZ apparently acted particularly on tonic seizures.

CONCLUSIONS

Our findings confirm that the empirical approach to drug treatment of the LGS is not adequate, leading to patients' receiving complex polytherapies with either over- or underdoses of drugs; seizure frequency remains high, and adverse reactions are frequent and severe.

Simplifying therapy and adjusting doses on the basis of drug plasma levels seemed to lead to an overall improvement of the clinical picture in most patients, with a small reduction in the mean number of seizures, but a definite reduction in the incidence of status epilepticus and a definite improvement in behavior (speech, motoricity, communication skills). Adaptation of therapy on the basis of individual drug plasma levels therefore appears to be valuable in patients with the LGS.

However, our findings also confirm that these patients show definite "resistance" to drug therapy even at satisfactory doses and plasma levels; the only patient who was completely free of seizures for a period of 5 months was classified in a subgroup of the LGS. Furthermore, the wide fluctuations in seizure frequency within patients during constant therapy suggest that the relation between drug therapy and clinical course should be critically assessed in patients with this particular type of epilepsy.

REFERENCES

Beaumanoir, A. (1976): *Les Épilepsies Infantiles. Problèmes de Diagnostique et de Traitement.* Roche, Bâle.

Gastaut, H., Dravet, C., Loubier, D., Giove, C., Viani, F., Gastaut, J. A., and Gastaut, J. L. (1973): Evolution clinique et pronostic du syndrome de Lennox-Gastaut. In: *Evolution and Prognosis of Epilepsies,* XIXème Reunion Européenne d'Enseignement Electroencephalographique, edited by E. Lugaresi, P. Pazzaglia, and C. A. Tassinari, pp. 133–154. Italseber, Milano.

Gastaut, H., Roger, J., Soulayrol, R., Tassinari, C. A., Regis, H., Dravet, C., Bernard, R., Pinsard, N., and Saint-Jean, M. (1966): Childhood epileptic encephalopathy with diffuse slow spike waves (otherwise known as "petit mal variant" or Lennox syndrome). *Epilepsia,* 7:139–179.

Gerna, M., Baruzzi, A., and Morselli, P. L. (1977): A simple GLC procedure for the determination of di-*n*-propylacetate and ethosuximide in human plasma samples. *(In preparation.)*

Gerna, M., and Morselli, P. L. (1976): A simple and sensitive method for the determination of clonazepam in human plasma. *J. Chromatogr.,* 116:445–450.

Hvidberg, E. F., and Dam, M. (1976): Clinical pharmacokinetics of anticonvulsants. *Clin. Pharmacokin.,* 1:161–188.

Lennox, W. G., and Davis, J. P. (1950): Clinical correlates of the fast and slow spike wave electroencephalogram. *J. Pediatr.,* 5:626–644.

McGee, J. (1970): Rapid determination of diphenylhydantoin in blood plasma by gas-liquid chromatography. *Anal. Chem.,* 42:421–422.

Morselli, P. L. (1973): Significato ed importanza della misura e del controllo delle concentrazioni plasmatiche dei farmaci nella terapia della epilessia. *Prospet. Pediatr.,* 3:523–541.

Morselli, P. L. (1977): Antiepileptic drugs. In: *Drug Disposition During Development.* Spectrum Publishers, New York *(in press).*

Morselli, P. L., Biandrate, P., Frigerio, A., Gerna, M., and Tognoni, G. (1973a): Gas-chromatographic determination of carbamazepine and carbamazepine-epoxide in human body fluids. In: *Proceedings of the Workshop of the Determination of Drugs in Body Fluids,* Nordwijkerhout, Netherlands, April 1972, pp. 169–175. Excerpta Medica, Amsterdam.

Morselli, P. L., Principi, N., Tognoni, G., Reali, E., Belvedere, G., Standen, S. M., and Sereni, F.

(1973*b*): Diazepam disposition in premature and full-term infants and children. *Perinat. Med.*, 1:133–141.

Viani, F., Bossi, L., Gerna, M., and Morselli, P. L. (1975*a*): Indicazioni del monitoraggio dei farmaci antiepilettici. *Gaslini,* 7:121–124.

Viani, F., Gerna, M., Riboldi, A., Rossotti, V., and Morselli, P. L. (1975*b*): Monitoraggio dei tassi plasmatici di alcuni farmaci (phenobarbital, difenilidantoina, carbamazepina) nella sindrome di Lennox-Gastaut e in altre forme di epilessia (parziale e generalizzata secondaria) dell'infanzia. *Riv. Neurol.,* 45:189–198.

Woodbury, D. M., Penry, J. K., and Schmidt, R. P. (Eds.) (1972): *Antiepileptic Drugs.* Raven Press, New York.

Epilepsy, The Eighth International Symposium,
edited by J. K. Penry. Raven Press, New York
© 1977.

Precise Adjustment of Phenytoin Dosage

A. Richens

St. Bartholomew's Hospital, London, EC1A 7BE, England

Since its introduction in 1938, phenytoin has found an important place in the treatment of major epilepsy, and in many countries it remains the most widely prescribed drug. Nevertheless, a number of problems arise in its clinical usage. It has a narrow therapeutic ratio such that the dose required to control seizures in some patients is only slightly below that which would produce intoxication; indeed, in some patients seizures are not adequately controlled despite the appearance of toxic symptoms. With chronic use, it causes a wide variety of adverse effects on almost every body system. Furthermore, it has been used badly in practice because the relationship between dosage and the resulting blood level has only recently been understood. The development of sensitive techniques for measuring drug levels in biological fluids has led to a rapid increase in our understanding of the pharmacokinetics of phenytoin, and a knowledge of these developments is essential if the clinician is to use the drug properly.

It has been realized that the prescription of standard doses of phenytoin results in a wide range of serum levels from one patient to another. In theory, it should be possible to tailor the dose of phenytoin to a patient's clinical response, namely, by increasing the dose of the drug until complete control of seizures is obtained or until toxic symptoms develop. In practice, however, the clinician tends to limit his prescription to a standard dose, usually one tablet or capsule three times daily, and this dose may produce a subtherapeutic level in one patient while causing intoxication in another. It is general experience that 300 mg daily produces a serum level below the optimum range of 40 to 80 μmoles/liter (Lund, 1974) in up to 50% of patients, and that adjusting the dosage to achieve a level within this range leads to effective control in a high proportion of patients. Routine monitoring of serum phenytoin levels may therefore enable the physician to achieve control with phenytoin alone in the majority of his epileptic patients (Reynolds et al., 1976).

The intersubject variation of serum levels produced by standard doses of phenytoin is mainly caused by genetic differences in the rate of hydroxylation of the drug by hepatic microsomal enzymes. These differences are, however, exaggerated by the fact that phenytoin metabolism is a saturable process, i.e., the hepatic enzymes have a limited capacity to handle the drug and above a certain dosage the liver is unable to increase the amount of drug handled in a given time.

139

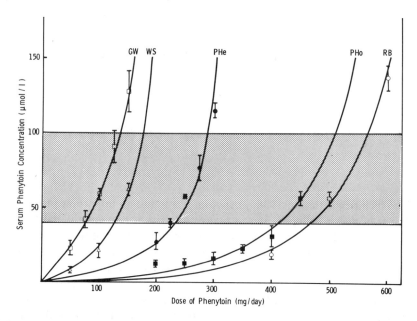

FIG. 1. Relationship between serum phenytoin level and drug dosage in 5 patients studied prospectively. Each point represents the mean and standard error of 3 to 8 separate estimations in the steady state. The hatched area represents the therapeutic range of serum phenytoin levels used in our laboratory (40 to 100 μmoles/l, i.e., 10 to 25 μg/ml). The curves were fitted by computer, using the Michaelis-Menten equation.

This situation can be described mathematically by the Michaelis-Menten equation (Mawer et al., 1974), but in practical terms there are several important implications for the clinician. Whereas with most drugs the relationship between the dose and serum level of a drug is a linear one, i.e., doubling the dose doubles the serum level, for phenytoin this is not the case. Within the therapeutic dosage range, successive increments in dosage produce a disproportionate increase in serum level, and the discrepancy becomes greater as the serum level rises to the upper end of the therapeutic range. This is illustrated in Fig. 1, in which the results of careful prospective studies in five epileptic patients are presented (Richens and Dunlop, 1975). Each patient was receiving phenytoin in combination with one or more other anticonvulsant drugs, and although the dose of the other drugs was held constant, the amount of phenytoin administered was either increased progressively (because lower doses had failed to control the patients' fits) or decreased (because of intoxication). Serum phenytoin was measured several times at each dose level after allowing 4 to 6 weeks for equilibration following a change in dose. In each case a nonlinear dose level relationship was found, and within the therapeutic range of serum levels a very steep relationship was found. This indicates that the dosage required to produce a therapeutic level was close to that which would have caused complete saturation of the enzyme system metabolizing the drug.

The steepness of the relationship between dose and serum level within the therapeutic range has a number of important implications in clinical practice:

1. Therapeutic levels are likely to be unstable because small changes in daily intake of the drug greatly alter the serum level. Drug intake is never completely under the control of the supervising physician because differences in biological availability (i.e., the amount of drug absorbed from a marketed preparation) and unreliable drug intake can occur without the physician's knowledge.

2. If serum phenytoin levels are used as a guide to phenytoin dosage, increments in dose should become smaller as the therapeutic range is approached. Intoxication will almost certainly result if the dose is increased by 100 mg or more in a patient whose serum level is approaching or is just within the therapeutic range. A nomogram has been devised for predicting dose increments in patients (Richens and Dunlop, 1975), but a simpler approach has been suggested by Professor George Mawer *(personal communication),* namely, that if the serum level is less than 20 μmoles/liter (5 μg/ml), an increment of 100 mg is permissible; if the level is 20 to 40 μmoles/liter (5 to 10 μg/ml), only 50 mg should be added; but if the level is just within the therapeutic range, say 40 to 60 μmoles/liter (10 to 15 μg/ml), the maximum increment allowable is 25 mg.

With available preparations, this recommendation is difficult to adhere to, but Parke-Davis in the United Kingdom is proposing to replace their 50-mg capsule with a 25-mg preparation, thus allowing more flexible dosage.

3. Because the enzyme which metabolizes phenytoin may be close to saturation, interactions with the drug are common and sometimes potentially hazardous to the patient. For example, sulthiame is a potent inhibitor of phenytoin metabolism, and the incidence of intoxication in patients on combined therapy is high. Many other drugs can inhibit phenytoin metabolism.

4. Because of the instability of phenytoin levels within the therapeutic range, the validity of the range needs reappraisal. Although the excellent work of Lund (1974) has supported the earlier claim (Buchthal et al., 1960) that a level of at least 40 μmoles/liter (10 μg/ml) is necessary to achieve adequate control, it is common experience that patients with relatively mild epilepsy may be fully controlled with serum levels below this value. It is important, therefore, that the clinician treat the patient rather than the serum level and not increase the dosage unnecessarily in order to achieve a theoretically desirable level. Drug level monitoring is valuable when used to supplement clinical observation, but it is no substitute for it. If a patient's epilepsy is adequately controlled by a serum level below 40 μmoles/liter (10 μg/ml), the stability of the level is likely to be much greater, and the danger of intoxication and adverse effects much less.

5. A knowledge of the pharmacokinetics of phenytoin together with the facilities for measuring serum levels will lead to much safer and more effective management of epileptic patients.

REFERENCES

Buchthal, F., Svensmark, O., and Schiller, P. J. (1960): Clinical and electroencephalographic correlations with serum levels of diphenylhydantoin. *Arch. Neurol.,* 2:624–630.

Lund, L. (1974): Anticonvulsant effect of diphenylhydantoin relative to plasma levels. A prospective 3 year study in ambulant patients with generalized epileptic seizures. *Arch. Neurol.,* 31:289–294.

Mawer, G. E., Mullen, P. W., Rodgers, M., Robins, A. J., and Lucas, S. B. (1974): Phenytoin dose adjustment in epileptic patients. *Br. J. Clin. Pharmacol.,* 1:163–168.

Richens, A., and Dunlop, A. (1975): Serum phenytoin levels in management of epilepsy. *Lancet,* 2:247–248.

Reynolds, E. H., Chadwick, D., and Galbraith, A. W. (1976): One drug (phenytoin) in the treatment of epilepsy. *Lancet,* 1:923–926.

Epilepsy, The Eighth International Symposium,
edited by J. K. Penry. Raven Press, New York
© 1977.

Has Carbamazepine-10,11-Epoxide an Independent Antiepileptic Effect in Man?

*Mogens Dam, ** Janne Sury, and † Johannes Christiansen

*Department of Neurology (University Clinic), Hvidovre Hospital, DK-2650 Hvidovre,
Denmark; ** Department of Psychiatry, Kommunehospitalet, DK-1399 Copenhagen K.,
Denmark; and †Department of Clinical Chemistry CL, Rigshospitalet (University
Clinic), DK-2100 Copenhagen Ø., Denmark*

Carbamazepine (CBZ)-10,11-epoxide has been found to be active against maximal electroshock in rats (Morselli et al., 1976). The plasma level of CBZ-10,11-epoxide in man varies relative to CBZ depending on whether CBZ is administered alone or in combination with diphenylhydantoin (DPH) or phenobarbital (PB) (Christiansen and Dam, 1975). It has been suggested that part of the clinical effect and the side effects of CBZ treatment might be caused by the epoxide (Dam et al., 1975).

The aim of the present retrospective investigation was to relate the antiepileptic effect to the plasma concentration of the epoxide when the patients were treated with CBZ alone or in combination with DPH, PB, or both, in order to investigate whether CBZ-10,11-epoxide has an antiepileptic effect of its own in man.

PATIENTS AND METHODS

We examined 132 epileptic patients with a mean age of 35 years (range 11 to 79) treated for 1 to 8 years with CBZ alone or in combination with DPH, PB, or both. The cases consisted of 118 patients with generalized tonic-clonic seizures (group A) and 57 patients with partial epileptic seizures with complex symptomatology (group B), all attending the outpatient clinic. Their seizure frequency and the plasma levels of CBZ and CBZ-10,11-epoxide were recorded during steady-state conditions. The patients were divided into three groups according to the severity of the disease: group 1 with seizures once a day to once a week; group 2 with seizures once a week to once a month; and group 3 with seizures less than once a month. After treatment with CBZ the patients were classified as improved or unchanged depending on shift from one severity group to another.

CBZ and CBZ-10,11-epoxide levels were determined by the TLC method described by Christiansen (1973).

RESULTS

Table 1 shows the results in the different groups of patients. There was a significantly greater number of improvements among the patients with generalized tonic-clonic seizures (group A) compared with the patients suffering from partial epileptic seizures (group B). As far as plasma concentrations are concerned, a significantly higher level of epoxide was found in patients on combined treatment compared with patients treated with CBZ alone. However, no significant difference could be demonstrated in the levels of CBZ or its epoxide between the improved and unchanged patients. This finding applied to both group A and group B.

DISCUSSION

The antiepileptic effect of CBZ was found to be superior in patients with generalized tonic-clonic seizures compared with patients suffering from partial epileptic seizures. These findings are in accordance with our previous results (Dam et al., 1975). The present study indicates that the better effect of CBZ in the patients with generalized tonic-clonic seizures is not due to a higher plasma level of the epoxide in these patients. As a matter of fact, almost identical patterns of the relative epoxide concentrations were found in the two groups of patients independent of improvement or unchanged status. It is a well-known clinical impression that the partial epileptic seizures are more resistant to antiepileptic treatment of any kind, and our results are in accordance with this experience.

The increased amount of epoxide in the groups on combined treatment is due to an accelerated metabolism of CBZ induced by DPH and PB, as previously shown by Christiansen and Dam (1975) and Schneider (1975). If the epoxide had an antiepileptic effect of its own in man, a better antiepileptic effect might be expected in the group of patients with a high relative plasma concentration of the epoxide, although these patients also may be particularly resistant to drug therapy as they need combination treatment. However, no significant difference was found in the effect in patients with a high or a low relative plasma concentration of the epoxide.

Recently Feigle et al. (1976) tried to distinguish between the anticonvulsant effect of CBZ and its epoxide in rats. They concluded that CBZ was a more potent anticonvulsant than the epoxide, and that CBZ possesses an activity of its own which may, however, be reinforced by the epoxide. In man it has not been possible to study the anticonvulsant effect of the epoxide *per se* as the substance is not available for clinical trials. The problem can therefore be studied only indirectly. The investigational design used in this study has not been able to reveal any additional effect of the epoxide in man.

SUMMARY

In a retrospective study of 132 epileptic outpatients treated for 1 to 8 years with carbamazepine alone or in combination with diphenylhydantoin, phenobar-

TABLE 1. Plasma concentrations of carbamazepine (CBZ) and carbamazepine-10, 11-epoxide (EPX) in the different groups of patients

| | Improved | | | | Unchanged | | | | |
| | mg/liter | | %[a] | | mg/l | | %[a] | | Total |
	CBZ	EPX	EPX	N	CBZ	EPX	EPX	N	N
A: Generalized tonic-clonic seizures									
CBZ alone	5.5 ± 1.6	1.1 ± 0.5	20 ± 5	12	8.0 ± 3.5	1.3 ± 0.8	16 ± 4	7	19
CBZ + DPH	4.8 ± 1.7	1.6 ± 0.7	32 ± 9	22	5.4 ± 1.0	1.7 ± 0.5	31 ± 8	11	33
CBZ + PB	6.0 ± 1.9	1.7 ± 0.6	30 ± 12	26	6.7 ± 0.8	1.9 ± 0.8	29 ± 10	10	36
CBZ + DPH + PB	4.3 ± 1.2	1.8 ± 0.6	41 ± 13	22	5.4 ± 2.1	2.3 ± 0.9	43 ± 13	8	30
B: Partial epileptic seizures with complex symptomatology									
CBZ alone	5.4 ± 1.9	1.1 ± 0.6	17 ± 4	8	6.7 ± 2.0	1.4 ± 0.7	20 ± 5	4	12
CBZ + DPH	4.6 ± 1.4	1.5 ± 0.6	31 ± 8	7	4.8 ± 1.0	1.5 ± 0.6	32 ± 11	9	16
CBZ + PB	6.6 ± 1.1	2.0 ± 0.6	31 ± 10	8	6.1 ± 0.9	1.7 ± 0.6	29 ± 11	4	12
CBZ + DPH + PB	4.2 ± 1.5	1.8 ± 0.5	45 ± 13	8	5.2 ± 1.6	2.2 ± 0.7	44 ± 13	9	17

[a] Carbamazepine-10,11-epoxide/carbamazepine ratio in percent.

bital, or both, we correlated the frequency of generalized tonic-clonic seizures (118 patients) and partial epileptic seizures with complex symptomatology (57 patients) with the plasma levels of CBZ and CBZ-10,11-epoxide.

The antiepileptic effect of CBZ was superior in patients with generalized tonic-clonic seizures compared with patients suffering from partial epileptic seizures. The better effect was not caused by a higher plasma level of the epoxide. The investigational design used in this study has not been able to reveal any additional effect of the epoxide in man.

ACKNOWLEDGMENT

We are grateful for discussion and technical comment from Professor Eigill F. Hvidberg.

REFERENCES

Christiansen, J. (1973): Assay of carbamazepine and metabolites in plasma by quantitative thin-layer chromatography. In: *Methods of Analysis of Anti-Epileptic Drugs,* edited by I. W. A. Meijer, H. Meinardi, C. Gardner-Thorpe, and E. van der Klein. Excerpta Medica, Amsterdam.

Christiansen, J., and Dam, M. (1975): Drug interaction in epileptic patients. In: *Clinical Pharmacology of Anti-Epileptic Drugs,* edited by H. Schneider, D. Janz, C. Gardner-Thorpe, H. Meinardi, and A. L. Sherwin. Springer-Verlag, Berlin.

Dam, M., Jensen, A., and Christiansen, J. (1975): Plasma level and effect of carbamazepine in grand mal and psychomotor epilepsy. *Acta Neurol. Scand. [Suppl.]*, 60:33–38.

Feigle, I. W., Feldmann, K. F., and Baltzer, V. (1976): Anticonvulsant effect of carbamazepine. An attempt to distinguish between the potency of the parent drug and its epoxide metabolite. *Proceedings from WODADIBOF III,* Exeter, England *(in press).*

Morselli, P. L., Rossi, L., and Gerua, M. (1976): Pharmacokinetic studies with carbamazepine in epileptic patients. In: *Epileptic Seizures—Behaviour—Pain,* edited by W. Birkmayer. Hans Huber Publisher, Bern, Stuttgart, Vienna.

Schneider, H. (1975): Carbamazepine: The influence of other antiepileptic drugs on its serum level. In: *Clinical Pharmacology of Anti-Epileptic Drugs,* edited by H. Schneider, D. Janz, C. Gardner-Thorpe, H. Meinardi, and A. L. Sherwin. Springer-Verlag, Berlin.

Epilepsy, The Eighth International Symposium,
edited by J. K. Penry. Raven Press, New York
© 1977.

Influence of Phenobarbital on the Serum Level of Phenytoin and Effect of Phenytoin on Primidone Metabolism

P. Ruf and R. Sauter

Swiss Institute for Epilepsy, 8008 Zurich, Switzerland

At the Swiss Institute for Epilepsy the estimation of antiepileptic drug levels has been routinely integrated into the therapy. The estimations of phenobarbital, phenytoin, and primidone are performed with the EMIT enzyme immunoassay, whereas gas chromatographic methods are used for some of the other antiepileptic drugs. Since this EMIT method is an easy assay to perform, it has been possible to collect more than 10,000 data values which are to be analyzed for the evaluation of interactions between antiepileptic drugs.

In the present study two examples of such an evaluation are presented.

INFLUENCE OF PHENOBARBITAL ON THE SERUM LEVEL OF PHENYTOIN

The problem of the influence of phenobarbital on the serum level of phenytoin has been discussed in many publications. However, there is no agreement among the authors on the change in phenytoin level to be expected after administration of additional phenobarbital. Kutt (1975) reviewed these publications and found that the authors had reported a decline in six clinical observations, a rise in five cases, and no effect in five cases.

Most of the publications so far include long-term studies with rather small groups of patients. This type of study is not suited to a statistical evaluation. Another commonly used kind of analysis, the linear regression of a plot of phenytoin levels versus phenytoin doses, was also rejected because both Sauter (1974) and Richens (1974) showed that this relationship is not linear.

METHODS AND RESULTS

In this study, we therefore compared only phenytoin levels within groups with similar phenytoin dosages. These "dose groups" were chosen from 0 to 2, 2 to 3, 3 to 4, 4 to 5, and 5 mg of phenytoin per kilogram body weight. For these dose groups the mean phenytoin levels of patients who received no phenobarbital and therefore served as control were 2.6 ± 0.3 (SEM, $N = 36$), 6.16 ± 0.81

($N = 54$), 7.82 ± 0.75 ($N = 97$), 10.51 ± 0.82 ($N = 83$),   and 12.59 ± 1.17 ($N = 72$), respectively.

The second approach was to compare—within these dose groups—the phenytoin levels to the phenobarbital levels. The influence of phenobarbital could be judged more easily this way, as will be shown by two different analyses of data.

Method of Mean Values

The phenytoin levels from patients within the same phenytoin dose group were divided into subgroups according to th.ir phenobarbital levels. These subgroups were 0 to 10, 10 to 20, 20 to 30, 30 to 40, and 40 to 50 μg/ml phenobarbital. The mean value of each of these subgroups was calculated. These mean values clearly show a tendency to increase with increasing phenobarbital levels. For example, for the group of patients receiving 3 to 4 mg/kg phenytoin, the corresponding phenytoin levels were 5.14 ± 0.81 (SEM, $N = 25$), 5.41 ± 0.74 ($N = 40$), 8.69 ± 0.75 ($N = 61$), 10.71 ± 0.76 ($N = 70$), and 13.43 ± 1.11 ($N = 36$). These values therefore prove an influence of the phenobarbital on the phenytoin levels. The above-mentioned value of the subgroup 40 to 50 μg/ml phenobarbital (13.43 with a standard deviation of 6.65) is higher than the lowest value of the subgroup 0 to 10 μg/ml with a significance of a 0.1% level.

This increase can be seen in all phenytoin dose groups, with the exception of the group 0 to 2 mg/kg. The changes in the mean values seem to point to a linear relationship in this plot. Additional analysis was therefore made with a second method.

Method of Linear Regression

The phenytoin levels of each dose group were plotted against the simultaneously measured phenobarbital level and a linear regression was made. The correlation coefficient varied for these groups from 0.29 to 0.58. This—with about 200 data points for each group—is a high level of significance for a linear relationship.

The regression lines as shown in Fig. 1 reveal a positive slope, indicating again a dependence of phenytoin levels on phenobarbital.

DISCUSSION

Comparison with patients receiving phenytoin alone shows an increase of phenytoin levels with high phenobarbital levels and a decrease with low phenobarbital levels. The highest value of the dose group 3 to 4 mg/kg previously mentioned is not only significantly higher than the lowest value, it is also higher than the control from patients without phenobarbital (7.82 ± 6.58, $N = 77$). The control values are equal to those of the patients with a phenobarbital level of 20

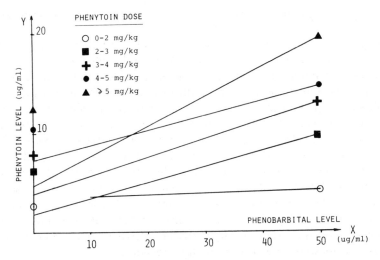

FIG. 1. Regression lines of phenytoin levels versus phenobarbital levels. The lines show a positive slope, indicating a dependence of phenytoin levels on phenobarbital. Comparison with patients receiving phenytoin alone (values on the y-axis) reveals an increase of phenytoin level with high phenobarbital levels against a decrease with low phenobarbital levels.

to 25 μg/ml. A high phenobarbital level therefore provokes a rise of the phenytoin level whereas lower phenobarbital levels provoke a decrease of the phenytoin in comparison to the control. A rise or a decrease of the phenytoin level depends primarily on the phenobarbital level.

The influence of the phenytoin level cannot be clearly deducted from the graph. However, it seems quite striking that there is an increase of the slope with increasing phenytoin doses.

The interaction of phenobarbital and phenytoin has been attributed in many publications to two opposite metabolic effects (Vree et al., 1975). On the one hand, phenobarbital accelerates the catabolism of the phenytoin by induction of the oxidizing enzymes in the liver and should therefore produce a decrease of the phenytoin level. On the other hand, phenobarbital is parahydroxylated by the same enzymes and competes therefore with the phenytoin.

The induction probably reaches a maximal value with a certain phenobarbital level. It is therefore not surprising that competition prevails at higher phenobarbital levels. The results, a decrease with low levels and an increase with high levels, are explainable or even predictable with this theory. This explains why analysis of patients with a great difference in their phenobarbital levels resulted in variations in the data (Buchanan and Sholiton, 1972), and why there is some contradiction in the table mentioned (Kutt, 1975). In those cases where the authors indicated a phenobarbital level at all, it was high when a rise was observed.

As opposed to many authors, we therefore conclude that under certain conditions—starting with high phenytoin levels and high phenobarbital levels—an augmentation of the phenobarbital dosage will provoke in most cases an increase in the phenytoin level, which might have serious consequences.

EFFECT OF PHENYTOIN ON PRIMIDONE METABOLISM

An opposite example represents the corresponding interaction on phenobarbital as metabolic product of primidone. Here, both induction—resulting in a higher conversion rate from primidone to phenobarbital—and competition in the catabolism result in an elevation of the phenobarbital. In the second study, it was therefore determined if the ratio of phenobarbital : primidone rises with phenytoin given concomitantly. This increase has been observed by many authors (Fincham et al., 1974). The results were sometimes contested because of the big standard deviation which results in the calculation of mean ratio (Reynolds, 1975).

With the assumption that the variation in the ratios was due mostly to a change of the phenobarbital level, it seemed possible to avoid the large standard deviation when plotting the ratio against the phenobarbital level. The regression lines were calculated for the group of patients receiving primidone alone and for the group of patients simultaneously receiving phenytoin. Positive slopes and high correlation coefficients were evident from both regression lines.

Two conclusions derived from this: first, the so-called mean ratio, which can be read about in most publications on primidone, cannot be generally accepted. The assumption that the phenobarbital level derived from primidone reaches a level three to five times greater than that of primidone is valid only within the most commonly used concentrations. It has to be pointed out that this ratio is a parameter which depends on the phenobarbital concentration.

The second conclusion concerned the influence of phenytoin. In the linear regression the slope of the line for patients with phenytoin was clearly greater than that for the controls. In monotherapy with primidone, the ratio, within the therapeutic range, varied from 1 to 7, whereas in patients who took phenytoin simultaneously, a ratio from 1 to 10 had been observed. This confirms the finding previously reported—which is to be theoretically expected—that phenytoin increases the relative phenobarbital concentration from primidone.

REFERENCES

Buchanan, R. A., and Sholiton, L. J. (1972): Diphenylhydantoin, interactions with other drugs in man. In: *Antiepileptic Drugs,* edited by D. M. Woodbury, J. K. Penry, and R. P. Schmidt. Raven Press, New York.

Fincham, R. W., Schottelius, D. D., and Sahs, A. L. (1974): The influence of diphenylhydantoin on primidone metabolism. *Arch. Neurol.,* 30:259–262.

Kutt, H. (1975): Interactions of antiepileptic drugs. *Epilepsia,* 16:393–402.

Reynolds, E. H. (1975): Interaction of phenytoin and primidone. In: *Clinical Pharmacology of Anti-Epileptic Drugs,* edited by H. Schneider, D. Janz, C. Gardner-Thorpe, H. Meinardi, and A. L. Sherwin. Springer-Verlag, Berlin.

Richens, A. (1974): Drug estimation in the treatment of epilepsy. *Proc. R. Soc. Med.,* 67:1227.

Sauter, R. (1974): Medizinischer Bericht. *Ber. Schweiz. Anst. Epil.,* 89:11-25.

Vree, T. B., Henderson, P. T., Van der Kleijn, E., and Guelen, P. J. M. (1975): Drug interactions at the metabolic level. In: *Clinical Pharmacology of Anti-Epileptic Drugs,* edited by H. Schneider, D. Janz, C. Gardner-Thorpe, H. Meinardi, and A. L. Sherwin. Springer-Verlag, Berlin.

Epilepsy, The Eighth International Symposium,
edited by J. K. Penry. Raven Press, New York
© 1977.

Automated Analysis of Prolonged EEG Recordings in Epileptic Patients

H. H. von Albert

Neurologischen Klinik des Bezirkskrankenhauses, D-8870 Günzburg, Germany

New equipment was developed in collaboration with Siemens-Erlangen (West Germany) for long-term EEG monitoring. With this electronic device, one can perform EEG needle recordings for up to 10 or 12 hr. An analyzing unit detects spikes, waves, or spike-and-wave (SW) combinations in the following conditions: (1) spikes are detected if a deflection of an amplitude more than 1.2 to 3.0 as high as in the averaged foregoing EEG takes between 15 and 55 msec; (2) waves are detected and counted if the amplitude of the foregoing EEG is lower in a proportion of 3:1 to 1.5:1 and frequency is under 6 cps; (3) spike-wave combinations are counted if within 300 msec after detection of a spike a wave is detected; in this case the amplitude of the spike can be lower than the amplitude of the foregoing average EEG.

Counted EEG signals are written at normal paper speed, also a time-compressed graphic demonstration is given by a trend recorder.

When one compares the results with usual EEG recordings or computer analysis of prolonged EEG recordings, an advantage is to be seen in the possibility of EEG recording and automatically analyzing for hours, using a not too expensive apparatus, resulting in pathological EEG signals expressed in numbers per hour. The possible error is now between 5 and 20%. EEG recordings can be reanalyzed, if necessary, from the tape.

Disadvantages are the error in counting, which is between 5 and 20%, and the fact that in some patients it is impossible to obtain a correct calibration of the analysis unit to the individual EEG, so that prolonged EEG recordings cannot be performed.

RESULTS

After a 2-year study with automatically analyzed prolonged EEG recordings, it is to be stated that:

1. Time of the so-called normal EEG recording is certainly too short to obtain representative information about the bioelectrical picture of brain function and/or seizures. In the patient whose tracing is shown in Fig. 1, a usual EEG

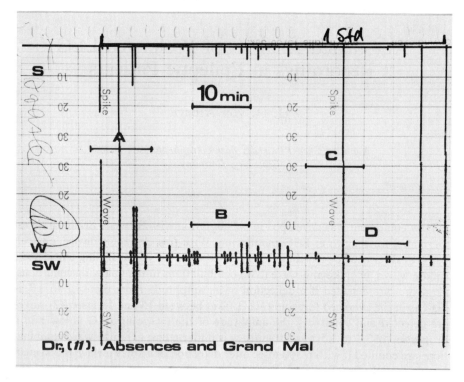

FIG. 1. Example of a time-compressed demonstration. S, spike; W, waves; SW, spike-and-wave combinations. Inhomogenous distribution of absences.

recording would give widely varying results, depending on the actual time of recording. In A, a pathological EEG is recorded with four long-lasting absences; during B recording only three short SW groups are seen; in C there is a long-lasting absence in an otherwise normal EEG; and in D the EEG recording could be analyzed as normal.

2. In patients with more than 20 to 40 pathological events per hour in prolonged EEG recordings, the new technique gives a better indication for drug therapy because it shows the actual EEG situation and is perhaps better and provides more information than serum levels of anticonvulsant drugs.

3. In patients with difficult differential diagnosis, prolonged EEG recordings are of great value to determine whether or not the patient is epileptic. In 10 patients the differential diagnosis could be cleared up, in 7 there were no spiking groups or other abnormalities in EEG recordings lasting between 3 and 5 hr.

4. For testing of new drugs or drug combinations, the quantification of EEG recordings by automatic analysis leads to better results.

5. Quantification of slow potentials, as delta waves, for instance, seems to be a good measuring of the state of cerebral coma or loss of consciousness, but further work is necessary.

Epilepsy, The Eighth International Symposium,
edited by J. K. Penry. Raven Press, New York
© 1977.

Relationship Between Quantitative EEG Measurements and Clinical State in Epileptic Patients

Peter Kellaway and James R. G. Carrie

Baylor College of Medicine and The Methodist Hospital, Houston, Texas 77030

In our recent work we have been examining several aspects of EEG monitoring of epileptic patients. These studies have involved quantitative measurement of variability of paroxysmal EEG abnormalities with respect to time, evaluation of EEG sampling and quantification procedures, and examination of correlations between clinical state and EEG findings.

METHODS

EEGs were recorded continuously during 36 hr in epileptic patients who were attached to the recorder by long leads and who, during the day, were permitted to sit in a chair, read, eat, talk, watch TV, and move around to a limited extent. The patients were continuously observed and recorded on closed-circuit (CC) TV.

Paroxysmal EEG abnormalities were quantified in two ways:

1. Visual analysis was performed following operational definition of criteria for visually detecting and manually measuring paroxysmal abnormalities. There was a high level of interobserver agreement for the awake EEG, and less satisfactory agreement for sleep EEGs.

2. Paroxysmal sharp transients occurring during overnight sleep were detected and quantified using a computer-assisted technique. This method is described in detail elsewhere (Carrie, 1976). There was a high level of interobserver agreement when this method was used.

Results for five patients, three with generalized and two with focal paroxysmal EEG abnormalities, are discussed in this chapter.

RESULTS

Variability of Paroxysmal EEG Patterns with Respect to Time

The first question which we have been investigating concerns the variability of paroxysmal EEG abnormalities with respect to time and can be stated thus: Does the amount of paroxysmal EEG abnormality show considerable quantitative variation, or does it vary only slightly in abundance, throughout prolonged time intervals?

If considerable variability in EEG characteristics with respect to time is found, there are two practical implications. First, relatively brief (approximately 1-hr) samples of EEG such as are obtained in a standard EEG recording are unlikely to provide measurements that show a good correlation with the overall prevailing clinical state of the patient. The findings of Browne et al. (1974) are relevant to this question. These workers concluded that only prolonged EEG monitoring can provide measurements that reliably estimate absence-seizure frequency in patients with absence epilepsy. Thus the lack of correlation between EEG findings and clinical state in epileptic patients that has long been noted by electroencephalographers may be due at least in part to inadequate sampling. We have been examining some quantitative aspects of this problem. Second, if there is substantial variability in EEG findings over time, anticonvulsant medication should be scheduled so as to provide maximal blood levels when the risk of occurrence of a seizure is greatest or when EEG abnormality is maximal if this is found to correlate with seizure hazard. Rowan et al. (1975) have reported findings in two patients that suggest that this may be a significant aspect of EEG monitoring. The first part of our research program has therefore been concerned with examining the extent to which measurements of paroxysmal EEG activity may vary throughout the day and night in the same patient, and with quantitatively evaluating the magnitude of the errors that may arise as a result of differences between measurements made on relatively small samples of EEG, such as the approximately 1-hr samples acquired during a routine clinical recording.

Figure 1 shows a time plot of the results from one patient. Although only generalized 3/sec spike-wave had been noted in the clinical EEG from this patient, examination of the 36-hr record revealed several types of paroxysmal abnormality. These different abnormalities responded differentially to treatment; this finding will be discussed in detail elsewhere. There was marked activation of paroxysmal activity during sleep, with suppression during REM in relation to an approximately 90-min cycle. There was a general similarity in the amount of abnormal activity observed during the two consecutive nights. However, this patient showed the greatest internight difference in respect of this measurement of all five subjects, possibly as a result of her wakefulness during the first night.

Figure 1 further shows that there was considerable variation in the amount of paroxysmal EEG activity per unit time during the awake state, suggesting that there might be considerable differences between measurements derived from short samples of EEG.

To quantitatively examine the variability between 1-hr EEG samples further, we tabulated the differences between the smallest and largest measurements derived from 1-hr EEG samples acquired under "steady-state" conditions (awake, unmedicated, or with steady blood levels of anticonvulsants). Inspection of these tables showed large differences between the smallest and largest measurements from 1-hr samples in all patients. The patient with generalized spike-wave

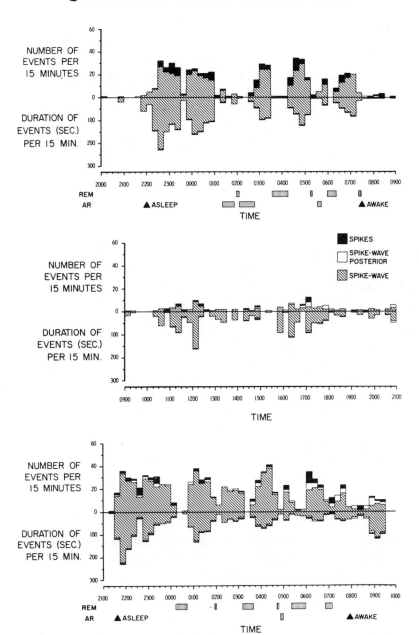

FIG. 1. Graphic plot showing results of visual analysis of 36-hr EEG of a patient with absence seizures and reported to show generalized 3/sec spike-wave in clinical EEG. Plot shows number and duration of paroxysmal abnormalities in consecutive 15-min intervals. Patient receiving no medication. AR, arousal, indicates when the patient was awake during the night.

who showed the largest difference between measurements from 1-hr samples had one spike-wave event with a duration of 2.1 sec during one 1-hr segment, and during another 1-hr sample had 38 spike-wave events with a total duration of 337.1 sec. One patient with focal spikes showed 113 discharges during one 1-hr sample and 1,749 during another. Further tables were constructed to examine the question of whether, by making measurements early in the morning and late in the evening, excessive variability between 1-hr samples was detected. These tables showed results from measurements obtained during the usual "working day" of most EEG labs (9 A.M. to 5 P.M.), and the interval between the starting times of the 1-hr samples with the largest and smallest measurement was noted to determine the interval between sampling that might be associated with large differences in the measurements of paroxysmal EEG activity. The patient with generalized spike-wave who showed the largest difference between the measurements for 1-hr samples had one spike-wave event with a duration of 2.1 sec during one 1-hr segment, and during another sample that started 2 hr later had 20 spike-wave events with a total duration of 314.1 sec. In one of the patients with a focal spike discharge, 222 and 1,749 spikes were observed during 1-hr samples whose starting times were separated by an interval of 4 hr.

Another way to examine the question of variability is to determine the maximum extent to which measurements derived from 1-hr samples differ from the mean calculated for the entire period of observation when the patient was awake. Tables displaying this information were constructed and it was found that there was a large range of variation in the measurements derived from 1-hr samples about the mean values. For example, the spike-wave measurements from 1-hr samples in one subject ranged from zero to over nine times the mean value for both the number of paroxysmal events and their total duration. Tabulations of data acquired during the 9 A.M. to 5 P.M. "working-day" period showed a smaller although large range about the mean values for samples that were in several instances closely spaced in time.

Overnight Samples of Paroxysmal EEG Activity

Since there is much variability in the measurements obtained from short samples of EEG, what methods of measurement can be used that provide more quantitatively stable results? It would appear that larger EEG samples are required. A method for quantifying generalized spike-wave EEG patterns by computer during prolonged recordings has been tested and will be described elsewhere (Carrie and Frost, *in press*). At present we have no information relating to the stability of paroxysmal EEG patterns from day to day. However, we have been examining the internight stability of the measurements obtained during the two consecutive overnight recordings during which observations are made in our 36-hr EEGs for the following reasons: First, sleep has long been recognized as a potent activator of abnormal patterns in the EEGs of epileptic patients. Second, overnight sleep monitoring provides a situation in which large samples of EEG can be acquired with relatively minor inconvenience to the patient. If it were to prove to be a method that provides a sample of EEG that gives a reliable estimate of the patient's clinical state, at least in some epileptics, recordings could be made on a portable tape recorder in the patient's home or transmitted from his or her home over the telephone lines. Third, we have been able to apply a convenient computer-assisted method for detecting and quantifying EEG sharp transients during overnight recordings.

The average percentage change from the smallest to the largest measurement for 1-hr samples and for the overnight samples (designating the smallest measurement in each pair as 100%) was computed. The average percentage change from smallest to largest measurement of number of events per hour for the five subjects was 1,231% for the 1-hr awake samples, 33% for the computer-assisted overnight measurements. It seems likely that internight stability of the measurements would be further improved if habituation to the recording conditions was allowed by recording for several consecutive nights (note the wakefulness of the patient during the first but not the second night in the analysis shown in Fig. 1; it is likely that the behavioral difference between nights reduced the internight stability of the measurements of paroxysmal activity).

Correlations Between Clinical State and EEG Findings

A further question that may be asked regarding EEG monitoring of epileptic patients is as follows: Suppose that we can develop methods for easily and conveniently acquiring EEG measurements that are stable while the patient is in a "steady-state" condition with respect to frequency of occurrence of seizures and blood levels of medication, to what extent do changes in these EEG measurements reflect (1) initiation of medication, (2) change of medication, and (3) change in clinical state of the patient? A third aspect of our research program has therefore been concerned with these questions, and we have some preliminary information.

In patients with absence epilepsy, reduction in the frequency of occurrence of seizures following the initiation of medication has been associated with a reduction in the amount of interictal spike-wave, both awake and during overnight sleep. However, in some patients with absence seizures, the EEG pattern shows several types of abnormality (e.g., the patient whose EEG time-plot is shown in Fig. 1), and the electrographic response to treatment is complex. These findings will be presented in detail elsewhere.

Two patients with epilepsy who showed focal paroxysmal EEG abnormalities have been studied. One of these patients was already receiving medication when first seen, and the dose of phenobarbital was increased between the first and second EEG studies. Seizures were eliminated, and there was a slight reduction in EEG spike frequency. In the second patient, phenobarbital treatment was started and the seizures ceased. The electrographic response to treatment was complex. The focal EEG spikes decreased in frequency, diminished in amplitude, and became more restricted topographically both when the patient was awake and during overnight sleep. Furthermore, relative augmentation of spike frequency occurred during REM sleep before treatment, but after initiation of medication spike frequency was reduced during REM.

CONCLUSIONS

1. Paroxysmal EEG abnormality shows such variability over time that 1-hr samples provide measurements that are poor indicators of the average amount of paroxysmal EEG abnormality or the frequency of occurrence of absence seizures.

2. Measurements of the number of paroxysmal events per hour derived from overnight EEG recordings using a computer-assisted method showed much greater agreement between samples than those obtained from 1-hr "routine" EEG records.

3. In patients with absence seizures, change in clinical state corresponds to the amount of interictal paroxysmal EEG activity, daytime and overnight, although we are now beginning to find evidence that even in patients with absence epilepsy the neurophysiological picture may not be entirely straightforward. In other types of epilepsy, complex relationships between clinical state, interictal EEG abnormality, and blood levels of anticonvulsant drugs have been observed. Clarification of the quantitative relationships between EEG patterns and clinical state in different types of epilepsy and in different epileptic patients is likely to be a substantial undertaking involving investigation of large numbers of subjects.

ACKNOWLEDGMENTS

This work was supported by U.S. Public Health Service Grant No. NS 11535 from NINCDS. The authors thank Ms. L. Aylor for expert technical assistance.

REFERENCES

Browne, T. R., Penry, J. K., Porter, R. J., and Dreifuss, F. E. (1974): A comparison of clinical estimates of absence seizure frequency with estimates based on prolonged telemetered EEG's. *Neurology (Minneap.),* 24:381–382.

Carrie, J. R. G. (1976): Computer-assisted EEG sharp-transient detection and quantification during overnight recordings in an epileptic patient. In: *Quantitative Analytic Studies in Epilepsy,* edited by P. Kellaway and I. Petersén. Raven Press, New York.

Carrie, J. R. G., and Frost, J. D., Jr. (1977): Clinical evaluation of a technique for detection and measurement of spike-wave paroxysms by computer. *Electroencephalogr. Clin. Neurophysiol. (in press).*

Rowan, A. J., Pippenger, C. E., McGregor, P. A., and French, J. H. (1975): Seizure activity and anticonvulsant concentration. *Arch. Neurol.,* 32:281–288.

ANTIEPILEPTIC DRUGS

Epilepsy, The Eighth International Symposium,
edited by J. K. Penry. Raven Press, New York
© 1977.

A Trial of Clonazepam in the Treatment of Severe Epilepsy in Infancy and Childhood

N. V. O'Donohoe and B. A. Paes

Our Lady's Hospital For Sick Children, Dublin 12, Ireland

In this study we attempted to assess the effectiveness of clonazepam used either singly or in combination with other drugs. In the trial, clonazepam was used to treat various types of epilepsy, many of them severe and intractable. Many of the patients had already been treated unsuccessfully with other drugs. The trial included 31 patients, all of whom were reviewed frequently during the first 12 weeks following introduction of the drug and thereafter depending on the clinical outcome. Drug levels were assayed at the end of the 1st, 4th, 6th, and 12th weeks after the introduction of the drug. Each patient had laboratory tests at the start of the trial, including full blood count, liver function tests, urea and electrolytes, and urinalysis, and these tests were repeated when possible during the first 3 months of the trial. The ages of the patients ranged from 1 month to 12.5 years, but over two-thirds of the patients were 6 years or younger (Table 1).

Nearly all the patients were suffering from generalized epilepsies, usually secondary generalized epilepsies. Ten were considered to have myoclonic epilepsy. These included patients having generalized myoclonic jerks, atonic-akinetic seizures associated with falling to the ground, sudden head-nodding, and salaam seizures involving flexion of the trunk. Mental retardation of variable degree was common in these patients, and some of them had permanent neurological abnormalities. The EEG abnormalities were variable, and some of the patients had the slow spike-wave patterns described by Lennox and Davis (1950).

In seven further patients, the myoclonic epilepsy was more severe. These patients had an early onset of epilepsy beginning with infrequent major seizures, and going on to the development of head-nodding attacks, atonic-akinetic attacks, atypical absences, and tonic-clonic seizures that were more frequent during sleep.

TABLE 1. *Age range of 31 patients*

Age (years)	No. of patients
0–3	16
3–6	7
6–9	4
9–13	4

159

Periods of prolonged minor epileptic status were common in these patients, and it was considered that they conformed to the clinical picture usually associated with the Lennox-Gastaut syndrome. The EEG patterns consisted of generalized disturbances, generalized slowing, and the typical slow spike-wave patterns associated with the syndrome.

Ten patients were suffering from infantile spasms and had the classic clinical picture and the classic EEG pattern associated with this condition. Of the ten patients, seven had symptomatic spasms and three had cryptogenic spasms.

The other four patients consisted of two patients with major tonic-clonic seizures, one with subacute sclerosing panencephalitis (SSPE), and one with the hemiplegia-hyperpyrexia-epilepsy (HHE) syndrome whose epilepsy following the acute episode was treated with clonazepam.

Of the 31 patients, 25 had previously been treated with other drugs, and 6 were having clonazepam as the drug of first choice. Of the 25 who had had other drugs, those with the Lennox-Gastaut syndrome were among those who had been particularly difficult to control, and 2 of these had had at least 20 other medications prior to being given clonazepam.

The arbitrary maximum dosage for infants under 1 year was 0.3 mg/kg/day, and for those over 1 year, 0.25 mg/kg/day. The drug was introduced slowly, usually beginning with 0.25 mg at bedtime in those under 1 year and 0.5 mg at night in the older group. Dosage was gradually increased every fifth day until the epilepsy responded to medication or until serious side effects were encountered. In some cases these side effects were severe enough to warrant stopping the drug.

The results were graded as follows (Table 2):

1. Excellent—i.e., those who responded extremely well with no subsequent relapse—6 patients.
2. Good—those patients whose control was rather better than adequate and who had occasional recurrences of attacks, i.e., better than 50% control—13 patients.
3. Moderate—those in whom improvement occurred, but the attacks were still frequent—4 patients.
4. Nil—i.e., no clinical improvement in the epilepsy—8 patients.

In the excellent group, the three patients with infantile spasms who were in this category were aged 4.5, 8, and 14 months. The 4.5-month-old belonged to the cryptogenic group, the 8-month-old developed spasms coincidentally with the administration of diphtheria immunization, and the 14-month-old developed spasms symptomatically in association with mild mental handicap. The patient with Lennox-Gastaut syndrome who had the excellent result was aged 9.5 years, and clonazepam produced an impressive control of his epilepsy following a failure of all other drugs. However, he had a mild recurrence and was reclassified in the "good" group. In general, EEG improvement correlated well with control of the epilepsy in those who had a satisfactory response to treatment.

TABLE 2. *Initial results after treatment with clonazepam*

			Type of epilepsy			
Result	Myoclonic	Infantile spasms	Lennox-Gastaut	HHE syndrome	Major tonic-clonic	SSPE
Excellent	1	3	1	1		
Good	7	3	2		1	
Moderate	1	1	2			
Nil	1	3	2		1	1

Although blood levels were estimated carefully in all patients treated, a review of the results showed no correlation between the antiepileptic effect of the drug and plasma levels, nor was it possible to demonstrate a relationship between the onset or severity of the various side effects and plasma concentrations of the drug. However, it did seem that steady-state concentrations of the drug resulted only after about 6 weeks of continuous therapy. An increase in dosage at any stage usually produced a rise in plasma concentration followed by fluctuations of the plasma level and a subsequent return to a steady state after a further 4 to 6 weeks of treatment. Other authors including Browne and Penry (1973) commented that there is a big scatter in blood levels and that the relationship to therapeutic efficiency was not as close as with other drugs. Of those cases categorized as having an excellent response, blood levels usually ranged between 20.4 and 74.8 ng/ml, and this range correlated well with that described by other authors (Reider, 1975).

The main side effect (Table 3) was drowsiness, which usually began soon after the introduction of the drug but was usually not a major problem if the drug dosage was slowly increased. Drooling associated with hypersecretion was noticed mainly in those patients with mental handicap. This particular side effect seemed to be dose related. One patient became severely ataxic and the drug was discontinued because of this. In five patients who were grossly hyperkinetic prior to the onset of therapy, the drug appeared to have a calming effect and the patients became more manageable. However, five other patients became overactive while on the drug and this overactivity increased as the dose was increased; in one such

TABLE 3. *Side effects of clonazepam*

Effect	No. affected
Early drowsiness	16
Drooling + hypersecretion	7
Ataxia	5
Hyperactivity	4
Attacks worsened by clonazepam	3
No side effects	5

patient this side effect led to the drug's being withdrawn. In three patients, the epilepsy became much worse while they were on treatment.

DISCUSSION AND CONCLUSION

Our results indicate that clonazepam is a useful drug in the treatment of the very serious varieties of epilepsy which occur in young children particularly. These patients constituted the majority of our series. Long-term follow-up is essential with this drug since some of the children who initially did well relapsed after a period of 1 or 2 months, and others who had a "good" response initially seemed to do better as time went on. In this series, either seizure control was complete or the seizures were significantly reduced in 19 out of 31 patients—initially a 61.3% success rate (comprising the "excellent" and "good" groups)—although on longer follow-up, seizure control had fallen to 17 out of 31 patients, 54.8% (Table 4).

TABLE 4. *Follow-up results 1–1.5 years after treatment with clonazepam*

	Type of Epilepsy					
Result	Myoclonic	Infantile spasms	Lennox-Gastaut	HHE syndrome	Major tonic-clonic	SSPE
Excellent	3	5		1	1	
Good	5	1	1			
Moderate	1	1				
Nil	1	3	6		1	1

Throughout the trial, clonazepam produced no significant hematological changes or other toxic effects.

ACKNOWLEDGMENTS

This study was carried out as part of the research program of the Children's Research Centre, Our Lady's Hospital For Sick Children, Dublin 12, and was supported by a generous grant from Roche Products, Ltd., of London.

REFERENCES

Browne, T. R., and Penry, J. K. (1973): Benzodiazepines in the treatment of epilepsy. A review. *Epilepsia,* 14:277.

Lennox, W. G., and Davis, J. P. (1950): Clinical correlates of the fast and slow spike-wave electroencephalogram. *J. Pediatr.,* 5:626.

Reider, J. (1975): Metabolism and pharmacokinetics of phenobarbital, diphenylhydantoin, ethosuximide and clonazepam in man. Presented to the Second Conference of the European Study Group on Child Neurology, Zurich, Switzerland, September 15–18.

Epilepsy, The Eighth International Symposium,
edited by J. K. Penry. Raven Press, New York
© 1977.

Treatment of Chronic Epilepsy for 1 to 2 Years with Clonazepam

R. N. Nanda, R. H. Johnson,* H. J. Keogh, D. G. Lambie,
I. D. Melville, and R. A. Shakir

*Department of Neurology, University of Glasgow, Institute of Neurological Sciences,
Southern General Hospital, Glasgow, Scotland*

At the Seventh International Symposium on Epilepsy we communicated the results of a double-blind crossover trial of clonazepam (Rivotril®, Roche Products Ltd.) in 30 patients whose epilepsy was poorly controlled (Nanda et al., 1976). The trial was for 9 weeks and we now report the results during the following 21 months of treatment in those patients who benefited. In addition, we report the effect of clonazepam therapy in 36 patients in whom the drug was introduced in an open trial for up to 22 months.

METHODS

Patients

Double-Blind Trial

We studied 30 patients, 22 males and 8 females, aged 11 to 40 years (mean, 26 years). Details of the types of epilepsy from which they suffered are given in Table 1. Twenty-five patients were receiving combinations of phenytoin, phenobarbital and primidone, and five were not receiving any medication.

Open Trial

The 36 patients in the open trial of clonazepam—19 males and 17 females, aged 11 to 44 years (mean, 27 years)—were treated and details are given in Table 1. All patients were receiving combinations of phenytoin, phenobarbital, and primidone.

---

* Present address: Department of Medicine, University of Otago, Wellington Hospital, Wellington, New Zealand.

TABLE 1. Results of treatment with clonazepam in the two trials

Type of epilepsy	No. of patients	Improvement in fit frequency (%)									
		Double-blind trial					After 20–22 months				
		100%	80%	50%	0–50%	Worse	100%	80%	50%	0–50%	Clonazepam withdrawn
Double-blind trial											
Myoclonic											
Jerks	3	3					3				
Jerks + tonic-clonic	12										
jerks		9	3				8[a]	3			
tonic-clonic		8		4			7		4		
Atypical absences	4	3			1			2			2
Frontotemporal											
Focal	7				7						7
Tonic-clonic	4			4			2	2			
Open trial											
Myoclonic											
Jerks + tonic-clonic	7	7									
Photosensitive	7	6	1								
Tonic-clonic	6	2		2	1	1					2
Frontotemporal	16			9	5	2					9

In those patients who did not benefit, clonazepam was withdrawn. 100%: no further attacks. Note that improvement was marked in patients with myoclonic and photosensitive epilepsies.
[a] One patient died.

Design of Trials

Before the trials all patients were assessed clinically and electroencephalographically. Further EEGs were obtained at the end of each part of the double-blind trial and during the open trial. In both the double-blind and open trials clonazepam was added to the existing anticonvulsant regimen. In the double-blind crossover trial the daily dose of clonazepam was 3 mg/day (1 mg in the morning and 2 mg at night). Matched placebo tablets were also used. In the open trial, the clonazepam dose was increased to an initial dose of 3 mg daily, and the dose later was increased or decreased as required. Those patients who benefited during the double-blind trial were also managed in the same way. All patients and relatives or hospital staff recorded the frequency of seizures and any side effects on specially prepared charts.

Blood samples were taken before and after clonazepam treatment for measurement of serum concentrations of anticonvulsants and for hematological examination and estimations of liver function, blood urea, and electrolytes. Measurements of phenytoin, phenobarbital, and primidone were performed by gas chromatography. Clonazepam was measured by a radioimmunoassay technique at the Psychoendocrine Centre, St. James's Hospital, Dublin (by courtesy of Dr. D. A. O'Kelly).

RESULTS

Seizure Frequency

The effect of clonazepam on seizure frequency for the patients in the double-blind trial, both during the trial and after 21 months, is shown in Table 1. The effectiveness of clonazepam therapy in the patients who improved was the same after 21 months as during the trial, but in four cases the clonazepam dose was increased to maintain effectiveness, doses of up to 12 mg daily (one patient) being given without side effects. It was possible to reduce or stop other anticonvulsants in four patients.

For the patients in the open trial, the effect of clonazepam on seizure frequency after 22 months is also shown in Table 1. As in the double-blind trial the drug was most effective in patients with myoclonic epilepsy and tonic-clonic seizures and also in those with photosensitive epilepsy.

Clonazepam was less effective in the patients with only tonic-clonic seizures and those with frontotemporal epilepsy.

Unwanted Effects

Of the 66 patients, 44 complained of drowsiness in the first week after clonazepam was given. In these patients drowsiness improved after the first week even though the dose of the drug was being increased slowly. After 2 to 3 weeks only six of the patients (all in the open trial) continued to complain of drowsiness.

These six patients were also ataxic, with hypotonicity of trunk and lower limb muscles. Clonazepam was reduced and then stopped in these patients. One patient in the open trial became depressed while on clonazepam and the drug had to be withdrawn. In another patient, a 12-year-old boy, a change of personality, with irritability and violent behavior, was reported and the drug was withdrawn. One patient reported excessive hair loss in the first month after starting clonazepam. This effect was transient and the patient continued to take the drug. At the end of 22 months none of those continuing treatment (45 patients) complained of any side effects.

Electroencephalograms

Ten patients with myoclonic epilepsy showed generalized polyspike-wave seizure discharges, and this paroxysmal activity was not recorded in seven patients during clonazepam therapy. The other patients with myoclonic epilepsy showed no EEG abnormalities. All patients with photosensitive epilepsy showed seizure activity with photic stimulation. Clonazepam therapy suppressed this photosensitive response in all EEGs recorded during the trial at monthly intervals. In all other patients EEGs were unchanged on clonazepam.

Observations on Blood, Anticonvulsant Concentrations, Hematology, and Biochemistry

Serum concentrations of phenytoin, phenobarbital, and primidone in the patients on the double-blind trial were not significantly altered by the addition of 3 mg of clonazepam daily for 4 weeks (Nanda et al., 1976). Serum concentrations of clonazepam in these patients ranged from 0.3 to 104 nM/liter (mean ± 39 nM/liter). In the open trial plasma clonazepam concentrations in patients whose epilepsy was well controlled on 2 to 12 mg of clonazepam daily ranged from 17 to 330 nM/liter (mean ± 134 nM/liter). Treatment with phenobarbital appeared to lower serum concentrations of clonazepam (Nanda et al., 1976). No biochemical or hematological abnormalities were noted during treatment with clonazepam.

DISCUSSION

The results of these trials indicate that clonazepam is effective in the treatment of generalized epilepsy with myoclonic jerks alone or with tonic-clonic seizures. This result is of considerable importance as this form of epilepsy has previously been difficult to treat (Van Woert and Sethy, 1976). The drug was also found to be particularly effective in photosensitive epilepsy. The value of the drug in epilepsy with associated myoclonus has been demonstrated in open trials, but the numbers of patients have been small, two trials only having five patients each with this condition (Huang et al., 1974; Goldberg and Dorman, 1976). In a double-blind trial in 1973 Edwards and Eadie showed that the drug is of value as a wide-spectrum anticonvulsant, but few of their patients had myoclonic epilepsy and there is no indication that any had photosensitive epilepsy. Our results for patients with atypical absences, tonic-clonic epilepsy, and temporal lobe epilepsy also indicate that clonazepam is sometimes of value in these forms of epilepsy.

In focal epilepsy our results in the patients in the double-blind trial suggested that the drug was of little value. It is possible that the daily dosage of 3 mg of clonazepam in our trial was insufficient for control of this type of epilepsy, as a higher dosage has been reported as being necessary in temporal lobe epilepsy (Huang et al., 1973). More satisfactory results were obtained in our open trial when the clonazepam dosage was increased (up to 10 mg daily) in the focal epilepsies.

Serum concentrations of clonazepam in our patients ranged from 0.3 to 330 nM/liter on a daily dose of 2 to 12 mg. It has previously been reported (Dreifuss et al., 1975) that after daily oral doses of 1.5 to 4 mg in patients taking clonazepam alone serum concentrations ranged from 40 to 240 nM/liter. We found that patients in the double-blind trial who showed clonazepam concentrations below 40 nM/liter were those who responded poorly to the drug.

Conflicting reports (Edwards and Eadie, 1973; Hara et al., 1976) have previously suggested that clonazepam may either raise or depress phenytoin or phenobarbital serum concentrations, but it has also been concluded (Huang et al., 1973) that there is no constant effect of clonazepam medication on serum concentrations of other anticonvulsants and that an increase in phenytoin concentrations might be due to more constant drug intake because of closer supervision. Our observations indicate that serum concentrations of phenytoin, phenobarbital, and primidone were not altered by the addition of 3 mg of clonazepam daily. It is also, however, possible that other anticonvulsants, particularly phenobarbital, taken in conjunction with clonazepam depress serum clonazepam concentrations and this may be of importance in therapy. We have found some evidence that the dose of clonazepam has to be increased with time in a few patients on long-term treatment. It remains to be defined whether this is due to tolerance to clonazepam or to accelerated metabolism of the drug.

SUMMARY

Patients who showed improvement (22) in a double-blind crossover trial of clonazepam in the treatment of 30 patients with chronic epilepsy have been followed for 21 months. In addition, 36 patients with various forms of chronic epilepsy have been studied in an open trial for up to 22 months. Observations have been made on seizure frequency, dosage, and serum concentrations of clonazepam necessary to maintain effective control. In both trials marked improvement occurred in patients with myoclonic epilepsy together with tonic-clonic convulsions and in patients with photosensitive epilepsy. Some patients with atypical absences or frontotemporal or tonic-clonic epilepsy also benefited.

The improvement in seizure control has been maintained (44 patients), although in four patients it has been necessary to increase the dose of clonazepam. Unwanted effects such as drowsiness and ataxia were initially common but only of short-term duration.

We conclude that clonazepam is particularly valuable in epilepsy with associated myoclonus and in photosensitive epilepsy. Patients with other forms of epilepsy may also benefit and the improvement initially seen has continued.

ACKNOWLEDGMENTS

We thank the patients for their cooperation and Roche Products Ltd., the Scottish Hospital Endowments Research Trust, and the Secretary of State for Scotland for support.

REFERENCES

Dreifuss, F. E., Penry, J. K., Rose, S. W., Kupferberg, H. J., and Sato, S. (1975): Serum clonazepam concentrations in children with absence seizures. *Neurology (Minneap.),* 25:255–258.

Edwards, V. E., and Eadie, M. J. (1973): Clonazepam—a clinical study of its effectiveness as an anticonvulsant. *Proc. Aust. Assoc. Neurol.,* 10:61–66.

Goldberg, M. A., and Dorman, J. D. (1976): Intention myoclonus: Successful treatment with clonazepam. *Neurology (Minneap.),* 26:24–26.

Hara, T., Inami, M., and Kaneko, T. (1976): The effect of clonazepam on plasma diphenylhydantoin level in epileptic patients. In: *Epileptology,* Proceedings of the Seventh International Symposium on Epilepsy, Berlin (West), 1975, edited by D. Janz, p. 152. Thieme/PSG, Stuttgart.

Huang, C. Y., McLeod, J. G., Sampson, D., and Hensley, W. J. (1973): Clonazepam in the treatment of epilepsy. *Proc. Aust. Assoc. Neurol.,* 10:67–74.

Huang, C. Y., McLeod, J. G., Sampson, D., and Hensley, W. J. (1974): Clonazepam in the treatment of epilepsy. *Med. J. Aust.,* 2:5–8.

Nanda, R. N., Keogh, H. J., Lambie, D., Johnson, R. H., Melville, I. D., and Morrice, G. D. (1976): The effect of clonazepam upon epilepsy control and plasma levels of other anticonvulsants. In: *Epileptology,* Proceedings of the Seventh International Symposium on Epilepsy, Berlin (West), 1975, edited by D. Janz, pp. 145–151. Thieme/PSG, Stuttgart.

Van Woert, M. H., and Sethy, V. H. (1976): Therapy of intention myoclonus with L-5-hydroxytryptophan and a peripheral decarboxylase inhibitor Mk 486. *Neurology (Minneap).,* 25:135–140.

Epilepsy, The Eighth International Symposium,
edited by J. K. Penry. Raven Press, New York
© 1977.

Clinical Observations on Clonazepam in Intractable Epilepsy

*A. D. Gregoriades and **E. G. Frangos

*Athens Child Guidance Unit, Athens, Greece; and **General Hospital for Mental
and Nervous Diseases, Athens, Greece

New medications are constantly being developed for clinical trial as anticonvulsants, the benzodiazepine derivatives seeming to be the most promising. After their development and use in various therapeutic indications, their anticonvulsant properties quickly attracted interest in their use as possible agents for the treatment of epilepsy. Animal experiments (Randall and Schallek, 1968) have shown that clonazepam, a new benzodiazepine derivative, possesses an anticonvulsant activity several times more powerful than that of nitrazepam, to which it is chemically similar. Since 1973, we have studied the effectiveness of clonazepam and we here report the results of this clinical trial.

PATIENTS AND METHODS

The preparation was given in 93 patients aged 4.5 to 50 years. They were divided into two major groups on the basis of their age. Each group was further subdivided according to the form of epilepsy present. (The types of seizures given in this chapter correlate with the Classification of the Epilepsies proposed by Gastaut in 1970.) Group A included patients up to 20 years of age who were treated by one of us (A.D.G.) on an outpatient basis. Group B consisted of patients from 21 to 53 years of age who were treated by one of us (E.G.F.) as inpatients at the General Hospital for Nervous and Mental Diseases, Athens, Greece.

Group A

Petit Mal

Twelve patients (ten males, 7 to 12 years; two females, 9 to 10 years) had petit mal. Three of the patients had frequent fits daily, three had a few fits daily, and the rest had many fits weekly. There were no neurological findings, mental retardation, or behavior disturbances. The EEGs in six patients showed typical 3 to 3.5 spike-wave discharges, and in the others it was diffusely abnormal with paroxysmal features.

Grand Mal

Three patients (two males and one female, 9 to 10 years) had grand mal. All patients had weekly fits. One patient had a history of perinatal brain damage with spasticity and severe mental retardation. The EEGs were diffusely abnormal in all cases.

Myoclonic Epilepsy

Ten patients (two males, 6 and 7 years; eight females, 5 to 14 years, including a pair of 8-year-old homozygotic twins) had myoclonic epilepsy. All patients had frequent fits, unaffected by previous treatment. There were no significant neurological findings. Mental retardation of mild degree was found in four patients. It was accompanied by behavior disturbances, severe in two, mild in the rest, which were also present in another case. All EEGs were typical of myoclonic epilepsy.

Infantile Myoclonic Encephalopathy (West Syndrome)

Six patients [two males, 4 and 6 years (residual case), and four females, 3 to 5 years] had West syndrome. The fit frequency was high in all patients. Mental retardation and neurological findings, mainly spasticity, were found in all, and behavior disturbances of various degrees were present in four patients. The EEGs were typical of hypsarrhythmia.

Astatomyoclonic Petit Mal (Lennox Syndrome)

Five patients (two males, 8 to 9 years, and three females, 9 to 10 years) were in this group. Four patients had frequent fits daily and one had weekly fits. Mental impairment, neurological findings, and behavior disturbances of various degree were present in three patients. All EEGs were typical, with slow spike-and-wave complexes.

Focal Seizures

Seven patients (five males, two brothers 8 and 10 years, and three others, 11 to 20 years) had focal seizures. The fits were mostly daily and of the motor type. The two brothers had rather severe behavior disturbances. The EEGs were diffusely abnormal, with disseminated spikes in some cases.

Group B

This group included 30 patients (18 males and 12 females, aged 21 to 53 years). They were selected from the 150 inpatients of our department at the General Hospital for Nervous and Mental Diseases because of their high fit frequency and severe mental disturbances which remained uncontrolled despite intensive treatment. Twelve patients had only one type of seizure (grand mal or psychomotor) and the other eighteen had mixed seizures. The etiology of the epilepsy could be traced in nineteen patients (four had a positive family history, nine perinatal brain damage, and six had suffered meningoencephalitis). The etiology was unknown in 11 patients. All EEGs were diffusely abnormal, with paroxysmal features.

Group C

Status Epilepticus

This group included 20 patients (8 males and 12 females, 25 to 48 years) with 31 episodes of status epilepticus. Of these, 13 patients (6 males, 7 females) had 22 episodes of status epilepticus with repeated generalized tonic-clonic seizures, coma, and autonomic disturbance. Seven patients (two males, five females) had nine episodes of absence status with the characteristic clinical and EEG findings.

TREATMENT

Because all patients had been previously seen and treated by us, a complete medical record was available for each of them, referring to the duration of the illness, the form and frequency of fits, the previous medication, and its effectiveness. Before treatment was initiated, pretherapy laboratory studies were performed, including a complete blood count, urinalysis, alkaline phosphatase, SGOT, bilirubin, and blood uric acid.

Except in the cases with status, clonazepam was administered orally as tablets. In the younger group A, the initial dosage was 0.25 mg t.i.d. This was increased by 0.25 mg every 2 to 3 days until satisfactory seizure control was obtained or side effects appeared, which precluded further increases. In the adults (group B), the initial dosage was 1 to 2 mg divided into three doses and the maintenance dose was 4 to 12 mg divided into three doses.

Previous anticonvulsant medication was continued after clonazepam was begun, then gradually decreased, and in some cases withdrawn. This was possible in four patients of the younger group A and two of group B.

Laboratory tests were repeated within 15 to 20 days after treatment was started. The outpatients were followed up every 1 to 3 months. Each patient recorded on a seizure calendar the type and frequency of fits and any other event relevant to the therapy with clonazepam. The duration of therapy ranged from 2 months to 2 years.

RESULTS

The effectiveness of a new anticonvulsant can be evaluated by its action on the fits and the general condition of the patient, particularly his mental condition and behavior disturbances, if they are present.

TABLE 1. *Effect of clonazepam on various forms of fits*

Seizure types	No. of patients	Very good	Good	None
Group A				
Petit mal seizures	12	8	3	1
Grand mal seizures	3	2	1	—
Myoclonic epilepsy	10	3	5	2
Infantile myoclonic encephalopathy with hypsarrhythmia (West's syndrome)	6	—	3	3
Astatomyoclonic petit mal (Lennox's syndrome)	5	1	3	1
Focal seizures	7	1	5	1
	43	15	20	8
Group B				
Grand mal seizures	6	—	2	4
Psychomotor seizures	6	1	1	4
Mixed seizures	18	3	9	6
	30	4	12	14
Total	73	19	32	22

In Table 1, the 73 patients of groups A and B are divided into three categories on the basis of their response to clonazepam. This was expressed as a percentage decrease in the frequency of fits occurring in the trial period compared with the frequency in the pretrial period. This result was considered as "very good" when complete control of fits was achieved, "good" when the fit frequency was reduced more than 50%, and "none" when it remained unchanged.

Group A

In petit mal seizures, improvement appeared in the first few days and reached its highest in 10 to 15 days at the latest.

Apart from the suppression of fits in two patients with myoclonic epilepsy, the severe behavior disturbances were significantly improved, which impressed the families of the patients.

A similar improvement occurred in two of the four patients with behavior disturbances in West's syndrome and in all patients with Lennox's syndrome. In two of the latter patients, the fit frequency quickly increased and behavior disorders worsened when the medication was temporarily stopped because the parents neglected to obtain a supply of the drug. These symptoms quickly subsided with the readministration of clonazepam.

Group B

It is significant to note that approximately two-thirds of the patients showing an improvement had mixed seizures.

The remarkable reduction of fit frequency was followed by a definite improvement in mental state of ten patients. This took the form of increased cooperation, alertness, greater concentration, elevation of mood, and a tendency toward less severe mood swings. The hyperkinetic activity, aggressiveness, destructiveness, and violent outbursts were generally improved to such an extent that three of them were discharged from the hospital and the others could be successfully employed in the occupational therapy department.

Group C

In all cases of status epilepticus, clonazepam was given intravenously. The effective dose was 1 mg. It was necessary to administer an additional 1 mg in four cases of generalized status and in seven of the absence status.

Of the 22 episodes of status epilepticus with generalized seizures, 13 were immediately controlled and the patients quickly recovered consciousness. In the remaining nine episodes, control was achieved in a few minutes.

In four of the nine episodes of absence status, the patients who had been stuporous for many hours began to speak and respond to questions after the injection and became entirely conscious in a few hours. In the five other episodes, the patients became conscious within a couple of minutes.

Effect on the EEG

A great amount of fast activity of 15 to 20 Hz of mostly low amplitude was recorded predominantly over the anterior regions, similar to but in greater amount than that appearing with the barbiturates. In group A, the EEGs showed an improvement in 36 patients and remained unchanged in 7 patients.

The greatest improvement was seen in nine cases of petit mal, in three of Lennox's syndrome, in two of myoclonic epilepsy, and in one of focal seizures, in all of which paroxysmal features were completely suppressed. In the remaining 14 cases, the paroxysmal features became less marked and a maturation of the basic rhythm was seen in some tracings. In group B, the EEG became normal in four, improved in ten, remained unchanged in nine, and deteriorated in seven patients. In group C, the EEG tracings changed abruptly and the typical paroxysmal features ceased entirely.

Side Effects

After starting treatment, many of our patients complained of tiredness, sleepiness, and lassitude. Symptoms of slight intoxication, such as ataxia, dysarthria, and dizziness were noted in four of the adults. In the younger group, side effects were milder except in two who had severe reactions. In all patients, the adverse effects were transient and gradually subsided, even if the administration of the drug was continued. Clonazepam had to be temporarily discontinued in two patients, one with a marked hypersalivation and another with a severe allergic reaction with an extensive rash covering the whole body. The drug was started again in both patients after 2 weeks in very small doses and was progressively increased without any reappearance of adverse effects. Regular monitoring of the blood and liver and kidney function showed no signs of organic damage.

DISCUSSION AND CONCLUSIONS

Our cases were carefully selected among epileptic patients treated because of the severity of their symptoms (fit frequency and behavior disturbances), which had remained unaffected by previous medication. This selection was intentional because we wished to investigate the wide spectrum of action of clonazepam that had been reported by others (Gastaut, 1970*b*; Groh and Rosenmayr, 1971; Martin and Hirt, 1973; Rett, 1973; Carson and Gilden, 1975). Our findings suggest that clonazepam is highly effective in treating primary petit mal and grand mal seizures. There appears to be a substantial effect in cases of myoclonic epilepsy, which is less marked in Lennox syndrome and focal seizures. It was effective in half of the patients with infantile myoclonic encephalopathy, with a reduction in fit frequency of up to 50%. In the older age group, best results were obtained in patients with mixed types of fits. It proved most effective in the treatment of status epilepticus. The excellent results obtained in all the episodes, the rapidity of action, and the absence of any side effects lend further support to the views of other writers (Gastaut, 1970*b*; Gastaut et al., 1971; Ketz et al., 1973) that clonazepam is at present the most effective agent available in the treatment of status epilepticus.

Another significant finding was its beneficial effect on mental state and behavior disturbances of our patients, particularly of the older group. This improvement was so marked in ten patients as to allow seven of them to be employed in the occupational therapy department of the hospital and three to be discharged from the hospital and live with their families. This action of clonazepam, which has also been noted by other writers (Caso Muñoz et al., 1971; Rett, 1971), is particularly interesting and needs further evaluation. It might be due to the anxiolytic and tranquilizing properties of the drug.

The main effect of clonazepam on the EEG was a definite decrease or complete elimination of generalized epileptic discharges, particularly of the spike-and-wave form.

Except in the cases of status, clonazepam was administered orally by very progressive dosage increases to prevent the occurrence of side effects. These were mostly transient and slight and did not cause undue distress. In two patients, they were severe in the sense that they necessitated the temporary withdrawal of the drug.

The findings of this trial are not always consistent with those of other authors. Various investigators (Lison and Fassoni, 1970; Gastaut, 1970*b*; Castroviejo, 1971; Groh and Rosenmayr, 1971; Rett, 1971, 1973; Martin and Hirt, 1973; Carson and Gilden, 1975) give different numbers and percentages of improvement in clinical symptoms and EEGs. This is probably the result of the different criteria for selection of their patients and the higher dosages administered. We may reasonably assume that if our patients had been randomly selected, our results would have been better.

In conclusion, clonazepam, by its wide spectrum of action and excellent effect on such a heterogeneous group of mostly refractory cases of epilepsy, is indeed a valuable addition to the therapeutic means at our disposal.

REFERENCES

Carson, J. M., and Gilden, C. (1975): Treatment of minor seizures with clonazepam. *Dev. Med. Child. Neurol.,* 17:306–309.

Caso Muñoz et al. (1971): Evaluation neuropsiquiatrica del Ro 5–4023 en 40 enfermos epilepticos. Paper III Congresso Panamericano de Neurologia, Sao Paulo, October 10–14.

Castroviejo, P. I. (1971): Experience sur 200 cas presentant devers genres d'epilepsie traités avec le Ro 5–4023. Paper, XIIIth International Congress of Pediatrics, Vienna, August 29–September 4.

Gastaut, H. (1970*a*): Clinical and electroencephalographical classification of epileptic seizures. *Epilepsia,* 11:102–113.

Gastaut, H. (1970*b*): Proprieties antiepileptiques exceptionelles d'une benzodiazepine nouvelle, le Ro 5–4023. *Vie Med.,* 51:5175–5188.

Gastaut, H., Courjon, J., Poire, R., and Weber, M. (1971): Treatment of status epilepticus with a new benzodiazepine more active than diazepam. *Epilepsia,* 12:197–214.

Groh, C., and Rosenmayr, F. W. (1971): Clonazepam (Ro 5–4023) ein neues Antikonvulsivum. *Wien Klin. Wochenschr.,* 83:334–337.

Ketz, E., Bernoulli, C., and Siegfried, J. (1973): Klinische und Hirnelektrische Prufung von Clonazepam (Ro 5–4023) unter besonderer Berücksichtigung des status epilepticus. *Acta Neurol. Scand.* [*Suppl.* 49], 53:47–53, and *Epilepsia,* 14:81–82 (Abstr).

Lison, M., and Fassoni, L. (1970): Estudo clinocoeletrencefalografico longitudinal en patientes epilepticos tratados com Ro 5–4023. *Arch. Neuropsiquiatr. (Sao Paulo),* 28:25–36.

Martin, D., and Hirt, H. R. (1973): Clinical experience with clonazepam (Rivotril) in the treatment of epilepsies in infancy and childhood. *Neuropädiatrie,* 4:245–266.

Randall, L. O., and Schallek, W. (1968): Pharmacological activity of certain benzodiazepines. In: *Psychopharmacology: A Review of Progress 1957–1967,* edited by D. H. Efron, pp. 153–184. Public Health Service Publication No. 1836, U.S. Government Printing Office, Washington, D.C.

Rett, A. (1971): Möglichkeiten und Crenzen der Clonazepam Therapie im Kindersalter. *Wien Klin. Wochenschr.,* 83:725–734.

Rett, A. (1973): Zwei Jahre Erfahrungen mit Clonazepam bei Zerebralen Krampfanfällen im Kindersaltern. *Acta Neurol. Scand.* [*Suppl.* 49], 53:109–116.

Epilepsy, The Eighth International Symposium,
edited by J. K. Penry. Raven Press, New York
© 1977.

Clinical Experience with Clonazepam in the Treatment of Posttraumatic Epilepsy

T. Syz and U. Spieler

Chirurgische Universitätsklinik B, Kantonsspital Zurich, Zurich, Switzerland

The anticonvulsant action of the benzodiazepine derivative clonazepam (Rivotril®) has been demonstrated in various forms of epilepsy of adults and children in many investigations (Gastaut, 1970; Blum et al., 1973; Ketz, 1973; Munthe and Strandjord, 1973). The good results of the various investigations, particularly in focal epileptic seizures, prompted us to use clonazepam. Instead of the medication previously used, clonazepam was clinically tested on a variety of patients with posttraumatic epilepsy following severe skull-brain injuries. Disappearance of epileptic seizures was the criterion of a good result.

PATIENTS

From 1974 to mid-1976, 23 patients with posttraumatic epilepsy were treated with clonazepam. Three patients died within 3 days of the initiation of therapy because of their severe concomitant injuries, so they could not be included in the assessment. Of the remaining 20 patients, only 13 had purely skull/brain injuries. The other seven had multiple injuries with severe damage to the thorax, abdomen, and extremities. In our accident clinic, 15 patients had skull operations and 5 were treated conservatively. All patients received prophylactic treatment against brain edema as soon as they entered the clinic.

The posttraumatic seizures started during hospitalization. These were focal motor seizures with or without generalization. The seizures first appeared clinically 1 to 48 days after trauma. In 14 patients, the epilepsy appeared in the first 10 days after the accident. The youngest patient in our clinic was 15, the oldest 72 years old.

METHODS

For all patients except one, treatment was started with clonazepam only. Because of the frequent occurrence of seizures or because of the very poor general condition of some of the injured, oral administration at the start of therapy was not possible. Initially, therapy began with 1 mg of clonazepam intravenously, after the appearance of epilepsy. This was followed by parenteral administration of 2 to 6 mg of clonazepam by slow drop infusion over 25 hr. This method was found to be very effective during our investigation. The dosage was varied according to the patients' individual clinical response and tolerance. As soon as possible, patients were transferred to oral therapy. The average maintenance dose was between 2 and 4 mg of clonazepam daily, it being necessary to effect dosage reductions slowly.

The type and frequency of seizures were recorded before and during the antiepileptic drug treatment. Whenever possible, an EEG was obtained before clonazepam therapy was started. Further EEGs followed on the 10th day and after 4 weeks. In severe cases, EEGs were also obtained at shorter intervals. For assessment of the EEGs, the accident surgeon received the help of Prof. Hess, Chief of the Institute for Encephalography at the University of Zurich. EEG evaluation later than 4 weeks after the first seizure was, unfortunately, not possible since most patients went for rehabilitation in other clinics.

RESULTS

All 20 patients treated with clonazepam were clinically seizure-free 4 weeks after the start of the epilepsy. In 40%, however, potentials suggestive of epilepsy could sometimes be found in the EEG, without the occurrence of frank seizures. An improvement in the EEG curve was attained in 50%. A normal EEG was achieved in only one case (5%), which, considering the grave skull injuries, must be counted as success. Twenty percent of the patients died during or shortly after our study because of their severe concomitant injuries.

Clonazepam was very well tolerated by these severely injured patients. It was observed that seizures could occur with sudden reduction of dosage, and that reduction of dosage must be slow. After an initially good response, epileptic seizures recurred in one patient on 6 mg of clonazepam. Therefore, clonazepam had to be combined with phenytoin. The phenytoin was given for 20 days, gradually tapered off, and therapy continued with clonazepam alone. Epilepsy potentials could not be confirmed in the later EEGS. The reason for this initial resistance to clonazepam is unclear.

The side effects of clonazepam were powerful sedation, hypersalivation, and a massive increase of bronchial secretions. The last symptom was especially troublesome to patients on long-term artificial respiration. These side effects could be significantly reduced by a decrease in dosage. In two elderly patients, we were forced to replace clonazepam by another medication because of respiratory complications resulting from the increased bronchial secretion.

CONCLUSION

In our investigation, which was limited to a maximum of 4 weeks, clonazepam proved very effective in the treatment of posttraumatic epilepsy. For surgeons, with limited experience in antiepileptic therapy, the medication is very advantageous because of its easy handling and the ease with which side effects can be overcome.

Considering the initial state of the individual patients and the final results that we achieved, we must consider the results obtained with clonazepam as very good. Because the patients were transferred to other clinics, a long-term investigation was not possible.

REFERENCES

1. Blum, J. E., Haefely, W., Jalfre, M., Polc, P., and Schärer, K. (1973): Pharmakologie und Toxikologie des Antiepileptikums Clonazepam. *Arzneim. Forsch.,* 23:377–389.
2. Gastaut, H. (1970): Propriétés antiépileptiques exceptionnelles d'une benzodiazépine nouvelle, le Ro 05–4023. *Vie Méd.,* 51:5175–5188.
3. Ketz, E. (1973): Status-epilepticus-Behandlung mit 'Rivotril.' *Schweiz. Med. Wochenschr.,* 103: 1134–1138.
4. Munthe, A. W., and Strandjord, R. E. (1973): Clonazepam in the treatment of epileptic seizures. *Acta Neurol. Scand.,* 49:97–102.

Epilepsy, The Eighth International Symposium,
edited by J. K. Penry. Raven Press, New York
© 1977.

Comparison of Sodium Valproate (Epilim®) and Clonazepam (Rivotril®) in Intractable Epilepsy

R. A. Shakir, R. H. Johnson,* H. J. Keogh, D. G. Lambie, and
R. N. Nanda

*Department of Neurology, University of Glasgow, Institute of Neurological Sciences,
Southern General Hospital, Glasgow, Scotland*

The introduction of new anticonvulsants requires their assessment both individually and comparatively. Although two newly introduced drugs, clonazepam (Roche Products, Ltd.) and sodium valproate (Epilim®, Reckitt and Colman, Ltd.), have now been subjected to several different trials independently, comparative assessment of their value is still needed. One comparative trial has been reported (Lance and Anthony, 1975), but it was carried out as an open trial, sodium valproate being given to patients in whom other drugs, including clonazepam, had not produced adequate control. The drugs were not therefore directly compared in the same patients. Thus we have carried out a crossover trial in the same patients, all of whom were initially poorly controlled. In addition, serum levels of other anticonvulsants were monitored to attempt to distinguish the direct effects of these drugs from the secondary elevation of other anticonvulsants by them. In particular, sodium valproate frequently increases serum phenobarbital levels in patients who are also receiving that drug (Richens and Ahmad, 1975). We therefore attempted to keep phenobarbital levels constant by reducing the dose of phenobarbital when indicated. The trial is still in progress, so we report the first part in which the drugs have been given for 8 weeks.

METHODS

Subjects

Thirty-two adult epileptic patients who were resident in Quarrier's Homes, Bridge of Weir, Renfrewshire, were studied. There were 15 males and 17 females aged 21 to 63 years (mean, 36 years). All the patients had a history of intractable epilepsy for 10 or more years, and none had evidence of a progressive disease.

---

* Present address: Department of Medicine, University of Otago, Wellington Hospital, Wellington, New Zealand.

The drugs being given to them were phenytoin (20), phenobarbital (17), primidone (14), carbamazepine (10), ethotoin (2), and pheneturide (1). The criteria of selection were that they were having more than five seizures per month for the preceding 3 months and that two estimations of anticonvulsants were carried out in that period, the values being within the usually accepted therapeutic ranges for phenytoin (40 to 80 μmoles/liter) or phenobarbital (40 to 160 μmoles/liter). Twenty-nine patients had frequent major seizures (generalized tonic-clonic fits), and these patients all had minor seizures as well (absences and focal attacks including adversive attacks, jacksonian attacks, and temporal lobe attacks). The patients showed a variety of electroencephalographic abnormalities. Thirteen of the patients had bilateral slow or spike-wave activities with no definite localization, nine had temporal lobe foci, five had other focal lesions, and two showed such lower voltage activity that focal lesions could not be identified. The remaining three patients had minor seizures only and the EEGs showed, respectively, centrencephalic, temporal lobe, and focal frontoparietal abnormalities.

Trial Design

The trial consisted of three consecutive periods each of 12 weeks, but as the last period has not been completed we now report the results from the first 8 weeks of each of them. Patients (32) who satisfied the criteria for selection given above were observed for 12 weeks during which serum concentrations of their anticonvulsants were estimated twice. The 32 patients were then divided into two groups each of 16 patients. One was given sodium valproate (400 mg four times daily, the dose being increased in four steps over a 2-week introduction period), and the other was given clonazepam (2 mg three times daily, this value being achieved over 2 weeks in three steps). In some patients, however, the dose of clonazepam was later reduced because of side effects (see Results). The serum concentrations of other anticonvulsants were kept constant in all patients by reducing their dosage if they showed an increase of more than 15%. After 12 weeks each group crossed over to the opposite drug over 6 weeks using a placebo matching the first additional drug they had received. The first drug was withdrawn over 2 weeks and the patient then continued to take the placebo for a further 4 weeks, in the latter 2 weeks of which it was withdrawn and the other drug introduced. Each group was then given the other drug for a further 12 weeks. There was therefore a period of 2 weeks during which the patients received placebo only, to reduce the possibility of interactions between the two drugs.

Serum anticonvulsant concentrations of phenytoin, phenobarbital, primidone, sodium valproate, and clonazepam were measured at 4-week intervals. The seizures were recorded by nursing staff as major and minor fits, as explained above. The reduction in seizure frequency was assessed using the number of seizures in each month, and the change was graded into good improvement (more than 75% reduction) and moderate improvement (50 to 75% reduction). Any reduction less than 50% was considered as no change. The significances of difference were assessed by the Wilcoxon signed-ranks test.

RESULTS

Twenty-five patients completed all parts of the trial. The remaining seven patients completed one part of the drug trial only, three patients completing the sodium valproate treatment period and four patients completing the trial with clonazepam. These seven patients left the trial for various reasons unrelated to the drug therapy. When the total number of seizures per month for sodium valproate and clonazepam were compared, each reduced the frequency of minor seizures significantly ($p < 0.005$ and $p < 0.05$, respectively), whereas major seizures were reduced with sodium valproate only ($p < 0.05$). These significant reductions in seizure frequency were obtained even though few patients had more seizures during treatment with both drugs. The changes are summarized according to the percentage improvement in Table 1.

Side Effects

The main side effect with both drugs was drowsiness (sodium valproate 25% of patients, clonazepam 65%), especially during the introduction periods. Ataxia also occurred (sodium valproate 17%, clonazepam 55%). Gastrointestinal symptoms (nausea, vomiting, and diarrhea) were noted in 10% of patients during sodium valproate treatment, but they were mild and transitory. In one patient in each group diplopia and mental changes were noted. Because of side effects the dose of clonazepam was reduced in 13 patients from 6 mg/day to 1 to 5 mg/day. Reduction of dose was not necessary for sodium valproate.

Effects on Other Anticonvulsant Serum Concentrations

During treatment with sodium valproate the doses of phenobarbital or primidone (in one patient) were reduced because of increase in serum phenobarbital concentration of more than 15% in six out of twenty-three patients (26%), so that the serum concentration returned to its original level. In one patient receiving sodium valproate there was an increase in the serum phenytoin of more than 15% and the dose was reduced. Similar changes were noted with clonazepam in four patients (17%) as the serum concentration of phenobarbital increased by more than 15% (three on primidone and one on phenobarbital). The doses were reduced similarly. These alterations did not significantly affect the seizure control.

The increase of serum phenobarbital concentrations appeared to be the main cause of drowsiness with sodium valproate, for reduction of the phenobarbital dose abolished drowsiness. The serum concentrations when steady doses had been achieved were 66.4 μg/liter (mean $\pm$ 24.5 SD) for sodium valproate and 23.3 ng/ml (mean $\pm$ 14.9 SD) for clonazepam.

TABLE 1. Reduction in seizure frequency: good improvement (> 75% reduction), moderate improvement (50 to 75% reduction), any reduction less than 50% (no change)

	Clonazepam				Sodium Valproate			
	Patients	> 75%	> 50%	No change	Patients	> 75%	> 50%	No change
Minor seizures								
Generalized	13	—	6	7	13	5	5	3
Temporal lobe	10	1	1	8	9	2	4	3
Focal	5	2	—	3	4	2	—	2
Unclassified	1	1	—	—	2	1	—	1
TOTALS	29	4	7	18	28	10	9	9
Major seizures								
Generalized	12	2	2	8	12	5	3	4
Temporal lobe	9	4	1	4	8	5	—	3
Focal	4	1	—	3	3	1	1	1
Unclassified	1	1	—	—	2	1	—	1
Totals	26	8	3	15	25	12	4	9

DISCUSSION

We have found that sodium valproate had a significant effect on control of both major and minor seizures. This is similar to the findings in other centers from both open and double-blind trials (Jeavons and Clark, 1974; Schafer and Kettner, 1974; Lance and Anthony, 1975; Richens and Ahmad, 1975). We also observed that the patients who responded best were those whose EEGs showed generalized abnormalities. In the present trial clonazepam was less effective, although some patients improved with it dramatically. We have previously shown that this drug is most effective in patients who have photosensitive epilepsy or associated myoclonus (Nanda et al., 1976; Nanda et al., 1977). The present trial was not designed to observe this effect.

The side effects and their frequency for the two drugs were as observed in the previously reported trials, the most severe problem being drowsiness with clonazepam which required the drug dose to be reduced. It has been observed that the side effects with clonazepam decrease with time (Nanda et al., 1976; Nanda et al., 1977), but the duration of our trial did not allow us to substantiate this. The drowsiness produced by sodium valproate appeared to be due to elevation of serum phenobarbital concentrations, a major complication in the use of this drug. We found, however, that a high proportion (74%) had little alteration of serum phenobarbital while receiving sodium valproate. Richens and Ahmad (1975) drew attention to elevation of phenobarbital and observed a mean increase of 27% in the seven patients studied. Our observations imply that the effect of sodium valproate on phenobarbital metabolism shows wide differences among patients. There is therefore need to investigate the causes for this, and work is in progress. The effects on phenytoin therapy were less marked, but they also require investigation. Although the effect of clonazepam on other anticonvulsants has been reported to be minor and inconsistent (Huang et al., 1973; Nanda et al., 1976; Nanda et al., 1977), in this trial we observed that four patients had increased phenobarbital levels during clonazepam therapy.

We conclude that sodium valproate was the more effective drug in this group of patients; it also had fewer side effects. Nevertheless, we observed major differences between individual patients in its effect on metabolism of phenobarbital and this requires further study.

SUMMARY

Thirty-two adult epileptic patients on multiple anticonvulsant drug therapy whose seizures were poorly controlled have been treated with sodium valproate and clonazepam in a crossover trial. Both drugs significantly reduced the frequency of minor seizures, with sodium valproate having a greater effect. The occurrence of major seizures was reduced significantly with sodium valproate only. In these patients with generalized epilepsy, sodium valproate appeared more useful and had fewer side effects than clonazepam. Drowsiness was a problem with clonazepam with the dose used. We conclude that in these patients with intractable epilepsy sodium valproate was the more effective drug, although clonazepam may be effective in a more restricted group of patients.

ACKNOWLEDGMENTS

We thank the patients and the staff of the Epilepsy Centre, Quarrier's Homes, Bridge of Weir, for their cooperation. We wish to thank Reckitt and Colman, Ltd., and Roche Products, Ltd., for support.

REFERENCES

Huang, C. Y., McLeod, J. C., Sampson, D., and Hensley, W. J. (1973): Clonazepam in the treatment of epilepsy. *Proc. Aust. Assoc. Neurol.*, 10:67–74.
Jeavons, P. M., and Clark, J. E. (1974): Sodium valproate in treatment of epilepsy. *Br. Med. J.*, 2:584–586.
Lance, J. W., and Anthony, M. (1975): Sodium valproate in treatment of intractable epilepsy: Comparison with clonazepam. *Proc. Aust. Assoc. Neurol.*, 12:55–60.
Nanda, R. N., Keogh, H. J., Lambie, D., Johnson, R. H., Melville, I. D., and Morrice, G. D. (1976): The effects of clonazepam upon epilepsy control and plasma levels of other anticonvulsants. In: *Epileptology,* Proceedings of the Seventh International Symposium on Epilepsy, Berlin (West), June 1975, edited by D. Janz, pp. 145–151. Thieme/PSG, Stuttgart.
Nanda, R. N., Johnson, R. H., Keogh, H. J., Lambie, D., Melville, I.D., and Shakir, R. A. (1977): Treatment of chronic epilepsy for 1 to 2 years with clonazepam. In: *Epilepsy: The Eighth International Symposium,* Dublin, September 1976, edited by J. K. Penry. Raven Press, New York.
Richens, A., and Ahmad, S. (1975): Controlled trial of sodium valproate in severe epilepsy. *Br. Med. J.,* 4:255–256.
Schafer, J., and Kettner, I. (1974): Dipropylacetate in the treatment of refractory adult cases of epilepsy. *Med. Welt,* 25:561.

Epilepsy, The Eighth International Symposium,
edited by J. K. Penry. Raven Press, New York
© 1977.

Sodium Valproate in Treatment of Children with Refractory Epilepsy

Ingrid Gamstorp

*Division of Child Neurology, Department of Pediatrics, University Hospital,
S–750 14 Uppsala, Sweden*

Sodium valproate (dipropylacetate) has been used as an antiepileptic drug on the continent for at least a decade and in Great Britain and Finland for at least 5 years. Good results and few side effects have been reported (Kugler et al., 1973; Völzke and Doose, 1973; Jeavons and Clark, 1974; Barnes and Bower, 1975; Simon and Penry, 1975; Sillanpää and Donner, 1976). The results have been particularly good in petit mal epilepsy, in which excellent or good results are reported in about 80% of the cases. In grand mal epilepsy and in temporal lobe seizures, excellent or good results have been described in about 60% of the patients. Lack of appetite, nausea, vomiting, loss of hair, change of hair-color, and impaired blood coagulation (Sutor and Jesdinsky-Buscher, 1974; Zwan, 1974) have been reported, but no serious or irreversible side effects. Several authors mention an increased wakefulness and increased attention span in at least some of the patients. With this background we started to use sodium valproate in June, 1975.

PATIENTS AND METHODS

Sodium valproate was tried in 27 children, 12 boys and 15 girls, aged 3 to 18 years at the start of the trial. In three girls the drug has been stopped because of lack of response and side effects. The seizure type was petit mal in five patients, myoclonic petit mal in one, myoclonic jerks in one, petit and grand mal in two, minor motor and grand mal in ten, temporal lobe seizures in three, and temporal lobe seizures and grand mal in four. The reason for trying sodium valproate was that conventional therapy gave unsatisfactory seizure control in nine patients, inpaired mental function in four, both in thirteen, and allergic reactions in one.

Sodium valproate was added to the previous medication except in the boy with allergic reactions to conventional therapy. The initial dose was 0.15 to 0.3 g twice a day. This dose was increased over 2 to 3 weeks to the final dose. The final daily dose varied from 25 to 70 mg/kg, given in two daily doses. In almost all the patients conventional therapy was reduced when the final dose of sodium valproate was reached; in responding patients conventional therapy was reduced considerably or stopped.

RESULTS

The effect on seizures and mental function is apparent from Table 1. Improvement of seizures means at least 75% reduction of seizure frequency; if the reduction was less, the patient was classified as unimproved. The effect of mental function was judged subjectively by the parents and at least one person outside the home, usually the child's teacher or preschool teacher. It is apparent from the table that nine patients became seizure-free and eight improved. The best results were obtained in children with petit mal alone or in combination with grand mal, as six of seven patients became seizure-free. The poorest responding group consisted of the patients with minor motor seizures and grand mal, but also in this group two became seizure-free, six improved, and only two were unimproved.

Sixteen patients improved mentally whereas eleven were unchanged. On the whole the same patients showed a decrease of seizure frequency and an improvement of mental function. One patient with petit and grand mal, who became seizure-free on sodium valproate without improvement of mental function, was normal before; he was allergic to other drugs. In most of the improved patients the increased alertness and better attention span came when the conventional therapy could be reduced or stopped. This was particularly apparent in the patients with petit mal, who had become seizure-free on ethosuximide but who complained of headache and fatigue and became slow learners at school. When, after introduction of sodium valproate, ethosuximide could be stopped without recurrence of the fits, considerable improvement in their mental capacity was seen. No patient showed improved mental function without better control of seizures and/or reduction of other therapy.

The observed side effects were severe tiredness in two patients, one of whom also became nauseated, loss of hair in one, and possibly an increased frequency of urination in two. The drug was stopped in the two patients with severe fatigue. The loss of hair, occurring in a girl of 11, prompted a reduction of the dose and

TABLE 1. *Effect of sodium valproate on seizures and on mental function*

Seizure type	Seizures			Mental function	
	Seizure-free	Improved	Unimproved	Improved	Unimproved
Petit mal	4		1	4	1
Myoclon petit mal			2		2
Myoclonic jerks		1		1	
Petit and grand mal	2			1	1
Minor motor and grand mal	2	6	2	8	2
Temporal lobe	1		2	1	2
Temporal lobe and grand mal		1	3	1	3

the administration of vitamin B. Some improvement of her hair occurred, but several weeks later she had another fit. The parents then increased her dose again and since then she has remained seizure-free. The parents of two children complained of an increased frequency of urination and deterioration of a previous existing enuresis. Routine urinalysis was normal in both. In one of the children the condition improved again without change of the medication.

Interaction with other antiepileptic drugs appeared likely in six patients, i.e., when sodium valproate was introduced children on ethosuximide complained of increased headache, children on primidone became more apathetic and sleepy, and children on phenytoin more ataxic. These side effects disappeared when the drugs mentioned were reduced with no change in the dose of sodium valproate; in two cases an increased level was measured of phenytoin and primidone, respectively.

The time of follow-up varied from 1 to 15 months. Of the nine seizure-free patients, five had been followed for less than 6 months and four for more, two of them for more than a year. Two relapses occurred; both children probably had too low a dose, and one again became seizure-free on a higher dose.

DISCUSSION

The findings are in general agreement with those previously reported, with excellent results in six of seven patients with petit mal with or without grand mal and in two of five with temporal lobe seizures. The side effects have also been reported before with the exception of the increased frequency of urination and enuresis noted at least temporarily in two patients; their connection with the administration of the drug remains questionable.

The dose used was slightly higher than that usually recommended (20 to 40 mg/kg) in the literature (Sillanpää and Donner, 1976). Three children had seizures on 25, 50, and 60 mg/kg, respectively, but became seizure-free when the dose was increased to 35, 70, and 70 mg/kg, respectively. Side effects have in some children started to come at 40 mg/kg, whereas others have tolerated 70 mg/kg. I have a personal, unreported experience from 1969 of trying sodium valproate in a few children at a dose of 15 to 25 mg/kg without improvement. A dose of 25 to 70 mg/kg thus should be tried before the drug is judged as ineffective.

SUMMARY

Sodium valproate was tried in a highly selected group of epileptic children, who either had not responded to conventional therapy or had side effects on it. Nine became seizure-free and eight had a considerable reduction of seizure frequency. Sixteen of them improved in their behavior and ability to learn. No serious or irreversible side effects were noted. Interaction with other antiepileptic drugs seemed common. The daily dose varied between 25 and 70 mg/kg. Time of follow-up was 1 to 15 months. In this limited material with a short follow-up, the drug appeared safe and well worth trying.

REFERENCES

Barnes, S. E., and Bower, B. D. (1975): Sodium valproate in the treatment of intractable childhood epilepsy. *Dev. Med. Child. Neurol.,* 17:175–181.
Jeavons, P. M., and Clark, J. E. (1974): Sodium valproate in treatment of epilepsy. *Br. Med. J.,* 1:584–586.
Kugler, J., Knörl, G., and Empt, J. (1973): Die Behandlung therapieresistenter Epilepsien mit Dipropylacetate. *Munch. Med. Wochenschr.,* 115:1103–1108.
Sillanpää, M., and Donner, M. (1976): Experiences on the use of dipropylacetate in the treatment of childhood epilepsy. *Acta Paediatr. Scand.,* 65:209–215.
Simon, D., and Penry, J. K. (1975): Sodium di-*N*-propylacetate (DPA) in the treatment of epilepsy. *Epilepsia,* 16:549–573.
Sutor, A. H., and Jesdinsky-Buscher, C. (1974): Gerinnungsveränderungen durch Dipropylessigsäure (Ergenyl®). *Med. Welt,* 25:447–449.
Völzke, E., and Doose, H. (1973): Dipropylacetate (Depakine®, Ergenyl®) in the treatment of epilepsy. *Epilepsia,* 14:185–193.
Zwan, Avd, Jr. (1974): Loss of hair caused by depakine. A report made during "Boerhave cursus voor Epilepsie," June 14, Leyden.

Epilepsy, The Eighth International Symposium,
edited by J. K. Penry. Raven Press, New York
© 1977.

Elimination of Carbamazepine in Children after Single and Multiple Doses

S. Pynnönen, *M. Sillanpää, E. Iisalo, and **H. Frey

*Departments of Pharmacology of Biomedical Institute, *Pediatrics, and **Neurology,
University of Turku, SF-20520 Turku, Finland*

Many clinical studies have shown that children need higher dosages of drugs per body weight than adults to achieve similar plasma levels (Svensmark and Buchthal, 1964; Iisalo et al., 1973). As a reason for this, a faster hepatic clearance has been proposed due to the relatively larger size of liver in childhood. We found relatively more of the epoxide metabolite (CBZ-E) of carbamazepine (CBZ) in children compared to adult patients (Pynnönen et al., 1977). In a group of 37 children and 13 adults the ratio of CBZ-E to CBZ was 0.26 in children and 0.17 in adults ($p < 0.01$). In the present chapter we have tried to clear up further the possible pharmacokinetic differences in 11 children and 13 adult volunteers.

PATIENTS AND METHODS

After chronic carbamazepine therapy (21.4 ± 18.0 weeks) in a daily dose of 10.0 ± 4.2 mg/kg, the medication of nine children was changed to another anticonvulsive drug because of therapy-resistant seizures. The change was done in hospital. In connection with other clinical samples, an extra 2 ml of blood was withdrawn into heparinized tube on 3 consecutive days. The calculations over the decline phase of CBZ were based on three plasma samples 13.4 ± 4.7, 34.4 ± 8.4, and 55.1 ± 8.4 hr from the last CBZ intake. Due to the low levels of CBZ-E, this metabolite could be measured only on five children for 2 days. Four of nine children had CBZ as a single drug, the remaining children received other anticonvulsive drugs in addition (Table 1).

The elimination kinetics after a single dose of CBZ was studied on two children (male, 1 year 7 months, and female, 4 years 10 months), whose partial seizures indicated CBZ therapy. After the single dose (male 9.3 mg/kg, female 11.1 mg/kg), three blood samples were taken at an interval of 12 hr, after which the continuous therapy was begun.

The acute elimination study of CBZ was carried out also on 13 male student volunteers (ages 19 to 21 years). The volunteers ingested as a single dose a 200-mg tablet, i.e., CBZ at 2.7 ± 0.3 mg/kg. The elimination phase was followed 12, 24, 36, 48, 72, and 96 hr after administration. One month after the single-dose study, nine of these volunteers continued the trial of chronic administration lasting 4

TABLE 1. Clinical and pharmacokinetic data after single and chronic administration of carbamazepine in 11 child patients and 13 adult volunteers

Age (yr : mo)	Sex	CBZ (mg/kg)	K_E (hr^{-1})	$T_{1/2}$ (hr)	V_d (liter/kg)	Cl (ml/min)	Cl (ml/kg/hr)
				Single Administration			
Volunteers:							
20	M	2.3	0.014	49.2	0.99	20.5	14.0
19	M	2.6	0.022	31.6	1.01	28.9	22.2
20	M	2.9	0.018	38.9	1.06	21.4	18.9
20	M	2.5	0.015	44.8	0.95	19.6	14.7
19	M	2.4	0.016	42.1	0.90	20.7	14.8
21	M	2.4	0.016	43.8	1.02	23.2	16.2
20	M	2.3	0.018	37.7	0.77	20.8	14.2
19	M	3.2	0.028	24.4	0.92	27.1	26.2
21	M	3.0	0.020	34.5	1.01	22.3	20.3
21	M	2.4	0.012	58.4	1.26	21.0	15.0
20	M	2.9	0.015	44.8	1.16	20.7	18.0
20	M	3.0	0.019	36.7	0.87	18.0	16.4
20	M	2.9	0.023	30.6	0.89	22.9	20.2
Mean		2.7	0.018	39.8	0.99	22.1	17.8
SD		0.3	0.004	8.8	0.13	3.0	3.7
Children:							
1 : 7	M	9.3	0.045	15.4	1.91	15.4	85.2
4 : 10	F	11.1	0.037	18.5	1.10	11.9	39.6
Mean		10.2	0.041	16.9	1.51	13.7	62.4
SD		1.3	0.005	2.2	0.57	2.5	32.2

Chronic Administration

Age (yr : mo)	Sex	CBZ (mg/kg/day)	Duration of therapy (weeks)	Observed C_{ss} (μmoles/l)		K_E (hr^{-1})		$T_{1/2}$ (hr)		Other drugs (mg/kg/day)
				CBZ	CBZ-E	CBZ	CBZ-E	CBZ	CBZ-E	
Volunteers:										
20	M	2.9	4	17.5	1.5	0.018	0.055	38.6	12.6	
20	M	2.9	4	16.0	1.7	0.025	0.043	27.5	16.0	
21	M	2.4	4	13.5	1.3	0.015	0.049	46.9	14.1	
20	M	2.9	4	14.0	2.0	0.017	0.025	39.1	27.8	
21	M	3.0	4	17.3	1.0	0.018	0.038	39.5	18.2	
19	M	2.4	4	17.5	1.2	0.016	0.075	44.7	9.3	
20	M	2.3	4	16.0	—	0.016	—	42.1	—	
19	M	2.6	4	14.0	1.2	0.017	0.017	41.9	41.0	
21	M	2.4	4	16.5	1.2	0.016	0.046	42.2	15.1	
Mean		2.6	—	15.8	1.4	0.018	0.044	40.3	19.3	
SD		0.3		1.6	0.3	0.003	0.018	5.5	10.3	
Children:										
0 : 2	M	5.3	5	6.0	0.4	0.019	—	36.2	—	Valproate 10.0
0 : 10	M	4.9	10	5.0	0.8	0.036	—	19.1	—	
1 : 1	F	9.2	54	20.5	4.2	0.027	0.043	25.4	16.0	Phenytoin 10.0
1 : 10	F	8.3	18	2.5	0.8	0.037	—	18.5	—	Phenemal 4.0
10	F	15.7	26	13.5	5.2	0.045	—	15.5	—	Diazepam 1.2
11	M	10.0	6	11.5	2.2	0.037	0.036	18.6	19.2	
13	M	9.9	2	17.0	5.0	0.041	0.054	16.9	13.0	
15	F	17.4	40	9.0	2.6	0.036	0.031	19.1	22.1	Nitrazepam 0.4 Primidone 11.0
15	M	9.0	32	14.5	2.9	0.039	0.073	17.5	9.5	Valproate 19.0
Mean		10.0	21.4	11.1	2.7	0.035	0.047	20.8	16.0	
SD		4.2	18.0	5.9	1.8	0.008	0.017	6.4	5.0	

weeks with a daily dose of CBZ at 2.6 ± 0.3 mg/kg (100 mg CBZ b.i.d.). The elimination of CBZ was followed at 12, 36, 60, 84, and 104 hr. The volunteers also had low concentrations of CBZ-E, and the calculation of this metabolite was based on the two values 12 and 36 hr after the last dose.

All the CBZ preparations used in this study, for both children and volunteers, were of the same manufacturer's batch (Ciba-Geigy, Basel, Switzerland). Thus the differences of disintegration of the commercial tablets were excluded.

The procedures in handling the samples and GLC analysis for CBZ were published recently (Pynnönen et al., 1976). The procedure for CBZ-E was analogous, but it was detected with an alkali flame ionization detector. The batch precision and the day-to-day reproducibility for CBZ-E were 16.0% ($N = 20$) and 19.5% ($N = 60$), respectively, if expressed as a coefficient of variation.

The elimination and the excretion of CBZ were assumed to follow the open one-compartment model proposed by Levy et al. (1975b) and Rawlins et al. (1975). The regression lines through the experimental data points were calculated by the method of least squares. The calculations of the overall elimination constant (K_E) and the half-life ($T_{1/2}$) were based on the slope of each regression line. The extrapolated plasma concentration at time zero was used for determination of the apparent volume of distribution (V_d). The total body clearance (Cl) was calculated with the equation $V_d \times K_E = Cl$.

RESULTS

The clinical and pharmacokinetic data are presented in Table 1. After a single 200-mg tablet of CBZ was given to 13 volunteers, the peak concentrations were obtained within 2 to 6 hr. Thereafter, the plasma levels declined monoexponentially in accordance with the open one-compartment model. The mean $T_{1/2}$ was 39.8 hr, the mean V_d, 0.99 liter/kg, and the mean Cl 17.8 ml/kg/hr. After one 200-mg tablet, our method was not sensitive enough to determine the kinetic parameters of CBZ-E. In two children after a single dose—assuming that the absorption was complete in 12 hr and the elimination had started in a monoexponential manner—the half-lives were 15.4 and 18.5 hr. The younger male infant had a larger V_d and faster Cl than the girl of nearly 5 years of age. In this acute trial a statistically significant difference of K_E and $T_{1/2}$ existed between adult volunteers and these two children ($p < 0.001$). V_d and Cl were not compared because of their wide variations in children.

When treated with 100 mg CBZ b.i.d. for 4 weeks, the nine volunteers achieved observed mean steady-state concentrations (C_{ss}) of 15.8 and 1.4 μmoles/liter for CBZ and CBZ-E, respectively. The mean half-life was 40.3 hr for CBZ and 19.3 hr for CBZ-E. In children after chronic CBZ therapy, the mean $T_{1/2}$ was 20.8 hr for CBZ and 16.0 hr for CBZ-E. The children had mean C_{ss} 11.1 and 2.7 μmoles/liter for CBZ and CBZ-E, respectively, after mean 21 weeks' therapy on mean dosage of CBZ at 10.0 mg/kg/day. Both K_E and $T_{1/2}$ were statistically and significantly different between children and adults after chronic administration of CBZ ($p < 0.001$). Contrary to this, the respective values of CBZ-E did not differ statistically and significantly from one group to another. Surprisingly, the volunteers and children did not differ statistically and significantly in their K_E and $T_{1/2}$ values between the acute and chronic administration of CBZ.

If we assume the fraction achieving the circulation (F) to be 1.0 for CBZ, the steady-state plasma concentrations can be predicted theoretically from the formula:

$$C_{ss} = \frac{F \times D}{V_d \times K_E \times T}$$

where D is the dose at an interval T (12 hr). From the mean values obtained in the single-dose experiments before, the theoretical C_{ss} of 29.3 μmoles/liter in children and 26.7 μmoles/liter in volunteers should be reached. The observed C_{ss} in children, 38%, and in volunteers, 59%, was, however, of the respective theoretical value.

DISCUSSION

The main finding of this study was that the children have a shorter $T_{1/2}$ and a higher K_E for CBZ than adults, after both a single and chronic administration. Thus children eliminated CBZ faster from plasma than adults. One boy, aged 1 year 7 months, had 4.8-fold faster clearance per body weight than the average adults. A girl of nearly 5 years had the respective value 2.2-fold. As the single administration of CBZ was possible to carry out in this connection only on two children, it is not certain that the clearance is age dependent. Because CBZ is almost totally metabolized and renal excretion of the parent drug is about 1% (Levy et al., 1975b; Faigle and Feldmann, 1975), the decreased clearance values with age were practically due to metabolic clearances. This agrees well with the fact that the relative size of the liver decreases with advancing age.

The apparent volume of distribution was also exceptionally large in this boy of 1 year 7 months mentioned above. This indicates more extensive tissue binding compared to older individuals. Other drugs, digoxin, for instance, have been found to have a high tissue uptake in infants, which is well in agreement with larger apparent volume of distribution (Gorodischer et al., 1976). A large apparent volume of distribution and an increased clearance rate have been presented as possible reasons for children needing higher drug dosages than adults in order to achieve the same therapeutic plasma level (Rane and Wilson, 1976). In the present study children with nearly four-fold daily dose of CBZ did not achieve the plasma level of volunteers.

The clearance values of CBZ in 13 volunteers were about ten-fold lower than generally found after lidocaine, nortriptyline, and propranolol, which all are extensively cleared by the liver and are subject to reduced bioavailability by "first pass" or presystemic hepatic metabolism. It was therefore unlikely that carbamazepine would be undergoing similar "first-pass" metabolism before reaching the general circulation. Furthermore, the clearances and the observed steady-state concentrations in volunteers exhibited low interindividual variations, which all are strange phenomena if the drug undergoes extensive "first-pass" metabolism.

The half-lives of CBZ did not differ significantly after single and chronic administration either in children or in adults. Thus, no enzyme induction could be assumed to take place according to our results. In their study, contrary to ours, Eichelbaum et al. (1975) found four epileptic adult patients to have the mean half-life decreased from 35.6 (elimination after a 200-mg tablet) to 20.9 hr (elimination after 3 weeks on multiple dosage of 10.5 mg/kg/day). This can partly speak for the dose-dependent kinetics of CBZ. The metabolic rate by using higher doses may be faster. The dosage used in the present study was four-fold lower than that used by Eichelbaum and colleagues.

Also in adults, the concentration ratio of CBZ-E to CBZ was higher in the study of Eichelbaum et al. than in ours, 0.15 versus 0.09. Although in this study the ratio of CBZ-E to CBZ was also higher in children (0.24) than in adults (0.09), the half-lives of the metabolite, CBZ-E, did not differ significantly between these groups. Even though only two data points were available to estimate the half-life of the epoxide metabolite, the data are comparable to those referred to in the literature (Eichelbaum et al., 1975; Morselli et al., 1975).

Until now no reports have been published involving intravenous administration of CBZ to man. Thus the fraction available in systemic circulation after oral administration is based on assumptions. In relevant literature the absorption of CBZ is assumed to be 100% because (1) ^{14}C-labeled CBZ has been found to be absorbed completely from human gastrointestinal tract (Faigle and Feldmann, 1975), and (2) the pharmacokinetic parameters have low interindividual variations (Rawlins et al., 1975). We found, however, a discrepancy between the observed and theoretical plasma values of CBZ. This might have been due to three factors. The first is enzyme induction during therapy when it had been started. The results in this chapter do not support this conception because the half-lives after acute and chronic administration were nearly identical. Secondly, the bioavailability of CBZ was not 100%. In experiments with monkeys in which intravenous and oral administration routes were compared, the bioavailability of CBZ ranged from 58 to 85% (Levy et al., 1975a). Thirdly, compliance by the patients and volunteers may have been incomplete.

In conclusion, our results show a larger distribution volume, a shorter half-life, a higher overall elimination rate constant, and a faster clearance of CBZ in children when compared to adults.

REFERENCES

Eichelbaum, M., Ekbom, K., Bertilsson, L., Ringberger, V. A., and Rane, A. (1975): Plasma kinetics of carbamazepine and its epoxide metabolite in man after single and multiple doses. *Eur. J. Clin. Pharmacol.,* 8:337–341.
Faigle, J. W., and Feldmann, K. F. (1975): Pharmacokinetic data of carbamazepine and its major

metabolites in man. In: *Clinical Pharmacology of Antiepileptic Drugs,* edited by H. Schneider, D. Janz, C. Gardner-Thorpe, H. Meinardi, and A. L. Sherwin, pp. 159–165. Springer-Verlag, Berlin.

Gorodischer, R., Jusko, W. J., and Sumner, J. Y. (1976): Tissue and erythrocyte distribution of digoxin in infants. *Clin. Pharmacol. Ther.,* 19:256–263.

Iisalo, E., Dahl, M., and Sundquist, H. (1973): Serum digoxin in adults and children. *Int. J. Clin. Pharmacol.,* 7:219–222.

Levy, R. H., Lochard, J. S., Green, J. R., Friel, P., and Martin, L. (1975a): Pharmacokinetics of carbamazepine in monkey following intravenous and oral administration. In: *Advances in Mass Spectrometry in Biochemistry and Medicine, Vol. 1,* edited by A. Frigerio and N. Castagnoli. Spectrum Publications, New York.

Levy, R. H., Pitlick, W. H., Troupin, A. S., Green, J. R., and Neal, J. M. (1975b): Pharmacokinetics of carbamazepine in normal man. *Clin. Pharmacol. Ther.,* 17:657–668.

Morselli, P. L., Gerne, M., De Maio, D., Zanda, G., Viani, F., and Garattini, S. (1975): Pharmacokinetic studies on carbamazepine in volunteers and epileptic patients. In: *Clinical Pharmacology of Antiepileptic Drugs,* edited by H. Schneider, D. Janz, C. Gardner-Thorpe, H. Meinardi, and A. L. Sherwin, pp. 166–180. Springer-Verlag, Berlin.

Pynnönen, S., Sillanpää, M., Frey, H., and Iisalo, E. (1976): Serum concentration of carbamazepine: Comparison of Herrmann's spectrophotometric method and a new GLC method for the determination of carbamazepine. *Epilepsia,* 17:67–72.

Pynnönen, S., Sillanpää, M., Frey, H., and Iisalo, E. (1977): Carbamazepine and its 10,11-epoxide in children and adults with epilepsy. *Eur. J. Clin. Pharmacol.,* 11:129–133.

Rane, A., and Wilson, J. T. (1976): Clinical pharmacokinetics in infants and children. *Clin. Pharmacokinetics,* 1:2–24.

Rawlins, M. D., Collste, P., Bertilsson, L., and Palmer, L. (1975): Distribution and elimination kinetics of carbamazepine in man. *Eur. J. Clin. Pharmacol.,* 8:91–96.

Svensmark, O., and Buchthal, F. (1964): Diphenylhydantoin and phenobarbital: Serum levels in children. *Am. J. Dis. Child.,* 108:82–87.

Epilepsy, The Eighth International Symposium,
edited by J. K. Penry. Raven Press, New York
© 1977.

Effectiveness of Daily Phenobarbital in the Prevention of Febrile Seizure Recurrences in "Simple" Febrile Convulsions and "Epilepsy Triggered by Fever"

Sheldon Mark Wolf

*Department of Neurology, Southern California Permanente Medical Group,
Los Angeles, California 90027*

Livingston (1954) divided febrile convulsions into two types: "simple" and "epilepsy triggered by fever." Seizures of the first type were brief and generalized, there were frequently relatives with febrile convulsions, and the electroencephalogram obtained a week after the child was afebrile was normal. Although there were some variations in criteria in different papers by Livingston (1954, 1958), in the "epilepsy triggered by fever" type, the convulsions were long or focal, epilepsy was present in the immediate family, and the electroencephalogram was abnormal.

Livingston (1968, 1972) has stated several times that continuous administration of phenobarbital is useless for the prevention of recurrent febrile convulsions in children who have had a "simple" febrile convulsion, but it is effective in decreasing febrile seizure recurrences in the "epilepsy triggered by fever" group.

The purpose of the present study was to test the theory that the effect of daily phenobarbital in the prevention of febrile convulsions is dependent on whether the initial febrile convulsion was or was not "simple," using Livingston's criteria.

PATIENTS AND METHODS

Three hundred and fifty-five children with an initial febrile convulsion seen at the Kaiser Foundation Hospitals in Southern California from 1970 to 1975 were randomized into three groups according to the last digit of the chart number. If the last digit was 1, 2, or 3 (group 1), continuous phenobarbital 3 to 4 mg/kg was prescribed, with an additional "load" of 30 mg/year up to a maximum of 120 mg at the onset of fever, followed by an increase in the dosage to 5 mg/kg for the duration of fever. If the last digit was 4, 5, or 6 (group 2), phenobarbital 5 mg/kg was prescribed, to be given at the onset and for the duration of fever, as well as an initial "load" of 30 mg/year to a maximum of 120 mg. If the last digit was 7, 8, or 9 (group 3), no phenobarbital prophylaxis was given. If the last digit was 0, the preceding digit was used. Fever was defined as a temperature over 100°F. The parents of all children in the study were instructed about the importance of quickly lowering the temperature with aspirin (60 mg/year) and cool water soaks. They were also asked to bring the child promptly to the emergency area if any fever occurred, so that bacterial infection, if present, could be treated with antibiotics.

With the use of life table methodology (Hill, 1971; Van den Berg and Yerushalmy, 1971) to adjust for the different lengths of inclusion in the study, we calculated the frequency of first febrile seizure recurrences for all children in the three treatment groups, for various intervals following the initial febrile convulsion. The duration of follow-up ranged from 6 to 70 months, with a mean of 28 months in all groups.

Children were designated as having "epilepsy triggered by fever" if the seizure was longer than 10 min (Livingston, 1958) or focal, if there was a history of epilepsy in parents or siblings, or if the EEG was abnormal 1 week after the febrile convulsion. If the seizure was less than 10 min, generalized, there was no history of epilepsy in the immediate family, and the EEG was normal, the child was included in the "simple" febrile convulsion group.

RESULTS

Of 290 children who could be classified according to these criteria, 216 (74.5%) were in the "simple" febrile convulsion group and 74 (25.5%) were in the "epilepsy triggered by fever" group. In the "simple" group, there were 62 children in group 1, 84 in group 2, and 70 in group 3. In the "epilepsy triggered by fever" cohort, there were 24 in group 1, 32 in group 2, and 18 in group 3. There were no significant differences in recurrence rates between groups 2 and 3 in either the "simple" or "epilepsy triggered by fever" categories. These were combined into one group for further analysis, which we called group 2 + 3.

There was a significant difference in the recurrence rate between group 1 and group 2 + 3, in both the "simple" and "epilepsy triggered by fever" children (Tables 1 and 2). Although in both groups the reduction in recurrence of febrile convulsions in children receiving daily phenobarbital reached statistical significance, the treatment effect was more pronounced in the "epilepsy triggered by

TABLE 1. *Febrile convulsion recurrences—initial febrile convulsion "simple"*

Months of follow-up	Group 1 (62) (%)	Group 2 + 3 (154) (%)	
6	3.5	7.8	ns
12	11.9	18.2	ns
18	11.9	23.8	$p < 0.05$
24	11.9	24.7	$p < 0.05$
36	11.9	28.6	$p < 0.01$

TABLE 2. *Febrile convulsion recurrences—"epilepsy triggered by fever"*

Months of follow-up	Group 1 (24) (%)	Group 2 + 3 (50) (%)	
6	5.3	16.0	ns
12	5.3	33.8	$p < 0.001$
18	5.3	41.6	$p < 0.0001$
24	5.3	44.6	$p < 0.0001$
36	5.3	44.6	$p < 0.0001$

fever" group. The difference in recurrence rates in both the "simple" and "epilepsy triggered by fever" groups was also statistically significant when group 1 was compared with groups 2 and 3 separately.

When the data were analyzed using either Livingston's 1954 criteria for "epilepsy triggered by fever" (seizure lasting longer than 1 hr or focal, epilepsy in the immediate family, abnormal EEG) or his 1958 criteria (seizure longer than 10 min or focal, abnormal EEG), the recurrence rate of febrile convulsions was significantly lower in group 1 than in group 2 + 3 in both the "simple" and "epilepsy triggered by fever" groups. Another criterion of "epilepsy triggered by fever" in the 1958 paper was age over 6 years, but there were no children in this study whose age at the time of the initial febrile convulsion was over 6 years.

In the continuously treated group (group 1), the recurrence rate of febrile convulsions was generally lower in the "epilepsy triggered by fever" group than in the children with "simple" febrile convulsions. This difference was not statistically significant.

In group 2 + 3, the febrile convulsion recurrence rate was higher in the "epilepsy triggered by fever" group than in the children with "simple" febrile convulsions, and the difference was statistically significant ($p < 0.05$).

Our results support Livingston's observation that the effectiveness of daily phenobarbital in reducing recurrent febrile convulsions is greater in children with features of "epilepsy triggered by fever" than in those with "simple" febrile convulsions. Our data disagree with his contention that daily phenobarbital is ineffective in the "simple" febrile convulsion group and show that this regimen produces a statistically significant decrease in febrile convulsion recurrences in both groups.

ACKNOWLEDGMENT

This work was based on a cooperative multicenter study done in the different Kaiser Foundation Hospitals in Los Angeles. The physicians who participated in the study were Drs. A. Carr, D. Davis, S. Davidson, E. Dale, E. Goldenberg, R. Hanson, G. Lulejian, M. Nelson, P. Treitman, and A. Weinstein. Computing assistance was obtained from the Health Sciences Computing Facility UCLA and supported by NIH Special Research Resources Grant RR-3. We wish to thank Dr. Alan Forsythe and Ms. Ellen Sommers for their expert assistance in data analysis.

REFERENCES

Hill, A. B. (1971): Life tables and survival after treatment. In: *Principles of Medical Statistics, 9th Ed.,* pp. 220–236. Oxford University Press, New York.

Livingston, S. (1954): *The Diagnosis and Treatment of Convulsive Disorders in Children.* Charles C. Thomas, Springfield, Ill.

Livingston, S. (1958): Convulsive disorders in infants and children. *Adv. Pediatr.,* 10:113–192.

Livingston, S. (1968): Infantile febrile convulsions. *Dev. Med. Child Neurol.,* 10:374.

Livingston, S. (1972): *Comprehensive Management of Epilepsy in Infancy, Childhood and Adolescence.* Charles C. Thomas, Springfield, Ill.

Van den Berg, B. J., and Yerushalmy, J. (1971): Studies on convulsive disorders in young children. II. Intermittent phenobarbital prophylaxis and recurrence of febrile convulsions. *J. Pediatr.,* 78: 1004–1012.

Epilepsy, The Eighth International Symposium,
edited by J. K. Penry. Raven Press, New York
© 1977.

Phenytoin-Induced Salivary IgA Deficiency and Gingival Hyperplasia

Johan A. Aarli

Department of Neurology, School of Medicine, University of Bergen, Bergen, Norway

Some epileptic patients on phenytoin treatment develop disorders of the immune system. The most frequent complication is serum IgA deficiency (Sorrell et al., 1971). IgA constitutes only a minor component of the serum immunoglobulins. IgA is, however, the predominant immunoglobulin in external secretions. Deficiency of serum IgA is frequently accompanied by a deficiency of secretory IgA (Ammann and Hong, 1973). The present study was therefore undertaken in order to investigate if phenytoin has a similar effect on salivary IgA as on serum IgA. The experimental work referred to in this chapter is described in detail in the article by Aarli *(in press)*.

PATIENTS AND METHODS

Groups of Individuals

The patients included 35 children (< 16 years) and 49 adults treated for epilepsy at the Departments of Neurology and Pediatrics. The control group consisted of 16 children and 15 adults.

Collection of Samples

Whole saliva was collected without flow stimulation. Samples were generally obtained 3 to 4 hr after breakfast and immediately frozen. Before use, the frozen saliva was quickly melted and cleared by centrifugation at $1,000 \times g$ for 20 min. Sera were obtained from the same individuals. Sera and saliva were stored at $-20°C$.

Quantitative Analysis of Immunoglobulins

Determination of the concentrations of immunoglobulins (Ig) and of albumin was performed by single radial immunodiffusion, using commercial equipment from Behringwerke (Behringwerke AG, Marburg/Lahn, West Germany).
Serum concentrations of IgA, IgG, and IgM were determined using Tri-Parti-

gen and S-Partigen IgA immunodiffusion plates. For salivary IgA and albumin, LC Partigen immunodiffusion plates were used. Standard human serum and standard Ig dilutions (IgG, IgA, IgM) obtained from Behringwerke served as references for all Ig determinations. The technical procedure was performed according to Aarli (1976).

The standard employed for quantitative analysis of IgA, in both serum and saliva, was 7S (serum) IgA. When a 7S IgA standard is used, the concentration of IgA in secretions will be underestimated approximately threefold (Tomasi and Grey, 1972). For saliva, values were therefore multiplied with a conversion factor of 3 (Brandtzaeg et al., 1970). By this method, and with the conversion factor, the lower limit for quantitative detection of salivary IgA is 2.4 mg/100 ml.

Preparative Ultracentrifugation

Preparative ultracentrifugation was performed as earlier (Aarli and Tønder, 1975). Sixteen successive fractions, numbered from the bottom, were obtained.

RESULTS

IgA Concentrations in Saliva and Serum

Children

The IgA concentration in saliva from healthy children was 16.44 ± 6.49 mg/100 ml (mean $\pm$ SD), and the range 3.3 to 25 mg/100 ml. IgA varied considerably in repeated samples from the same individual, but values below 3.3 mg/100 ml were not detected.

Serum concentrations of IgA from healthy children ranged between 0.8 and 3.0 mg/ml. IgA levels were normal in sera and saliva from children with epilepsy in samples taken before any drug treatment was given.

The IgA concentration in saliva from children taking antiepileptic drugs was 7.23 ± 5.93 mg/100 ml (range 0 to 28 mg/100 ml). The difference from the normal group is statistically significant ($p < 0.01$). Thirteen patients had salivary IgA concentrations ≤ 3 mg/100 ml. Two patients had extremely weak precipitation lines in double diffusion experiments on agar against anti-IgA antiserum. Both patients had serum concentrations of IgA < 0.05 mg/ml.

Adults

The IgA concentration in saliva from healthy adults was 19.48 ± 6.56 mg/100 ml (range 9 to 32 mg/100 ml). Serum IgA levels in healthy adults varied from 0.7 to 3.0 mg/ml. The IgA concentration in saliva from adult epilepsy patients was 13.53 ± 12.76 mg/100 ml (range 0 to 60 mg/100 ml). The difference is statistically significant at a 2% level.

Eleven patients with low serum IgA (< 0.6 mg/ml) showed salivary IgA $\gtrless 3$ mg/100 ml. The concentration of albumin was determined in seven of these samples. The values ranged from 2 to 46 mg/100 ml, giving a low IgA: albumin ratio. The normal or even increased salivary IgA in these patients is therefore partly the result of either concentration of saliva or transudation of serum proteins through inflamed gingiva. Salivary IgG and IgM were therefore determined.

Salivary Concentrations of IgG and IgM

The IgG concentration in saliva from normal controls seldom surpassed 1.5 mg/100 ml. Of 21 epilepsy patients taking phenytoin, 11 had IgG concentrations in saliva of ≥ 1.5 mg/100 ml. There was a high ($p < 0.01$) correlation between high salivary concentration of IgG and salivary IgA.

The correlation between high salivary IgA and high salivary albumin was at the same level of significance. Furthermore, highest concentrations of IgA were found in saliva from patients with gingival inflammation.

Raised IgM levels were found in saliva from some epilepsy patients, but this was infrequent, and a low salivary IgA was seldom accompanied by compensatory increase of IgM.

Salivary IgA in Gingival Hyperplasia

Six patients had phenytoin-induced gingival hyperplasia. Five of these patients had low serum IgA; the concentration was normal in one patient. The salivary IgA concentration was low in five patients, high in one. The high IgA was matched by an increase of salivary IgG, which again correlated with inflammatory changes of the gingiva (Table 1). After ultracentrifugation of saliva from

TABLE 1. *Serum and salivary IgA, salivary IgG, IgM, and albumin in patients with gingival inflammation and hyperplasia*

| Patient No. | Serum IgA | Salivary concentrations of | | | | Gingival | |
		IgA	IgG	IgM	Albumin	Hyperplasia	Inflammation
1	0.18	3.0	2.0	0	6.2	I	+
2	0.02	0	1.5	ND	ND	II	+
3	0.10	2.4	0.4	0	3.0	II	+
4	0.08	0	0.3	0.5	5.2	I	+
5	0.72	2	0.3	0.7	1.9	I	+
6	0.31	10.5	3.0	1.0	6.1	III	+++
Normal mean	1.17[a]	16.44	1.44[b]	0.21[b]	—	—	—

ND, not done.
[a] Aarli and Tønder, 1975.
[b] Brandtzaeg et al., 1970.

this patient, IgA was detected only in fractions 8 and 9, whereas secretory component occurred mainly in fractions 9 through 11. For comparison, we also performed ultracentrifugation with secretory IgA-containing saliva. Here, SC and IgA were demonstrated in fractions 5 and 6, SC also in 9 through 11. The findings indicate that the high salivary IgA from the patient with gingival hyperplasia (Table 1, No. 6) mainly represents serum-derived IgA.

Several patients with subnormal and even undetectable salivary IgA showed no signs of gingival hyperplasia.

DISCUSSION

The normal adult mean concentration of secretory IgA in whole saliva was approximately 19.5 mg/100 ml. This figure is in accordance with data obtained by other workers (Waldman et al., 1968; Brandtzaeg et al., 1970). IgA concentrations in saliva of patients taking phenytoin were, however, considerably lower than normal. The salivary IgA concentration was normal in epileptic patients before phenytoin treatment. Phenytoin can induce a fall in the serum concentration of IgA (Aarli, 1976). We can now conclude that phenytoin treatment induces a fall also of salivary IgA in some epileptic patients.

Patients with selective IgA deficiency have no increase in the incidence of gingival inflammation (Brandtzaeg et al., 1970). This is commonly ascribed to the increased transfer of IgM into their secretions (Brandtzaeg, 1971). The present study shows that patients with phenytoin-induced depletion of salivary IgA have frequently no compensatory IgM increase. Patients lacking IgA may therefore manifest an increased susceptibility to gingival inflammation when oral hygiene is insufficient. In some patients, however, a high concentration of salivary IgA was found. Ultracentrifugation data showed that this increase can be ascribed to the presence of 7S IgA. An increase of salivary IgA was accompanied by an increase of salivary IgG. The salivary concentration of IgG is mainly a function of tissue fluid leakage through mucous membranes and is significantly increased in periodontal inflammation, which is also accompanied by raised salivary concentrations of IgA (Brandtzaeg et al., 1970).

Gingival inflammation in phenytoin-treated epilepsy patients is intimately connected with gingival hyperplasia. There is a significant relationship between the severity of gingival hyperplasia and the grade of clinically visible gingival inflammatory symptoms (Aas, 1963). Presumably, meticulous oral hygiene is sufficient to prevent the development of more severe gingival hyperplasia, even when salivary IgA is deficient. But when local IgA deficiency is combined with poor oral hygiene, the first line of defense of the gingiva is out of function and gingival inflammation can occur. IgG and IgA may transude from the blood, but this is insufficient to eliminate the inflammation. The organism will repair the chronic inflammation by repair processes, and the phenytoin-accelerated fibroblast proliferation results in gingival hyperplasia.

ACKNOWLEDGMENTS

This work was supported by the Norwegian Research Council for Science and the Humanities and in part by a grant from Norske Hoechst AS.

REFERENCES

Aarli, J. A. (1976): Drug-induced IgA deficiency in epileptic patients. *Arch. Neurol.,* 33:296–299.
Aarli, J. A. (1976): Phenytoin-induced depression of salivary IgA and gingival hyperplasia. *Epilepsia,* 17:283–291.
Aarli, J. A., and Tonder, O. (1975): Effect of antiepileptic drugs on serum and salivary IgA. *Scand. J. Immunol.,* 4:391–396.
Aas, E. (1963): Hyperplasia gingivae diphenylhydantoinea. *Acta Odontol. Scand. [Suppl.],* 34:1–142.
Ammann, A. J., and Hong, R. (1973): Selective IgA deficiency. In: *Immunological Disorders in Infants and Children,* edited by E. R. Stiehm and V. A. Fulginiti. W. B. Saunders, Philadelphia.
Brandtzaeg, P. (1971): Human secretory immunoglobulins. II. Salivary secretions from individuals with selectively excessive or defective synthesis of serum immunoglobulins. *Clin. Exp. Immunol.,* 8:69–85.
Brandtzaeg, P., Fjellanger, I., and Gjeruldsen, S. T. (1970): Human secretory immunoglobulins. I. Salivary secretions from individuals with normal or low levels of serum immunoglobulins. *Scand. J. Haematol. [Suppl.],* 12:1–83.
Sorrell, T. C., Forbes, I. J., Burness, F. R., and Rischbieth, R. H. (1971): Depression of immunological function in patients treated with phenytoin sodium (sodium diphenyhydantoin). *Lancet,* 2:1233–1235.
Tomasi, T. B., and Grey, H. M. (1972): Structure and function of immunoglobulin A. *Prog. Allergy,* 16:81–213.
Waldman, R. H., Mann, J. J., and Kasel, J. A. (1968): Influenza virus neutralizing antibody in human respiratory secretions. *J. Immunol.,* 100:80–85.

Epilepsy, The Eighth International Symposium,
edited by J. K. Penry. Raven Press, New York
© 1977.

The Influence of Phenytoin and Carbamazepine on Endocrine Function: Preliminary Results

K. Lühdorf, P. Christiansen, J. M. Hansen, and M. Lund

Department of Neuromedicine, KAS Glostrup, 2600 Glostrup, Denmark

Impotence has been described as a complication of epilepsy, especially temporal lobe epilepsy (Hieron and Saunders, 1966; Taylor, 1969). Recently an uncontrolled study by Christiansen, Deibjerg, and Lund (1975) indicated an unsuspected high frequency of impotence among male epileptic patients. Furthermore, a correlation between low 17-ketosteroid excretion and impotence was observed. These findings raised the suspicion that impotence might be drug induced.

PATIENTS AND METHODS

On the above-mentioned background, a study group called the Copenhagen Study Group of Side Effects of Antiepileptic Drugs[1] is now running a prospective study. In this study are included previously untreated male epileptic patients under the age of 45 years. Also 10 normal subjects have been included. All patients are screened before the initiation of any medical treatment and following 2 weeks and 3 months of treatment. The drugs of investigation are phenytoin and carbamazepine, the patients being randomized to treatment with either drug. The initial 24-hour dosage of phenytoin is 6 mg/kg body weight, whereas the 24-hr dosage of carbamazepine has been 600 mg, increasing to 1 g following 3 days of treatment.

Each screening includes evaluation of liver enzyme function, as well as testicular, adrenal, thyroidal, hypothalamic, and pituitary function. Furthermore, calcium and folate metabolism are being investigated.

RESULTS AND DISCUSSION

Preliminary results concerning some of the parameters investigated will be presented. At the present time 10 normal subjects and 7 epileptic patients have finished the first and second screenings.

---

[1] Members of the group are E. P. Bennett, C. Christiansen, P. Christiansen, J. M. Hansen, A. Holm, S. G. Johnsen, J. P. Kampman, K. Kjaersgård, S. Micic, J. F. Larsen, N. Larsen, M. Lund, K. Lühdorf, J. Naestoft, P. Runing, L. Skovsted, and B. Svenstrup. Gentofte Hospital: Dept. of Neuromedicine; Glostrup Hospital: Dept. of Clinical Chemistry, Laboratory of Clinical Chemistry, Dept. of Clinical Pharmacology, and Dept. of Neuromedicine; Herlev Hospital: Dept. of Gynecology, Dept. of Medicine. Statens Seruminstitut Hormone Dept.

Serum Concentration of Phenytoin and Carbamazepine

Nine patients received phenytoin. The mean serum phenytoin level was 10 mg/liter (range 6 to 14). Eight patients received carbamazepine. The mean serum carbamazepine was 10 mg/liter (range 8 to 14).

Liver Enzyme Function

As phenazone metabolism is known as a good indicator of liver enzyme function (Conney, 1967; Vesell and Page, 1969; Andreasen et al., 1974), the liver enzyme induction caused by the two drugs has been evaluated by measurement of phenazone half-life and clearance following the intravenous injection of 1 g of phenazone.

Phenazone half-life decreased significantly during both phenytoin and carbamazepine treatments. The mean values were (1) with phenytoin the half-life decreases from 543 to 344 min ($p < 0.05$, $N = 7$); (2) with carbamazepine the half-life decreases from 590 to 375 min ($p < 0.01$, $N = 8$). A corresponding increase in clearance was observed. The mean values were (1) with phenytoin clearance increases from 58.1 to 87.4 ml/min ($p < 0.05$, $N = 7$); (2) with carbamazepine clearance increases from 52.0 to 76.1 ml/min ($p < 0.02$, $N = 8$). (Wilcoxon test for pair differences.) These results indicate that both drugs are liver enzyme inducing to the same degree.

Cortisol Metabolism

As free cortisol urinary 24-hr excretion appears to be the best single test in the evaluation of adrenal cortical function (Hsu and Bledsoe, 1970), this parameter has been measured. Free cortisol excretion increases during both phenytoin and carbamazepine treatment. With phenytoin excretion increases from 88 to 172 μg ($p < 0.01$, $N = 9$). With carbamazepine·excretion increases from 126 to 200 μg ($p < 0.05$, $N = 8$). (Wilcoxon test for pair differences.)

Also, the excretion of 17-ketogenic steroids has been measured. As carbamazepine interferes with this analysis, measurements during carbamazepine treatment are not available. The 17-ketogenic steroid excretion decreases slightly during phenytoin treatment, the mean measurements at the first and second screenings being 11.4 and 7.9 mg ($p < 0.01$, $N = 9$). (Wilcoxon test for pair differences.)

These results are in agreement with the results of other investigations concerning phenytoin (Costa et al., 1955; Choi et al., 1971). Werk, MacGee, and Sholiton (1964) found during phenytoin treatment highly increased excretion of 6-hydroxycortisol, a metabolite which is not a 17-ketogenic steroid. This observation has been interpreted as the result of liver enzyme induction by phenytoin, and this is in agreement with the knowledge that steroid hormones are metabolized by hydroxylating inducible liver enzymes (Conney, 1967; Kuntzman, 1968). Whether the increase in 6-hydroxycortisol can alone explain the described changes in cortisol metabolism must await the accumulation of further results.

Androgens, Follicle-Stimulating, and Luteinizing Hormones

The 24 hr excretion of fractionated 17-ketosteroids (17-KS) has been measured. 17-KS excretion decreases during both phenytoin and carbamazepine treatment. The mean values from the first and second screenings are total 17-KS excretion: (1) phenytoin 39 and 23 μmoles ($p < 0.01$, $N = 9$), (2) carbamazepine 54 and 26 μmoles ($p < 0.01$, $N = 8$); androsterone excretion: (1) phenytoin 16 and 7 μ moles ($p < 0.01$, $N = 9$), (2) carbamazepine 20 and 8 μmoles ($p < 0.01$, $N = 8$); ethiocholanolone excretion: (1) phenytoin 12 and 9 μmoles (ns, $N = 9$), (2) carbamazepine 17 and 9 μmoles ($p < 0.01$, $N = 8$). (Wilcoxon test for pair differences.)

During dexamethasone suppression the mean values of total 17-KS, androsterone, and etiocholanolone excretion (first and second screenings) were total 17-KS excretion: (1) phenytoin 15 and 13μmoles ($p < 0.05$, $N = 9$), (2) carbamazepine 18 and 12 μmoles (ns, $N = 7$); Androsterone excretion: (1) phenytoin 7 and 5 μmoles ($p < 0.01$, $N = 9$), (2) carbamazepine 8 and 4 μmoles ($p < 0.02$, $N = 7$); and etiocholanolone: (1) phenytoin 7 and 6 μmoles (ns, $N = 9$), (2) carbamazepine 8 and 5 μmoles ($p < 0.05$, $N = 7$). (Wilcoxon test for pair differences.) These results indicate decreased excretion of both adrenal and testicular derived androgens.

Serum concentrations of testosterone have been measured by radioimmunoassay. Mean serum testosterone increases slightly during phenytoin treatment, the values from the first and second screenings being 466 and 623 ng/100 ml ($p < 0.05$, $N = 8$). Serum testosterone remains unchanged during carbamazepine treatment, the mean values from the first and second screenings being 378 and 426 ng/100 ml (ns, $N = 9$). The reference for normal males aged 20 to 50 years is 285 to 907 ng/100 ml.

Serum concentrations of follicle-stimulating hormone (FSH) and luteinizing hormone (LH) have been measured, but they remain essentially unchanged during both phenytoin and carbamazepine treatment. The mean values (first and second screenings) are (1) phenytoin: FSH 8 and 10 second international reference preparation of human menopausal gonadotropin (IRP-HME)/ml, LH 9 and 10 second IRP-HMG/ml; (2) carbamazepine: FSH 6 and 9 second IRP-HMG/ml, LH 10 and 11 second IRP-HMG/ml.

A depressive effect of the two drugs on the hypothalamic-pituitary system or the testes is unlikely. Why 17-ketosteroid excretion decreases is open to discussion. Liver enzyme induction causing the formation of large amounts of androgen metabolites not measured as 17-ketosteroids is a possible explanation.

Thyroidal Parameters

Serum triiodothyronine (S-T$_3$), serum thyroxine (S-T$_4$), and triiodothyronine resin uptake (T$_3$ test) have been measured. Free T$_3$ and T$_4$ index an approximation to the concentration of free hormone has been calculated. It is apparent from Table 1 that there is a decrease in all parameters. The decrease in S-T$_4$ during

TABLE 1. *Mean thyroidal parameters before and after 2 weeks of treatment*

Parameter	Phenytoin			Carbamazepine		
	S1	S2	p	S1	S2	p
S-T$_3$ ng/100 ml	168	147	<0.02	169	158	ns
S-T$_4$ μg/100 ml	7.1	5.9	ns	7.7	6.3	<0.01
T$_3$ test	1.10	1.00	<0.02	0.99	0.91	<0.02
Free T$_3$ index	183	143	<0.01	167	144	<0.02
Free T$_4$ index	7.69	5.74	<0.01	7.58	5.70	<0.01
N		9			8	

S1, First screening; S2, second screening,
S-T$_3$, serum triiodothyronine by radioimmunoassay.
S-T$_4$, serum thyroxine by displacement method.
T$_3$ test, Triiodothyronine resin uptake test.
Wilcoxon test for pair differences.

phenytoin treatment and the decrease in S-T$_3$ during carbamazepine treatment are not significant. The decrease in free T$_3$ and T$_4$ index is, however, significant for both drugs.

Other investigators examining phenytoin have obtained similar results (Chin and Schussler, 1968; Hansen et al., 1974). As has been proposed in previous studies concerning phenytoin, the most likely interpretation of the results described is enhanced thyroidal hormone metabolism due to liver enzyme induction (Mendoza et al., 1966; Hansen et al., 1974).

CONCLUSION

Both phenytoin and carbamazepine are potent liver enzyme inductors. 17-ketosteroid excretion decreases, whereas serum FSH, LH, and testosterone levels remain essentially unchanged. The mechanism by which phenytoin and carbamazepine acts on these parameters is still unknown. A significant increase in cortisol 24-hr urinary excretion has been found for both drugs. How this is brought about is not fully clarified, but liver enzyme induction is probably involved. Finally, a significant decrease in free T$_3$ and T$_4$ index has been demonstrated, this decrease being most likely due to liver enzyme induction.

No differences between the two drugs have been found. To our knowledge, results concerning the influence of carbamazepine on adrenal, testicular, and thyroidal function have not previously been available.

REFERENCES

Andreasen, P. B., Ranek, L., Statland, B. E., and Tygstrup, N. (1974): Clearance of antipyrin-dependence of quantitative liver function. *Eur. J. Clin. Invest.*, 4:129–134.
Chin, W., and Schussler, G. C. (1968): Decreased serum free thyroxine concentration in patients treated with diphenylhydantoin. *J. Clin. Endocrinol. Metab.*, 28:181–186.

Choi, Y., Thrasher, K., Werk, E. E., Sholiton, L. J., and Olinger, C. (1971): Effect of diphenylhydantoin on cortisol kinetics in humans. *J. Pharmacol. Exp. Ther.,* 176:27–34.

Christiansen, P., Deibjerg, J., and Lund, M. (1975): Potens, fertilitet og Konshormonudskillelse hos yngre mandlige epilepsilidende. *Ugeskr. Laeger.,* 41:2402–2404.

Conney, A. H. (1967): Pharmacological implication of microsomal enzyme induction. *Pharmacol. Rev.,* 19:317–366.

Costa, P. J., Glaser, G. H., and Bonnycastle, D. D. (1955): Effects of diphenylhydantoin (Dilantin) on adrenal cortical function. *Arch. Neurol. Psychiatr.,* 74:88–91.

Hansen, J. M., Skovsted, L., Lauridsen, U. B., Kirkegård, C., and Siersbaek-Nielsen, K. (1974): The effect of diphenylhydantoin on thyroidal function. *J. Clin. Endocrinol. Metab.,* 39:785–789.

Hieron, R., and Saunders, M. (1966): Impotence in patients with temporal lobe lesions. *Lancet,* 2:761–763.

Hsu, T. H., and Bledsoe, T. (1970): Measurement of urinary free corticoids by competitive protein-binding radioassay in hypoadrenal states. *J. Clin. Endocrinol. Metab.,* 30:443–449.

Kuntzman, R. (1969): Drugs and enzyme induction. *Ann. Rev. Pharmacol.,* 9:21–36.

Mendoza, D. M., Flock, E. V., Owen, C. A., and Paris, J. (1966): Effect of 5,5-diphenylhydantoin on the metabolism of L-thyroxine-131 J in the rat. *Endocrinology,* 79:106–118.

Taylor, D. C. (1969): Sexual behavior and temporal lobe epilepsy. *Arch. Neurol.,* 21:510–516.

Vesell, E. S., and Page, J. G. (1969): Genetic control of phenobarbital-induced shortening of plasma antipyrin half-lives in man. *J. Clin. Invest.,* 48:2202–2209.

Werk, E. E., MacGee, J., and Sholiton, L. J. (1964): Effect of diphenylhydantoin on cortisol metabolism in man *J. Clin. Invest.,* 43:1824–1835.

Epilepsy, The Eighth International Symposium,
edited by J. K. Penry. Raven Press, New York
© 1977.

Effect of Diphenylhydantoin on Serum Cholesterol and Triglyceride Levels in Patients with Epilepsy

Mauri I. Reunanen and Eero A. Sotaniemi

Department of Neurology and Clinical Research Unit, University of Oulu, Finland

Long-term treatment with anticonvulsants is often associated with various metabolic disorders (Reynolds, 1975).

Compounds such as diphenylhydantoin (DPH) and barbiturates have a strong inducing effect on enzymatic reactions carried out in the liver, and it is widely believed that metabolic side effects associated with anticonvulsant therapy are due to this phenomenon. The biosynthesis of cholesterol and triglycerides is catalyzed by liver enzymes, which are known to be influenced by various drugs such as barbiturates and exogenic hormones. It may be assumed that anticonvulsant treatment may also change the lipid metabolism of epileptics. This study was undertaken to evaluate this problem.

PATIENTS AND METHODS

Subjects

We investigated 18 consecutive epileptics (10 females and 8 males) who were chosen for DPH therapy. The mean age was 29.5 years (range 15 to 67 years). None of them had been previously treated with anticonvulsants or any other drug known to induce hepatic enzyme system. The patients were collected during a long-term period to avoid the possible seasonal effect on the results. They came from a limited area where dietary habits varied little. During follow-up the patients were asked to continue their usual diet. All patients were able to carry on their daily duties after DPH therapy was begun.

Methods

The epileptic fits were controlled by the administration of diphenylhydantoin. The daily dose was 200 to 350 mg per patient. The serum drug levels were monitored during the follow-up period, and the DPH content, analyzed by gas-chromatography, varied from 0.8 to 24.0 μg/ml.

The serum cholesterol and triglyceride levels were estimated before the institution of DPH treatment and then 1, 3, and 6 months after and at 6-month intervals thereafter during the follow-up period. Eighteen patients were followed-up for 3 months, fourteen for six, and thirteen for 30 months.

The blood samples were taken between 8 and 10 a.m. after a 12-hr fast for analysis of the lipid levels by a standard analyzer system (Technicon). Statistical analyses were performed by calculating the significance of the difference between the means of any correlating samples.

RESULTS

Figures 1 and 2 depict the individual and mean (± SD) values of serum cholesterol and triglyceride levels before and during the trial.

Cholesterol

The mean serum cholesterol before treatment was 6.39 ± 1.19 mmoles/liter and after 1 month 7.45 ± 1.45 mmoles/liter; the increase was significant ($p < 0.005$). During follow-up the mean serum cholesterol remained at this elevated level varying from 6.92 ± 1.55 mmoles/liter to 7.61 ± 1.41 mmoles/liter.

Triglycerides

The mean serum triglyceride level was 1.39 ± 1.00 mmole/liter before treatment, and after 1 month it was 1.79 ± 1.28 mmoles/liter; the increase was

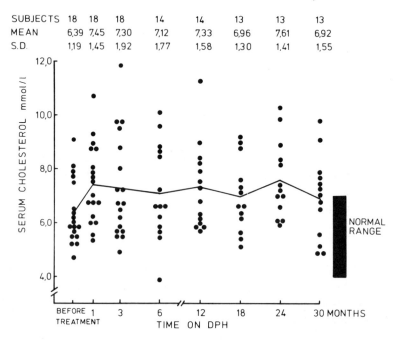

FIG. 1. Individual and mean (± SD) serum cholesterol values during DPH therapy.

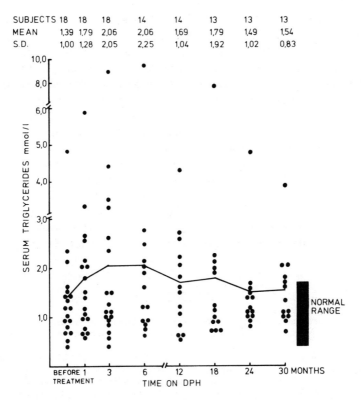

SUBJECTS	18	18	18	14	14	13	13	13
MEAN	1,39	1,79	2,06	2,06	1,69	1,79	1,49	1,54
S.D.	1,00	1,28	2,05	2,25	1,04	1,92	1,02	0,83

FIG. 2. Individual and mean (± SD) serum triglyceride values during DPH therapy.

significant ($p < 0.05$). During the follow-up period there was marked individual variation on the response of the serum triglyceride levels, but the mean change was not statistically significant.

Timing of the Changes

The timing of maximal changes of cholesterol and triglyceride values varied individually after the beginning of DPH therapy. The maximal triglyceride level was reached on the average after 5.5 months and that of cholesterol after 13.2 months.

DISCUSSION

This study demonstrates that therapy with diphenylhydantoin has an effect on serum lipid levels. There was a significant increase in serum cholesterol and triglyceride levels after 1 month of treatment. The serum cholesterol level remained constantly elevated, whereas the increase in serum triglycerides was a temporary phenomenon.

The mechanism by which DPH increases the serum cholesterol level is not known, but some explanations may be discussed on the basis of the known pharmacological effects of the drug. One of them could be the possible phenobarbital-like effect of DPH on hepatic microsomal enzymes, by which it could stimulate cholesterol synthesis (Jones and Amstrong, 1965). At the same time, the intestinal absorption of cholesterol may be increased after an increased formation of bile acids (Redinger and Small, 1973). Also, the increase of serum cholesterol could be due to subclinical hypothyroidism based on the decreasing effect of DPH on the circulating thyroid hormone levels (Mølholm Hansen et al., 1974). An explanation for the transitory increase in triglyceride levels remains at least as obscure as that of cholesterol. The hepatic synthesis could be increased. The action of DPH on the pancreatic beta cells causing an inhibition of insulin release has been considered to play some role (Kizer et al., 1970).

Since the elevated levels of serum lipids, cholesterol and triglycerides, are regarded as a risk factor in relation to atherosclerosis and ischemic heart disease, it seems reasonable to check regularly the serum lipid levels during treatment with DPH.

REFERENCES

1. Jones, A. L., and Amstrong, D. T. (1965): Increased cholesterol biosynthesis, following phenobarbital induced hypertrophy of agranular endoplasmic reticulum in liver. *Proc. Soc. Exp. Biol. Med.,* 119:1136–1139.
2. Kizer, J. S., Vargas-Cordon, M., Brendel, K., and Bressler, R. (1970): The in vitro inhibition of insulin secretion by diphenylhydantoin. *J. Clin. Invest.,* 49:1942–1948.
3. Mølholm Hansen, J., Skovsted, L., Birk Lauridsen, U., Kirkegaard, C., and Siersbaek-Nielsen, K. (1974): The effect of diphenylhydantoin on thyroid function. *J. Clin. Endocrinol. Metab.,* 39:785–789.
4. Redinger, R. N., and Small, D. M. (1973): Primate biliary physiology. VIII. The effect of phenobarbital upon bile salt synthesis and pool size, biliary lipid secretion, and bile composition. *J. Clin. Invest.,* 52:161–172.
5. Reynolds, E. H. (1975): Chronic antiepileptic toxicity: A review. *Epilepsia,* 16:319–352.

Epilepsy, The Eighth International Symposium,
edited by J. K. Penry. Raven Press, New York
© 1977.

Variation of Therapeutic Plasma Concentrations of Phenytoin and Phenobarbital with the Type of Seizure and Co-Medication

D. Schmidt

*Abteilung für Neurologie, Klinikum Charlottenburg, Freie Universitat Berlin, 1000
Berlin 19, Germany*

We reported earlier that the therapeutic plasma concentrations of phenytoin and phenobarbital are related to the severity of epilepsy (Schmidt and Janz, *in press*). Patients who needed high therapeutic concentrations had a more severe form of epilepsy than those with lower therapeutic levels. We called the epilepsy severe when more than four grand mal seizures had occurred previously and/or the seizure-free period was shorter than 1 year in more than 10 years of intensive medical treatment. It is, however, conceivable that other factors, such as the type of seizure, could also determine the severity of epilepsy. Therefore, we studied whether the therapeutic plasma concentrations are different for grand mal seizures as compared to partial seizures. Furthermore, we were interested in determining whether the therapeutic concentration of phenobarbital is independent of co-medication with phenytoin. If co-medication influences the therapeutic level, it would drastically limit the concept of the therapeutic concentration for patients treated with more than one drug.

PATIENTS AND METHODS

Plasma concentrations were estimated by enzyme immunoassay or gas-liquid chromatography in patients with epilepsy receiving phenytoin alone or in combination with other antiepileptic drugs (Schmidt, 1976). The therapeutic plasma concentration was determined in 15 patients with phenytoin alone and in 18 patients with co-medication of phenytoin and primidone by gradually increasing the dose and estimating the steady-state plasma level at which the patient became free of seizures, as described earlier (Schmidt and Janz, *in press*). The seizure-free period for both groups averaged 10.9 and 11.8 times longer, respectively, than the individual interval between seizures in the year prior to complete seizure control. Patients with signs of toxicity were excluded. For complete control of seizures in patients with co-medication, the dose of phenytoin was increased in six patients. Primidone was increased in five patients, and there was no change of dose in seven patients.

RESULTS

The therapeutic concentrations of phenytoin and phenobarbital did not differ significantly with grand mal or partial seizures (mostly complex partial seizures) (Table 1). Of twenty patients with both grand mal and partial seizures, only five needed a higher therapeutic concentration for complete control of partial seizures than for grand mal seizures. In two patients, a 41% higher concentration of phenytoin was necessary. In three patients, partial seizures persisted despite therapeutic levels for grand mal.

TABLE 1. *Therapeutic plasma concentrations after treatment with phenytoin, primidone, or both*

	Plasma concentration (μg/ml)	
Seizure type	Phenytoin	Phenobarbital
Treatment with phenytoin or primidone		
Grand mal	14.3 ± 7.5, $N = 6$	40.1 ± 15.8, $N = 7$
	ns	ns
Partial seizures	17.2 ± 3.9, $N = 10$	39.0 ± 17.0, $N = 8$
Treatment with phenytoin and primidone as compared to primidone alone		
Grand mal and partial seizures	—	39.5 ± 15.9, $N = 15$
Grand mal and partial seizures	17.0 ± 14.2, $N = 18$	26.6 ± 10.2[a], $N = 18$

[a] $p < 0.01$; Student's *t*-test.
The therapeutic plasma concentrations of phenytoin and phenobarbital are similar for grand mal and partial seizures. Co-medication with phenytoin decreases the mean therapeutic concentration of phenobarbital.

It is rather difficult to prove that the therapeutic concentrations were influenced by antiepileptic co-medication. When regarding interpatient differences, one cannot be quite sure that the additional drug is really necessary for complete seizure control unless one reduces it. This has not been done. We chose a different design. We selected patients who were becoming seizure-free with increasing concentrations of either phenytoin or phenobarbital (PB) or both drugs. So it may be concluded that both drugs were necessary for seizure control. With these difficulties in mind, we found that 18 patients needed a significantly lower mean therapeutic level of phenobarbital as derived from primidone when phenytoin was at mean therapeutic levels as previously described for single-drug therapy with phenytoin (Schmidt and Janz, *in press*) (Table 1). Complete seizure control was reached with higher DPH and lower PB levels in six patients; seven patients had lower DPH and higher PB levels; whereas five patients showed higher levels of both drugs as compared to their own subtherapeutic levels.

DISCUSSION

The therapeutic concentrations of phenytoin and phenobarbital were similar for grand mal or partial seizures (Table 1). The therapeutic concentration of phenytoin may differ with the type of seizure in some patients. This obviously presents a limitation for the general use of the concept of therapeutic concentrations. On the positive side, however, it is encouraging that for some patients therapeutic plasma concentrations emerge as an investigative tool to study the epileptic process in its different clinical manifestations.

The possible influence of co-medication on the therapeutic concentration is difficult to prove. One may argue that comparison of two groups of patients implies the danger of comparing epilepsies of varying severity. We found that mean therapeutic levels of phenobarbital are lower with phenytoin co-medication as compared to the levels established by similar criteria in patients on one drug only (Schmidt and Janz, *in press*). A considerable variation of therapeutic levels of phenobarbital and phenytoin in individual patients on co-medication has been shown.

It may be concluded that it is not useful to extrapolate therapeutic concentrations from patients treated with one drug to those on co-medication. This limits the use of this concept for practical clinical purposes as the majority of patients still receive more than one antiepileptic drug. Apart from pharmacokinetic interaction between both drugs, a pharmacodynamic interdependence has to be considered.

REFERENCES

Schmidt, D. (1976): Measurement of diphenylhydantoin and phenobarbital by enzyme immunoassay and gas-liquid chromatography. *J. Neurol.*, 213:41–46.
Schmidt, D., and Janz, D. (1977): Therapeutic plasma concentrations of phenytoin and phenobarbitone. In: *Proceedings of the Third Workshop on the Determination of Antiepileptic Drugs in Body Fluids* (WODADIBOF III) Pitman Medical, London. *(in press)*.

Epilepsy, The Eighth International Symposium,
edited by J. K. Penry. Raven Press, New York
© 1977.

WODADIBOF III: Third International Workshop on the Determination of Antiepileptic Drugs in Body Fluids

Christopher Gardner-Thorpe

Department of Neurology, Royal Devon and Exeter Hospital, Exeter, England

The Third International Workshop on the Determination of Antiepileptic Drugs in Body Fluids was held in Exeter, England, in August, 1976.

In 1972, a group of chemists, pharmacologists, and clinical doctors met in Heemstede, The Netherlands, to discuss the problems they had encountered in the determination of antiepileptic drugs in body fluids. The workshop, which was concerned particularly with methodology, provided the opportunity to resolve problems by discussion rather than by the written word alone.

The 1972 meeting enabled collaboration and friendship to develop, and this opportunity was renewed in 1974 at the second workshop held in Bethel, West Germany, where papers were concerned more particularly with the pharmacology of antiepileptic drugs. At that time, interest had shifted slightly from phenytoin and phenobarbital to carbamazepine, clonazepam, and sodium valproate.

The theme of the third workshop was essentially clinical, although, as on previous occasions, the papers and discussion ranged from methodology and pharmacology to clinical topics.

Thirty-two papers were presented in 2 days. From the philosophical aspects of drug therapy to the use of the EMIT system, quality control schemes, problems of administration, and absorption of antiepileptic drugs, the subjects ranged to animal experiments and the effects of drugs on the electroencephalogram, to long-term monitoring and the choice of single- or multiple-drug therapy, to differences in prescription patterns and in metabolism of drugs in different countries, to interactions, toxicity, and immunoglobulin disturbances.

The wide range of drugs in use in the control of epilepsy in different countries was emphasized, since at least eight drugs (phenytoin, phenobarbital, primidone, carbamazepine, clonazepam, sodium valproate, phensuximide, and methsuximide) were considered in detail. Almost all of the papers were concerned with studies in man.

The following general conclusions may be drawn from the workshop:

1. Gas-liquid chromatography is the most popular method of estimation and generally has supplanted thin-layer chromatography and spectro-

photometry. EMIT is becoming popular on account of its speed and simplicity in use, but it is more expensive.

2. Quality control schemes have contributed significantly to the improvements in techniques of estimation, although financial considerations (of a different kind) are also important in this sphere.

3. Although consideration of protein-binding is important in the research sphere, the methods of analysis generally available are insufficiently precise to encourage the measurement of anything other than the total content of drug in plasma or serum. Salivary studies may be useful, but cerebrospinal fluid studies are of less clinical value.

4. Further advances in knowledge of metabolism in man have been made in the last few years. Ethnic differences also seem to exist.

5. The introduction of methods for the estimation of antiepileptic drugs has led to improved control of seizures in the populations studied. However, the value of monitoring individual patients, except in special circumstances, is harder to quantify.

It would not be appropriate to attempt to summarize further the contributions of individual workers at WODADIBOF III. The proceedings will be published soon and will deal with the three topics—methodology, pharmacology, and clinical aspects.

It is planned that WODADIBOF IV will be held in Sandvika, Norway, in 1979. Prospective participants will be encouraged to take part in a planned research program of topics where the gaps in knowledge of antiepileptic drug therapy seem to be greatest. The semiformal atmosphere of a workshop provides a good forum for the sharing and development of ideas and research.

The WODADIBOF meetings seem to play a useful part in the multidisciplinary evaluation of antiepileptic drug monitoring.

BEHAVIOR MODIFICATION AND REHABILITATION

Epilepsy, The Eighth International Symposium,
edited by J. K. Penry. Raven Press, New York
© 1977.

Behavior Modification and Rehabilitation of Patients with Epilepsy

Olaf Henriksen

Statens Senter for Epilepsi, 1301 Sandvika, Norway

Psychological factors may play an important role in precipitating seizures. This is demonstrated by the observation that seizure frequency often is remarkably reduced after admission to the hospital when the medication is unchanged.

In the following I shall discuss some of the factors producing psychosocial problems and adverse behavior and present some of our experiences in modifying behavior, mainly in children, in our attempt to rehabilitate them.

The common psychosocial problems in patients with epilepsy are often due to the way they were brought up by their parents. We frequently see children who at the age of 3 to 4 years are extremely difficult to handle. They show outbursts of rage, refuse to go to bed, refuse to eat, and complicate all ordinary daily activities. They develop temper tantrums or even go into fits if their demands are not fulfilled. This behavior seems to start early in life because of the uncertainty in the parental attitude. Parents tend to be less firm when bringing up a handicapped child than they are with a normal child. They are apt to spoil the child, but what is more important, they try to avoid anything that may precipitate a seizure or unwished behavior. A child is quick in sensing these things and soon becomes able to rule the parents and the whole home. A vicious circle is created in which the behavior problem can be greater than the seizure problem.

In some cases, however, the psychiatric symptoms and behavior disturbances seem to be directly related to brain damage. This is stated by Rutter et al. (1970) who in their study of the children on the Isle of Wight showed that psychiatric disorders are considerably more common in children with psychomotor fits than in children with other varieties of epilepsy. It is suggested that this is due to a specific neurophysiological mechanism in direct relationship to the epileptogenic lesion of the temporal lobe. Also, when compared with children with chronic physical disorders without brain damage, the children with epilepsy have an increased rate of psychiatric disorders. According to Rutter and his collaborators this is determined by neurological, intellectual, educational, and sociofamilial factors. Although specifically neurological symptoms to some extent are responsible for the development of emotional and behavior disorders, the authors stress that the psychological factors associated with psychiatric disorders in children with epilepsy largely are the same as in children in general. The mechanisms involved in the development of psychiatric disorders are probably similar in both groups.

Our experience is in agreement with this. Like Rutter et al. (1970), we find (Fossen Daae et al., 1971) no specific syndromes in the group of children with epilepsy. The fact, however, that the child has its handicap and the parents constantly feel the threat of an oncoming seizure increases the chances that the parents give up against the child's normal testing out. This special relationship between the child who has epilepsy and his parents may be one of the reasons why these children have a greater susceptibility to psychiatric disorders.

Still it is an open question why children with psychomotor epilepsy are found to have a high rate of psychiatric disorder, as stated by many authors (Nuffield, 1961; Ounsted et al., 1966; Rutter et al., 1970). A neurophysiological mechanism seems most likely, but states of partial consciousness so typical of psychomotor seizures may well be more psychologically threatening to a child than a total loss of consciousness. Rejecting attitudes from those associated with the patient may also be strong when people do not recognize that he is unaware of what he is doing.

The effect of antiepileptic drugs is another factor of importance. There is evidence that various types of behavioral disturbances may occur from the use of antiepileptic medication. Well known is the symptom of hyperactivity in children treated with phenobarbital. Occasionally, psychiatric reactions are provoked by benzodiazepines. Special behavior disturbances are also seen in connection with phenytoin intoxication. High doses of phenobarbital may cause considerable behavioral disturbances. Sporadic cases of psychotic reactions may also be seen during treatment with most antiepileptic drugs. An exception is perhaps carbamazepine, which probably is the anticonvulsant that most persistently has been given credit for a positive psychotropic effect. In spite of several works on this topic, this still remains to be proved. Although it is generally agreed that the behavioral disturbances are reversible, Valerta et al. (1974) assert that serious deterioration associated with chronic phenytoin intoxication may be irreversible. It is evident that our knowledge of psychopharmacology of antiepileptic drugs is unsatisfactory because of inadequate and unsophisticated reporting of behavioral change and because of the common problem of polypharmacy. More accurate observations are needed on less heterogenous groups of patients.

Factors that may cause psychiatric disorders in connection with epilepsy are shown in Table 1.

The factors indirectly responsible for the psychiatric disorders are mostly related to the organic brain lesion and treatment with anticonvulsant drugs. It is therefore difficult to keep the two groups apart. Most of the factors in the second group would have a strong psychological effect on any human being —young or old, epilepsy or no epilepsy.

In handling children with epilepsy and psychiatric disorders, it is usually impossible to evaluate the organic factors exactly. A thorough diagnostic evaluation of both the neurological deficits and the psychological symptoms is impor-

TABLE 1. *Factors that may cause psychiatric disorders in patients with epilepsy*

I. Direct
  1. Organic brain lesion
    Depending on: Type of lesion
                  Location
                  Extent
                  Multiple locations
                  Epileptogenic activity
  2. Anticonvulsant drugs
    Depending on: Side effects
                  Intoxication
II. Indirect
    Psychological effects of the interation between patient and environment
    Caused by: Low IQ
              Retarded language
              Retarded reading—dyslexia
              Physical handicaps
              Having fits
              Side effects of drugs
              Family problems
              School problems
              Vocational problems
              Marital problems

tant, and adequate treatment must be given whenever possible. After treatment with anticonvulsant drugs has been started, it may be most rewarding to treat the psychiatric problems. To demonstrate this I would like to present a case report on a 4-year-old girl who was admitted to us with a behavior disorder as her main problem.

This girl was the youngest of five siblings. Without known etiology she had her first epileptic attack—a grand mal seizure—when she was 7 months old. In spite of antiepileptic medication her epilepsy developed into a severe form, the EEG indicating hypsarrhythmia. She was successfully treated with ACTH and had no great seizure problem when admitted to us. Grand mal seizures were provoked by fever only occasionally. For more than a year she had been treated with primodine and phenytoin. It was obvious to the parents that her language was retarded, while she seemed intelligent and adequate otherwise for her age. She could say only a few words at the age of 4 and went into a rage when she was not understood. Her behavior had become increasingly problematic. She refused to cooperate in daily activities such as getting dressed, eating her meals, and going to bed. She was mentally strong and persistent and could scream for hours, day or night, and bang her head if her demands were not met. The whole family, but especially her parents, were completely exhausted and at a loss in bringing up the child.

On admittance, no neurological symptoms were found except for her retarded language, which she seemed aware of and which frustrated her. The EEG was within normal limits. We kept the parents in the hospital for a week and had daily sessions in the kindergarten with the child and the parents. Together with the psychologist, our experienced preschool teacher guided the parents in the handling of their child. She was met with a consistent attitude from the whole staff. Negative behavior was neglected and positive behavior rewarded. After several weeks in the hospital the child calmed down and was easier to handle. We could then concentrate more on the organic factor—the dysphasia. Eventually her language improved during the treatment given by the speech therapist. She became seizure-free by adjusting the original medication to adequate levels, and she was discharged 2 years later with the same medication. Her behavior had been greatly improved, and today the child is living at home, has developed a language, and attends normal school.

That the relationship between child and parents played a great role in producing the secondary psychiatric problems was demonstrated in this case when she went home on vacation after functioning well in the hospital for many months. She took up her previous behavior and reigned over her parents as before. Breaking the old pattern was a long and hard process for the parents.

This case illustrates a child with speech retardation caused by an organic brain lesion and with tremendous secondary behavioral problems that eventually dominated the whole clinical picture.

Probably her epileptic seizures initially made the parents surrender to the child's behavior. Before starting treatment of the main problem—the dysphasia—it was necessary to reduce the behavior problems. Only then was it possible to evaluate the degree of organic speech therapy required. Initially it was impossible to quantify the importance of the organic brain lesion. This also was found to be of less importance as one proceeded with psychotherapy. This case demonstrates that it is not necessarily the epileptic brain lesion as such which causes a psychiatric disorder, but a complicated mixture of factors. The case report stresses what we feel is a general rule: the secondary—psychological—disturbances will be the most rewarding to treat, and only if this is done can the patient receive the full benefit from other types of treatment.

In the adult population of patients with epilepsy, the factors contributing to behavior problems are about the same. In addition, the chance of brain damage caused by repetitive seizures is greater and this may cause progressive dementia and secondary psychosocial problems. The side effects of long-standing medication may play a great role. Finally, the psychological influence of the society's reactions toward "an epileptic" is enhanced by rejection from family and friends, inability to get a job, and the epileptic's the frightful Democles' sword of knowing that wherever he is, he may suddenly pass out and do things that are out of his control.

Many authors have dealt with the psychosocial problems of patients with epilepsy. Through the years there have been different opinions concerning the "epileptic personality." In the last decades, however, there seems to have been general agreement that most people with epilepsy have normal personality and intellect; there is no specific epileptic character. It seems adequate today to quote Guerrant et al. (1962) who say that if defects of personality or intellect do occur, they may vary from one person to another, and they are due to one or more of the following factors: (1) structural brain disease, (2) uncontrolled seizures, (3) anticonvulsant drugs, or (4) psychological reactions to family and social isolation and rejection.

It is necessary to stress again that defects of personality or intellect do occur more frequently in patients with epilepsy than in the normal population. Rutter et al. (1970) found five times as many children with psychiatric disturbances in the epilepsy group compared to the control group.

There seems to be less agreement as to whether patients with psychomotor epilepsy have a higher incidence of psychiatric disorders than those with the remaining types of epilepsies. Rutter et al. (1970) and Gudmundsson (1966) in their materials consisting of children and adults, respectively, all found twice as many cases with psychiatric disorders in the group with temporal lobe epilepsy as in those with the other types of epilepsy. This has been challenged by Small et al. (1962) who suggest that there are few if any differences between patients with psychomotor epilepsy and other adult epileptics. Guerrant et al. (1962) failed to prove a higher incidence of psychiatric problems in the group with psychomotor epilepsy. In their work in 1958 Vislie and Henriksen concluded that the extent rather than the site of the lesion had a greater influence on psychiatric disturbances.

The consequence of these data is that a substantial group of patients with epilepsy are multiproblem cases. In Norway we have a population of approximately 4 million, and we estimate that about 16,000 have active epilepsy (Krohn, 1961). About 25% of these, i.e., 4,000, live outside institutions—integrated in the society—but more or less incapacitated by psychosocial problems. Mainly patients from this group are referred to the Epilepsy Center in Sandvika, the only one if its kind in Norway. It should be stressed that about 60% of the patients with active epilepsy function well in society (Krohn, 1961). During the last decade neurological as well as pediatric and psychiatric services have been strengthened throughout the country. This means that the patients now referred to us represent the most difficult of the 4,000 multiproblem cases. We receive a select group of patients with a high percentage of severe brain damage and an even higher percentage of psychosocial problems. This is confirmed by the following data concerning 100 consecutive discharges from our pediatric department. Data on etiology and neurological diagnostic work have been left out, since our goal was to show how much one can achieve through milieu therapy and family therapy combined with drug therapy.

Of the 100 patients, 5 were younger than 3 years, and the rest were between 3 and 15 years old. The intellectual capacity was within normal range in 23% of the patients, whereas the remaining 77% were more or less mentally retarded. In addition to seizure problems, the children had behavior disturbances and

TABLE 2. *Result of medical treatment and milieu therapy of 100 children with epilepsy*

	Unchanged	Moderate but definite improvement	Marked improvement
Seizure problems	29	31	40
Behavior disturbances and character disorders	33	24	43
Family problems	14	35	51
School problems	39	23	38

character disorders, family problems, and school problems. Of the 100 patients, 82 had a serious seizure problem whereas 18 had a slight or no seizure problem. Only 10 had an intact character and no behavior problem. All 100 had family problems and 90 had school problems.

The results of treatment were assessed at the time of discharge by several members of the team. A remarkable improvement was found in all four groups (Table 2).

These figures show clearly how rewarding it can be to direct the therapy on all four problem categories. Even in the most severe cases improvement in several aspects was seen.

Often vicious circles develop in which the seizures trigger the family problems, the family problems induce behavior problems and character disturbances, which often cause school problems, and these secondary problems may provoke more seizures.

Treatment of any of these factors may have a positive influence on the other factors. We find that most of our patients have developed such serious secondary symptoms that the symptoms do not disappear by treatment of the seizures only. The secondary problems have become independent, self-sufficient. In our group of severely handicapped children in which all four types of problems were attacked, improved behavior and rehabilitation as well as reduction of the seizure problem were achieved.

These results are obtained by teamwork between people from many professions. The multiprofessional team attached to each of our two pediatric units with 20 children each consists of eight nurses, ten nurse-aids, three maids, one preschool teacher, two preschool teacher's assistants, one psychologist, and one physician. One speech therapist, one social worker, and one physiotherapist are shared between the two units.

We do not apply behavior modification therapy in the current meaning of the word, but use rather a great variety of techniques adjusted to each case after a thorough diagnostic work-up. This diagnostic work is also the result of teamwork between the nursing staff, the teachers, the psychologist, and the physician. At the weekly staff meetings plans are made for each child to help him with his main problems. Social training in the broadest sense of the word often plays an important role. In some cases individual psychotherapy is needed and in other cases individual therapy by both the psychologist and the physiotherapist or the speech therapist may be beneficial.

An important part of the therapy is the evaluation by specially trained teachers, since a child may be relieved of many problems if an adequate school situation can be arranged. Of the greatest importance, however, is to establish a good contact with the parents. All parents need information and counseling, and often it is necessary to have frequent sessions with them. If the patients live far away, they may come and stay at the hospital for a week or more for intensive family therapy. This is time consuming for the staff but always very rewarding.

When a child is discharged, a follow-up at home is always necessary. Our information to the home milieu is of the greatest importance. Teachers and other people of importance for the patient in his local milieu are sometimes called to the hospital for staff meetings, or some of the staff members may visit the home. On such visits opportunities are used to spread information about epilepsy.

More than half of the people with active epilepsy are able to function in their jobs. Krohn (1961) has investigated factors related to vocational problems: only 35% of the patients with normal IQ and serious behavior problems were able to work, although 71% of those with frequent intractable seizures but normal IQ and no behavior problems were able to work. This demonstrates that behavior problems may be more incapacitating than the seizures. It is therefore important not only to treat the seizures with anticonvulsant drugs but also to treat the behavior problems. In the adult group this treatment will follow very much the same principles as are used with children. In addition, many patients need vocational training and rehabilitation, which in Sandvika is taken care of by a specialized team. Time does not allow me to discuss this important part of the treatment.

Some psychotherapeutic methods of breaking the vicious circles have been mentioned. It is not possible to give a complete survey of this complicated matter. For instance, I will not discuss neurosurgery or the techniques of biofeedback. However, one important method in behavior modification cannot be left out, namely, treatment with anticonvulsant drugs. Successful drug treatment making the patient seizure-free may abolish the secondary psychosocial problems. Even moderate reduction of seizure frequency may diminish the secondary problems. Cases with intractable seizures, however, may require high dosages of a combination of several drugs, which may create additional problems of side effects and intoxication. Such side effects as psychiatric disturbances, lethargy, and reduced mental capacity are too often seen. Gingival hyperplasia and hirsutism may cause secondary psychiatric symptoms. Thus side effects may cause more secondary problems than the seizures themselves, and in many cases it is preferable to have some seizures rather than the intolerable "behavior modification" of being over-drugged.

We have seen remarkable improvement of behavior after switching from a complicated medication to a simple one consisting of sodium valproate only.

A 12-year-old boy was discharged after 4 months in our neuropediatric ward. In spite of treatment with all available drugs, his seizures, which started at the age of 4, persisted. For the preceding couple of years he had been incapacitated by frequent grand mal seizures as well as severe side effects from his complex medication. His behavior disturbances were progressive, creating problems intolerable for all the members of the family. The year before his admission, his problems were so great that he could not attend school and had to have private lessons at home. On admittance he was dull, lethargic, and mentally retarded with behavior disturbances and a disagreeable character. He had frequent grand mal seizures when he was started on sodium valproate. After 3 weeks he was seizure-free, and all other drugs were stopped. The EEG became normal, and the patient improved in all aspects. The lethargy disappeared and he became more interested and sociable, and eventually was a popular patient. His school performance improved, and on psychological tests (WISC) the verbal IQ increased from 66 to 84, and the performance IQ increased from 58 to 76 (comparison done with the psychological test performed 2½ years prior to admittance). When he was home on vacation he was like a new boy, and the behavior and family problems were greatly reduced. He was discharged after we found an adequate school for him and arranged an appointment with the local child psychiatry services.

SUMMARY

I will again draw attention to the list of factors contributing to psychiatric problems in patients with epilepsy (see Table 1). All these factors are important, but in various degree from case to case. The group of patients is heterogenous, and the number of factors multiple with a complicated interaction. It is therefore difficult to find any specific correlation between the primary and secondary factors and the behavior disorder.

In conclusion, I want to stress that after a neurological diagnosis and work-up, information and prophylactic guidance should be given together with adequate medication. It is important to remember that about 25% of the patients with epilepsy have or will develop psychosocial problems for which they will need help from a multiprofessional team.

REFERENCES

Fossen Daae, A., Ringstad Fossum, T., and Munthe-Kaas, A. W. (1971): Psykologiske aspekter ved barne-epilepsi. *Nord. Psykiatr. Tidsskr.,* 25:440–447.

Gudmundsson, G. (1966): Epilepsy in Iceland. *Acta Neurol. Scand.* [*Suppl.*], 25:43.

Guerrant, J., Anderson, W. W., Fischer, A., Weinstein, M. R., Jaros, R. M., and Deskins, A. (1962): *Personality in Epilepsy.* Charles C. Thomas, Springfield, Ill.

Krohn, W. (1961): A study of epilepsy in Northern Norway, its frequency and character. *Acta Psychiatr. Neurol. Scand.* [*Suppl. 150*], 36:215–225.

Nuffield, E. J. (1961): Neurophysiology and behaviour disorders in epileptic children. *J. Ment. Sci.,* 107:438–458.

Ounsted, C., Lindsay, J., and Norman, R. (1966): *Biological Factors in Temporal Lobe Epilepsy.* Clinics in Developmental Medicine No. 22. The Spastics Society Medical Education and Information Unit in association with W. Heinemann, London.

Rutter, M., Graham, P., and Yule, W. (1970): *A Neuropsychiatric study in Childhood.* Lavenham Press Ltd., Lavenham, Suffolk.

Small, J. G., Milstein, V., and Stevens, J. R. (1962): Are psychomotor epileptics different? *Arch. Neurol.*, 7:187–294.

Valerta, J. M., Bell, D. B., and Reichert, A. (1974): Progressive encephalopathy due to chronic hydantoin intoxication. *Am. J. Dis. Child.*, 128:27.

Vislie, H., and Henriksen, G. F. (1958): Psychic disturbances in epileptics. In: *Lectures on Epilepsy,* edited by A. M. Lorentz de Haas Elsevier, Amsterdam.

Epilepsy, The Eighth International Symposium,
edited by J. K. Penry. Raven Press, New York
© 1977.

Psychological Intervention with Parents of Children with Epilepsy

J. Clausen

Clinical Psychologist, Statens Center for Epilepsy, Sandvika, Norway

As Dr. Henriksen pointed out in his chapter, there is a close connection between the attitudes and insight of parents and their children's possibility to develop optimally according to their resources. This applies to all children, but is more important when a given child has more than the usual obstacles to struggle with.

I will touch only briefly on what kinds of parent-child relations may be problematic, and then describe some of the approaches we use at the State Center for Epilepsy in Norway.

Parents who have a child with a handicap are usually afraid that their handling of the child may do additional harm to the child. They often find that they receive too little help and support in this area. Paradoxically, parents of children with medium-sized handicaps may feel this stronger than parents of severely handicapped children.

Insecurity in the parents may be coupled with feelings of guilt, aggression, resentment, or even repulsion. The time does not allow me to go into details here, and I will talk about the parents of children with epilepsy as one group, even if this is a simplification.

When a child enters one of our pediatric wards, we always have some kind of contact with the parents. I will now describe the minimum amount of contact the families receive at the ward. As the child is admitted, one or preferably both of the parents accompany the child. Then they go through the anamnestic interviews with the physician, the social worker, the teacher, and the psychologist. For the psychologist it is important then to form an impression of the parents' attitudes toward the child—special reactions to the first seizure, to the diagnosis of epilepsy, etc.

Normally the parent stays at the hospital for 4 to 7 days if the child is 4 years old or older. If the child is younger, we like the parent to remain with the child during the whole stay if possible.

During the parents' stay they are encouraged to be present at the ward and have contact with the nurses and the nurses' aides, to inform the staff of the daily habits of the child, and also to observe how the staff handles seizures and behavioral problems.

This is repeated during visits—and as the time of discharge approaches.

Through this we have ample opportunity to get to know the parents and vice versa. This enables the parents to listen to our advice on different problems. If emotional security is not instilled in the parents, any kind of lasting effect of treatment is impossible. We must realize that when we tell parents how to treat their children, we are dangerously near threatening their self-esteem.

Therefore, the procedure described above in many instances is not sufficient. Often there is need for more directly problem solving and therapeutically oriented intervention.

I will now describe a procedure that we have found useful with parents whose relationship with their child severely decreases the child's chances of development and severely influences the family patterns.

In these cases we have the parents—both if at all possible—stay at the hospital for 1 week. It is prearranged that the parents accompany the child most of the day in the ward, in school or kindergarten, and to any other appointment the child has. In all these situations the different members of the staff are instructed to show the parents how they deal with difficult situations. They convey to the parents their understanding of the child and help the parents to be able to try alternative behavior toward the child. In addition, the psychologist talks with the parents at least once each day. The parents' reactions to the different situations can then be brought forth and discussed. It is extremely important that the psychologist is informed by the staff about significant episodes or that one of the staff is present because we often see resistance in parents against exposing their difficulties. This must be understood in close relation to their despair over their handicapped child, their feelings of helplessness and shortcomings as parents. Therefore, it is important to help the parents expose their feelings and deal with them. Afterwards, the parents can try new ways of handling the problems and can come back and discuss their success or failure. We are then able to start a process, and it is important that the parents can develop ideas, try them, discuss them, formulate new ideas, etc.

The parents' resistance to change is sometimes so great that new learning can not take place. In these instances we have to treat this problem first and only afterwards is it possible to change the parents' behavior toward their children.

The procedures described have been tried with several parents and have proved useful. Our experience shows that this method has more lasting effect than if our contact with the parents has not been as systematic and intensive as described.

We often see that families that have a child with behavioral problems become enmeshed in vicious circles and their problems increase if left untreated. We do not know if the child always is the cause of the family difficulties because we see, as in family therapy in general, that the family pattern is dependent on mutual interaction among the family members, and the symptom bearer is often the one referred to us.

The procedures described are of course costly of time and resources; nevertheless, we find they are of such great value that they are justified. As this kind of counseling also contains much general enlightenment on child-rearing problems, we believe that it may prevent some problems for younger siblings.

If problems are deep rooted, the above-described program will not be sufficient alone. It may still be of value, but in addition other kinds of psychotherapy are required depending on the possibilities and kinds of problems.

What has been said so far relates only to patients who are admitted in the State Center for Epilepsy in Sandvika. The children admitted there usually have had previous contact with health services and usually have serious problems in more than one area of functioning. It is of great importance to contact the parents at an early stage to prevent the development of some of the problems we meet in Sandvika.

For this reason several of the professional groups in Sandvika take an active part in parent courses arranged by a humanitarian organization. These courses last for 2 weeks, and all the expenses including travel are paid by the organization (with state support). During the last few years fathers have begun to participate in these courses, but the majority are mothers. The fathers who lose wages for this time have this loss covered by the social security system.

The mother or parents bring the child with epilepsy, and the children are taken care of when the parents attend the course. The content of the course is related to the many different sides of epilepsy, such as somatic, social, educational, vocational, and psychological aspects. The lectures are relatively short with plenty of time for questions and answers afterwards.

The parents are divided into groups of six to eight. These groups are under the leadership of a psychologist or a social worker. The groups meet for four sessions and the parents are encouraged to tell each other about their difficulties and frustrations and also their successes and pleasures.

These group sessions often allow the participants to talk frankly about their feelings toward the child for the first time, and they have a chance to be listened to and taken seriously. Many of the parents we meet in these courses feel that nobody else has the same kinds of problems as they, and to experience that this is not so is of great importance. We often find that after participating in such a course many parents become active initiative-takers in the local branches of the League Against Epilepsy.

I do not have time to go into more detail on these courses. Dr. Henriksen has pointed out the importance of visiting the home milieu. We find that parents behave more naturally and feel more secure when we visit them in their natural surroundings than when they visit the hospital. The child is in his natural environment, and it is of great value for the total assessment to make an observation under these conditions. Obviously, contact must have been established before the visit if the feeling of an inspection visit is to be avoided.

To sum up, then, I claim that psychological intervention with the parents is imperative in the treatment of children with epilepsy. We have seen in Sandvika that it is impossible to rely on somatic treatment alone for many of our child patients.

It would be preferable to be able to engage more in prophylactic work with parents. We know that parents who receive news that their child is mentally retarded, has physical handicaps, or both experience a shock reaction. During this phase their feelings should be uncovered, be allowed to be felt, and be worked through. In this way it may be possible for the parents to deal with their own reactions instead of freezing them. This kind of work should not be limited to an epilepsy center—or any other center—but should be a natural and evident part of any pediatric hospital or ward.

Epilepsy, The Eighth International Symposium,
edited by J. K. Penry. Raven Press, New York
© 1977.

Behavior Therapy for Seizure Control

D. I. Mostofsky

Department of Psychology, Boston University, Boston, Massachusetts

"It is a truism that the mind does not exist apart from the brain, yet the practice of categorizing diseases as 'neurological' and 'psychiatric' suggests otherwise" (Pincus and Tucker, 1974).

Throughout the various discussions on epilepsy there is embedded the surfacing suggestion that environmental conditions external to the epileptogenic tissue may be a major source of potentiating the seizure disorder. In support of this thesis, anecdotal reports abound, and the reports include descriptions of unusual circumstances where seizures are triggered and situations where seizures rarely occur. For the most part, both medical and mental health specialists have tended to restrict their concern to the sequelae—the profound personal and interpersonal disturbances—which seizure disorders frequently create. Only infrequently have there been serious attempts to directly control or modulate seizure problems by any form of psychotherapy or behavior modification.

THE VARIETY OF TECHNIQUES

At the outset, it is reasonable to assume that any of the standard techniques developed as part of the general armamentarium in behavior modification may be applied to the control of seizure disorders. In general, this assumption seems to obtain. The various reports of therapeutic procedures (subsuming 12 procedural or technique strategies) appear to be clustered into three major distinct categories. For the most part, these designations represent styles, formats, and qualitatively describable orientations rather than rigorously definable differences, either in operation or in theoretical implication. The categories represent, at best, convenient frames of reference for describing the *therapist's* activities and *presumed rationale* for reducing the seizure disorder. Most often, the classifications are not mutually exclusive of one another; indeed, it is not uncommon to incorporate more than a single category of procedure in a given therapy program.

I. Reward Management: Protocols 1 Through 6

1. Denial of reward. When praise, attention, etc. are commonplace, this paradigm requires that the occurrence of a seizure is not followed by a display of care, concern, or attention. The seizure is ignored—as one might ignore some other undesirable behavior such as a tantrum—and the expectation is for continued nonrecognition of this behavior to lead to its extinction.

2. Penalty program. In this procedure, when the patient has a seizure he is asked to enter a "time-out room" or "special-care ward," an environment in which he does not have access to reinforcement. Rather than the passive approach of ignoring the behavior, this procedure requires that the observer intervene and react to the patient. In an institutional setting this may involve moving a patient from an open ward setting to a less open setting or denying the patient visits or off-ground privileges. In a home or school setting with a child this might take the form of denying the child a recess period, a favorite game, or activity. It is explained to the patient that such action is being taken so that he will no longer be in any danger, and when his condition improves he will be able to return to his previous situation (to the open ward or to a particular activity).

3. Relief (avoidance) program. In this procedure an aversive stimulus, such as shock or putrid medicine, is administered and is continued until the subject demonstrates a reduction in either the clinical or electrical manifestations of the seizures.

4. Punishment program. In this program a seizure is immediately followed by the administration of a noxious stimulus. This may take the form of shouting at the patient, using overcorrection, administering an annoying electric shock, or presenting an unpleasant noise or flash of light.

5. Overt reward program. Following totally seizure-free periods or following a particular time period in which there is a significant decrease in seizure rate, rewards or tokens are administered. For example, starting at 10-min intervals, praise, tokens, or privileges are administered providing that no seizure occurs. The criterion time is gradually extended to hours and days. Another method is to set a goal for the maximum number of seizures per day. If the goal is met, the patient receives the specified reward. The criterion is gradually set at lower numbers of seizures for the particular patient.

6. Covert reward program. Seizure-provoking and non-seizure-provoking scenes are suggested to the patient while he is in a relaxed state. These scenes are immediately followed by imagined scenes of appropriate reward and nonreward. No tangible token, privilege, praise, or punishment is given; only the imagined representation is suggested to the patient.

II. Self-Control: Protocols 7 Through 10

7. Relaxation. The patient is instructed in progressive muscle relaxation, without any added overt rewards, and is told to induce the relaxation whenever stress or prescience of the seizure appears.

8. Desensitization/hypnosis. While relaxed, the patient is instructed to visualize or think of seizure-provoking scenes.

9. Traditional (dynamic) psychotherapy. The patient is seen in group or one-to-one traditional psychotherapy sessions and is given guidance to understand

and to combat underlying anxieties and conflicts, and he is supported to resolve them at a conscious level.

10. Self-control. This category includes a variety of techniques often developed by patients themselves, which they feel are helpful in preventing a seizure, diminishing its severity, or stopping the seizure once it has begun. Examples include a patient's report that she shakes her head vigorously from side to side to stop a seizure. Some patients report that by concentrating and "trying to talk themselves out of having the seizure" they can prevent one by saying such things as, "Oh no, I am not going to have a seizure," or "You can't get the best of me."

III. Psychophysiological Techniques: Protocols 11 and 12

11. Habituation or extinction. When seizures are sensory precipitated (e.g., trigger sensitivity to light flash), the stimulus is presented below threshold and the intensity or frequency is gradually increased until the stimulus loses its evocative capability.

12. Biofeedback. The patient is instructed to generate a bioelectric pattern or waveform. Correct matches are appropriately fed back or are actively rewarded (e.g., by a light or sound signal or even monetary rewards) or punished (e.g., by a slight electric shock).

The preceding list of treatment techniques is not meant to be an exhaustive list of possible therapeutic tactics; rather, it represents a summary of the different procedures that have already been reported as successful in the management of seizure disorders. In addition, the separate programs or procedures are not intended to suggest that they need be mutually exclusive. It is not unusual for more than one of these techniques to be used serially or concurrently with the same patient. In addition, one cannot exclude the possibility that elements such as progressive relaxation or reward and punishment *always* accompany any behavioral program. The labels for this taxonomy were chosen to convey as clearly as possible the particular essence, art, and style of the procedures, and they are not meant to provide a rationale for technical definition or assumptions about any underlying theory.

SOME THEORETICAL SPECULATIONS ON THE DYNAMICS OF SEIZURE CONTROL

There is compelling evidence that epileptic seizures are not easily explained simply by invoking the presence of scarred neuronal tissue or an improper biochemical environment. The problem has been eloquently stated by Rodin (1968, p. 343):

> The great majority of neurophysiological and neurochemical investigations still deal with the "epileptic focus" or the properties of the "epileptogenic neuron." These are important studies, but they are likely to be insufficient in providing the final answer to the problem. [One should also ask] What are the factors that are responsible for

the spread of abnormal electrical activity in this particular patient? Even more important would be the question: How does the patient's condition differ on the five days of the week when he is seizure-free from that of the sixth day when he has an attack?

This review tried to organize the various attempts involving an engineering of the patient's environment which are designed to control seizures through behavioral interventions. If the results are convincing, as I think they are, they reassert the role of psychosomatic mechanisms in central nervous system functioning. To be sure, the presumed underlying causal agents may indeed be only accidentally related to the assumptions that underlie the stated procedures and techniques. At least three such possibilities of pseudo-treatment can be considered: (1) placebo effects; (2) biorhythmic effects; and (3) spurious, contaminated, and insufficient data.

Perhaps the loudest cry against the validity of the behavior therapies is raised when EEG data do not confirm a diagnosis of seizures. One reply is that even if seizures are not real, they are of serious concern to the patient and to the physician, and often result in additional and unnecessary medication. Also, a definable percentage of the "normal" population is found to have EEG abnormalities and does not suffer from seizure disorders, and it is not at all uncommon to hear reports of an improved clinical picture while the EEG seems to deteriorate, or the converse. In short, the dictum to treat the patient, not the EEG, pointedly reminds one that the EEG must be evaluated as one of the many measures in the total perspective of the patient's symptomatic profile.

But, as Melzack (1975) has noted, there remains the need to satisfy other criteria before an experimental research protocol can be regarded as a valuable, ethical, and preferred therapeutic procedure, viz.: a demonstration that (1) the effect of the treatment procedure is greater than the placebo effect; (2) the therapy produces changes of sufficient magnitude and duration to have clinical significance; (3) the procedure is transferable from the laboratory or hospital milieu to the normal day-to-day environment; (4) once acquired, the effect lasts long enough to be meaningful. In varying degrees these criteria are in fact satisfied, as this review has shown. To be sure, our acquaintance with "what works" and under which conditions anything works best is fragmentary and incomplete, but the implications for theory development in both behavior and neurophysiology are powerful indeed.

SUMMARY

The empirical evidence, viewed even with the strongest conservatism, suggests much promise for the application of behavioral treatment protocols in epilepsy therapy. The greatest gain would be expected with those patients who are experiencing many and severely disrupting seizures and for whom surgery is not possible and/or for whom pharmacological management has proven ineffective. It is quite likely that even among the more normative and "controlled" seizure patients, relief from seizures and potential reduction of anticonvulsant drug dependency may be realized by such adjunct treatment programs. These findings can be completely contained in existing theory. But more important, they may provide the basis for refining and extending behavior theory and neurophysiological hypotheses and thereby enable a better appreciation of the age-old pathophysiology which is epilepsy and its imbrication with the behavioral sciences.

The modern expression of these views is evident in Forster's (1967) summary of his pioneering and important studies: "We believe that the area of physiology opened by Ivan Petrovich Pavlov is pertinent and relevant to the field of epilepsy, and that there is a need to take a longer and harder look at these psychophysiological processes in epilepsy."

ACKNOWLEDGMENTS

I am indebted to my colleague Barbara Balaschak for the sustained support of our clinical efforts and for her contributions to this chapter, which will appear as part of an expanded critical review ("Psychobiological Control of Seizures," D. Mostofsky and B. Balaschak, *Psychological Bulletin,* July, 1977). I also acknowledge the support of Cesare Lombroso, who has been responsible for much of the development of our Behavioral Neurology Program at The Children's Hospital Medical Center in Boston.

REFERENCES

Forster, F. M. (1967): Conditional reflex therapy in epilepsy. *Georg. Med. Bull.,* 21:69–76.
Melzack, R. (1975): The promise of biofeedback: Don't hold the party yet. *Psychol. Today,* 9:22–81.
Pincus, J. H., and Tucker, G. J. (1974): *Behavioral Neurology.* Oxford University Press, New York.
Rodin, E. A. (1968): *Prognosis of Patients with Epilepsy.* Charles C Thomas, Springfield, Ill.

Epilepsy, The Eighth International Symposium,
edited by J. K. Penry. Raven Press, New York
© 1977.

Behavior Disturbance and Type of Epilepsy in Children Attending Ordinary School

G. Stores

University Department of Psychiatry, and Park Hospital for Children, Oxford, England

Above-average rates of disturbed behavior have consistently been reported in people with epilepsy both in childhood and during adult life. Most studies, however, have been carried out on selected groups of patients attending specialized centers. The Isle of Wight survey (Rutter et al., 1970) was unusual in attempting to screen a whole population of children but, although the findings in that study confirmed that children with epilepsy tend to be more disturbed than their nonepileptic counterparts, no real attempt was made to discover how this generalization might apply to the different types of childhood epilepsy.

Among the few investigations in which this question has been considered, one preliminary study carried out some years ago by Nuffield (1961) did suggest that, of epileptic children seen in a neuropsychiatric center, those with 3/sec spike-and-wave EEG patterns were characteristically shy, retiring, or neurotic, whereas others with temporal lobe abnormalities tended to be aggressive. More recently, Flor-Henry (1972) has argued that different patterns of behavior are seen in adult patients with temporal lobe lesions depending on which hemisphere is primarily affected. The present study was designed to measure various aspects of behavior in a relatively unselected group of schoolchildren with epilepsy made up of four separate EEG subgroups.

PATIENTS AND METHODS

From a 3-year series of records in the EEG Department of the Park Hospital for Children in Oxford, a group was compiled which consisted of 70 children with epilepsy who were still of school age between the years 1973 and 1975. Each child had undergone several recordings over a varying period of time, allowing the characteristic EEG features to be defined. Most of these children were under the care of pediatricians in Oxfordshire and neighboring counties, and few had been referred for specialized neurological or psychiatric assessment. To minimize the possible behavioral effects of low intelligence or other handicaps leading to special education, we confined the study to children attending ordinary state primary or secondary schools.

This total epileptic group was made up of the following four subgroups defined

245

in terms of the type of EEG abnormality shown in repeat recordings usually over a period of years:

1. A *3/sec spike-and-wave* subgroup ($N = 17$) including children whose EEGs consistently contained bursts of generalized, relatively well-organized, bilaterally synchronous spike-and-wave activity of about 3 cps without focal spike discharges in any recording.
2. An *irregular spike-and-wave* subgroup ($N = 17$) with recurrent bursts of generalized, bisynchronous, but poorly organized spike-and-wave activity without focal spike discharges in any recording.
3. A *right temporal spike* subgroup ($N = 16$) in which a consistent spike focus was seen in the temporal or immediately adjacent areas of the right hemisphere.
4. A *left temporal spike* subgroup ($N = 20$) consisting of children with a persistent spike focus in the temporal or nearby areas of the left hemisphere.

These subgroups were similar in age (mean age 10.1 to 11.3 years), and all four contained about equal numbers of boys and girls.

For comparison, 103 nonepileptic children were studied, all of whom were also attending local state primary or secondary school and, like the epileptic children, whose backgrounds represented the whole socioeconomic range.

Each child's behavior at school was assessed by means of Connors' Teacher Rating Scale (Connors, 1969). This consists of 39 items of disturbed behavior at school which are rated by the teacher as applying in varying degrees to each child. The scale has a high degree of test-retest reliability and has been shown to consist of the following five factors (Werry et al., 1975): (1) conduct problem (or antisocial behavior), (2) anxiety, (3) inattention, (4) overactivity, and (5) social isolation from other children.

The scale was completed by the teachers for every child in the study. From the ratings on individual items, one can derive scores for each child on each of these five factors. Comparisons were made of these factor scores between the nonepileptic children and the epileptic group or subgroup. Chi-squares were calculated from 2×2 contingency tables which showed the number of epileptic children scoring at or below the median score or above the median score of the nonepileptic group.

RESULTS

When the epileptic children as a whole were compared with the nonepileptic group of children, the former were found to be significantly more anxious and inattentive ($p < 0.001$ in both cases) but not significantly different from the nonepileptic children in other respects.

Each EEG subgroup was then compared separately with the nonepileptic group for individual factor scores. The results of this analysis indicated that

TABLE 1. *Factors on which EEG subgroups score significantly higher than nonepileptic children*

Subgroup	Factors
	Sexes combined
3/sec spike and wave	Anxiety,[a] inattention[b]
Irregular spike and wave	Anxiety,[b] inattention,[b] social isolation[c]
Right temporal spike	Anxiety[a]
Left temporal spike	Anxiety,[b] inattention,[b] social isolation,[b] overactivity[c]
	Boys only
3/sec spike and wave	Anxiety,[a] inattention[c]
Irregular spike and wave	Anxiety,[b] inattention,[b] social isolation[b]
Right temporal spike	Anxiety,[a] inattention,[c] social isolation[c]
Left temporal spike	Anxiety,[a] inattention,[b] social isolation,[b] overactivity[c]

[a] $p < 0.001$.
[b] $p < 0.01$.
[c] $p < 0.05$.

distinct patterns of disturbed behavior seemed to be associated with each EEG subgroup. Table 1 shows the factors on which each EEG subgroup scored significantly higher than the nonepileptic children with both sexes combined. In no instance was there a significant difference in conduct problem scores, but, as regards the other factor scores, the subgroups appeared to form a series from the children with a right temporal spike focus who scored significantly higher only on anxiety, to the left temporal lobe subgroup who were the most disturbed of all with significantly higher scores on anxiety, inattention, social isolation, and overactivity.

The same type of analysis was then carried out for boys and girls separately, and this produced quite different results. The most striking effect concerned sex differences themselves. When girls in each subgroup were compared with nonepileptic girls, the only significant difference seen was that girls with 3/sec spike-and-wave patterns were more inattentive and overactive than their nonepileptic counterparts; otherwise, epileptic girls were generally no different from nonepileptic girls.

The findings for epileptic boys were in contrast, and Table 1 also shows that boys in all four subgroups were significantly more anxious, inattentive, and socially isolated than nonepileptic boys except for those in the 3/sec subgroup who were not more socially isolated. The left temporal subgroup is additionally the only one with significantly higher overactivity scores, making it overall the most disturbed subgroup of the four.

DISCUSSION

The results of this preliminary study suggest that for the purposes of identifying characteristic patterns of behavior in different forms of childhood epilepsy, a classification based on consistent EEG findings is of value but also that sex differences are particularly important.

However, the behavior of epileptic children can be affected in many ways, and factors other than EEG type of seizure disorder have to be considered. Small but significant positive correlations were found between age and all the factor scores except inattention, but the subgroups are no different from each other or from the nonepileptic children as far as age is concerned. Each epileptic child's seizure frequency in the preceding 2 years was assessed since frequent seizures seem likely to disrupt behavior, but no relationship between frequency of seizures and factor scores was found. Finally, children with generalized seizure discharge (especially the 3/sec spike-and-wave subgroup) tended to be taking ethosuximide, whereas the most common drug prescribed for the temporal lobe subgroups was phenytoin. There was, however, considerable overlap in the type of treatment taken, and, in any case, no difference was found between the disturbance scores of the drug groups considered separately.

The much higher rates of disturbance found in epileptic boys in this study are in keeping with the general tendency for boys to be apparently more vulnerable than girls to various types of stress in life (Rutter, 1971). Nuffield's (1961) contrast between 3/sec spike-and-wave children and those with temporal lobe abnormalities gains a little support from the present findings, but a close correspondence would not have been expected, as Nuffield's population was drawn from a neuropsychiatric clinic and the children in this investigation are largely unselected in this way. In addition, Nuffield's study was based on a retrospective analysis of hospital notes, whereas the present findings are derived from a teachers' questionnaire concerning children's behavior at ordinary school. They imply that, at least in epileptic boys, various behavioral difficulties may exist depending on the type of seizure disorder. Although these difficulties may not be sufficient to lead to psychiatric referral, it is possible that they affect progress at school adversely. Indeed, there is some evidence that the reading skills of epileptic boys with a left temporal lobe spike focus are particularly impaired (Stores and Hart, 1976). That conduct problems are not more common in the children with epilepsy may be because that type of disturbance more than any other leads to psychiatric referral and removal from ordinary school.

These findings suggest that the behavioral difficulties and the needs of children with epilepsy attending ordinary school can be identified with some precision. This can best be achieved, however, by avoiding general statements and examining well-defined types of seizure disorders separately when quite different patterns of disturbance can be expected to emerge.

ACKNOWLEDGMENTS

This study was kindly supported by the Research Fund of the British Epilepsy Association and the Mental Health Trust and Research Fund, to both of which

I am most grateful, as well as to the teachers and, of course, the children who were involved in the investigation.

REFERENCES

Connors, C. K. (1969): A teacher rating scale for use in drug studies with children. *Am. J. Psychiatry,* 126:884–888.
Flor-Henry, P. (1972): Ictal and interictal psychiatric manifestations in epilepsy: Specific or non-specific? *Epilepsia,* 13:773–783.
Nuffield, E. J. A. (1961): Neuro-physiology and behaviour disorders in epileptic children. *J. Ment. Sci.,* 107:435–457.
Rutter, M. (1971): Parent-child separation: Psychological effects on the children. *J. Child Psychol. Psychiatry,* 12:233–260.
Rutter, M., Graham, P., and Yule, W. (1970): *A Neuropsychiatric Study in Childhood. Clinics in Developmental Medicine,* No. 35 and 36. Spastics International Medical Publications and Heinemann, London.
Stores, G., and Hart, J. A. (1976): Reading skills in children with generalised or focal epilepsy attending ordinary school. *Dev. Med. Child Neurol.,* 18:705–716.
Werry, J. S., Sprague, R. L., and Cohen, M. N. (1975): Connors' Teacher Rating Scale for use in drug studies with children—an empirical study. *J. Abnorm. Child Psychol.,* 3:217–229.

Epilepsy, The Eighth International Symposium,
edited by J. K. Penry. Raven Press, New York
© 1977.

Long-Term Casework Support with Epileptic Patients

Rachel Tavriger

The National Hospital for Nervous Diseases, London, England

Patients with epilepsy who are referred to the psychiatric social work department of the hospital where I work tend to fall into four main categories of social maladjustment, as shown in Table 1.

Patients in Groups I and II have primarily medical problems and do not really come within the scope of this chapter. Obviously, uncontrolled fits give rise to work, accommodation, and other allied problems, often leading to depression and anxiety if support is not available, or, as in Group II, if behavioral patterns associated with brain damage or low IQ create practical and relationship difficulties. However, I would like to concentrate on the comparatively neglected Groups III and IV, particularly bearing in mind Kendell's paper, "The Concept of Disease and Its Implications for Psychiatry," in the *British Journal of Psychiatry,* October, 1975.

Over the past years, I have accumulated a very varied clientele of patients in these two groups, including those still attending the hospital for neurological supervision and those whose medication is now monitored by the family doctor.

Many patients whose seizures are not completely controlled complain that their fits are often more frequent at times of social stress, and they appear to derive some degree of comfort and support from the knowledge that their social worker is available for regular discussion and additional crisis interviews. Most of these patients have had intensive social work contact at the onset of medical treatment, several of them having daily interviews while inpatients and graduating to weekly and then monthly outpatient appointments, sometimes over a period of years. The ultimate aim is to reduce contact to the level of an annual Christmas card, as a reassurance that someone is still interested in their progress and the knowledge that if things do go wrong, they can return for renewed support and help. Parents often find this of great benefit, and it is not unusual to receive a telephone call from the mother of a child seen at, for example, age 10, when the time for leaving school approaches or adolescent problems of adjustment, often unrelated to seizures, appear.

There is, in addition, a further group of patients whose fits are well controlled but whose personality problems remain unsolved. Neurologists feel that epilepsy is not the basic problem, whereas psychiatrists stress the epileptic component and

TABLE 1. *Patients referred to Psychiatric Social Work Department (Maida Vale Hospital)*

Group	Description
I	Social difficulties because of fits
II	Behavioral problems associated with epilepsy and brain damage
III	Exacerbation of normally controlled fits because of social stresses
IV	Personality disorders and epilepsy (seizures adequately controlled)

feel that social problems or problems of relationships do not constitute a treatable illness.

To illustrate the sorts of patients in these two groups, I would like to give two case histories of patients who have received casework support with, I hope, some good result.

CASE HISTORIES

Anna, age 23, belongs to Group III (see Table 1), patients who suffer an exacerbation of usually adequately controlled fits when confronted with social stresses and relationship problems. She was first seen as an inpatient, having been admitted for control of frequent petit mal attacks and occasional grand mal attacks. Her epilepsy had started at age 12, and although of good average intelligence she had achieved little at school, leaving at age 17 without any qualifications. She came from a wealthy country family, and although she had had every material advantage, her childhood, and especially her adolescence, had been extremely traumatic. Her father was an alcoholic and her mother had divorced him when Anna was 10 years old. Her mother had remarried 2 years later to a second alcoholic, and when I met Anna, her mother was about to embark on a third marriage to a third alcoholic. Anna had kept in touch with her own father who had continued to give her financial support, but this was irregular and Anna was in debt. She had left home when she was 21, following a broken engagement, and was sharing a flat with a girl she disliked and distrusted. Work was even less successful. She had had a series of dull, routine jobs, from most of which she had been let go for poor time keeping or for her aggressive behavior toward other members of the staff on her own level.

In the hospital, Anna responded well to a new regimen of medication but was reported to be unfriendly and snobbish with the other patients. She admitted to being worried about her mother and depressed about the future. When I saw her, she told me she could see little hope of any real change. She had had several hospital admissions in the past and had left the hospital with her fits well controlled, only to find herself lonely and bored, and the whole circle starting again. She admitted that every grand mal attack she had had over the last 4 years had been the result of her failure to take her tablets when she was "fed-up."

We had daily interviews for the 10 days she remained in hospital, during which time we held a joint family interview to discuss training and jobs. Her parents agreed to pay for a crash course at a receptionists' school, and Anna tackled this with enthusiasm. Both she and I felt it was important that the contact be maintained and I arranged to see her weekly in the evenings after she had started work. That was over 2 years ago. The first year was one of many crises, including two grand mals, when a love affair went wrong, and she again "forgot" to take her tablets. She also had a period of 3 weeks of frequent minor attacks when she quarreled with another girl at work. At her request, I saw her employer, who was most supportive and helped Anna to sort things out. Our meetings gradually tailed off until she phoned me after a gap of about 6 months to ask for an appointment, since her fits seemed to be becoming more frequent again. At this interview she told me she had recently learned that her father was dying of cancer, and we had several meetings to help her work through her feelings about this. During this period she was able to continue in her job and to maintain the relationships she had built up. I have not heard from her now for some months, but I am quite sure that if stresses she cannot tolerate arise, she will contact me for further support.

Group IV

Jenny is typical of (see Table 1), patients who have personality disorders *and* epilepsy, the seizures being controlled for all practical purposes. Patients falling into this group are, I think, more difficult both to help and to assess improvement. Jenny is aged 38, married, with three daughters, aged 14, 12, and 9. Her husband is a commercial artist, a rather passive man with many problems of his own. Jenny had attended the hospital for some years for routine supervision of medication for minor attacks, thought to be of temporal lobe origin, but which occurred very infrequently and did not cause loss of consciousness. She came to the attention of the Psychiatric Department, having arrived at the hospital in great distress following a row with her husband, whom she had threatened with a bread knife! Jenny had had a somewhat unorthodox childhood. Her father was a petulant hypochondriac and her mother a complaining martyr. Jenny had been sent to a progressive boarding school, which seemed to have encouraged her to emulate both her parents, instead of helping her to develop some sort of structure or guideline for more acceptable social behavior.

I have been seeing Jenny for an hour a week, sometimes with her husband, but mostly on her own, for over 2 years. During this period, she has had only two episodes of minor fits which neither she nor her family see as part of the problem. Her childish, attention-seeking behavior continues, but the family is still intact, and the girls are gradually creeping through adolescence. Although Jenny remains an extremely difficult woman, she is now at least aware of her behavior and has some insight into the impossible demands she makes on everyone. We have recently switched to a behavior therapy approach in which we rehearse the coming week's stressful events and decide how she should deal with them. If she does not carry out the prescribed behavior, I see her for only 10 min the following week, just long enough for me to set her a task in self-control for the coming week. Because of the relationship we have built up over the past 2 years, this approach, so far at least, looks promising as long as we do not set our goals too high. She is beginning, I think, at long last to understand the need for self-imposed limits, and her family has voiced some appreciation of this.

DISCUSSION

I think it quickly becomes obvious from these histories that the severity of the epilepsy bears little relation to the severity of the patient's difficulty in coping with his problems. The aim of casework, therefore, must be to effect a modification not only of the patient's environment but also of his personality so that adjustment to real life regardless of the epilepsy can be achieved. This involves a psychotherapeutic approach on a long-term basis. I do not believe this to be an uneconomic proposition in terms of more complete control of seizures, and even more importantly, in terms of the constructive social functioning of the patient so that he can realize his potential to become a fully independent member of the community.

I am not suggesting that such casework techniques are peculiar to the setting in which I work, and, indeed, I suspect that many social workers, given the access to similar cases and the needed time, would follow the same pattern of working. I would, therefore, make a plea for a realization from our medical colleagues that such a service can be available, and that control or partial control of fits by medication is not always sufficient in the long term. The needs of young people in particular must not be overlooked if they are to avoid developing deeply entrenched behavior difficulties in later life. I would urge that not only patients with practical difficulties be referred to social work departments, but also those patients who show signs of emotional disturbance, even when seizures appear to be satisfactorily controlled.

SUMMARY

Patients with epilepsy tend to be referred to the social work department only if the frequency or severity of their seizures produces overt social problems such as loss of work, unsuitable housing, or lack of mobility. Although these are accepted as important problems, there are many patients suffering from less severe forms of epilepsy whose areas of stress lie in the field of personality and the inability to make satisfactory relationships. Intensive and ongoing casework has an important part to play in helping such patients to become more fully operative members of the community, and also in helping them to maintain better control of their seizures. Two case histories are outlined to illustrate this concept and to demonstrate some of the techniques involved. A plea is made for the recognition by the medical profession of social malfunction as a condition treatable by casework.

REFERENCE

Kendell, R. E. (1975): The concept of disease and its implications for psychiatry. *Br. J. Psychiatry,* 127:305–315.

Epilepsy, The Eighth International Symposium,
edited by J. K. Penry. Raven Press, New York
© 1977.

Personality Traits in Epilepsy

*P. Bech, **K. Kjaersgård Pedersen, †N. Simonsen, and
**M. Lund

*Psychochemistry Institute, Rigshospitalet, Copenhagen, Denmark; and Departments of
** Neurology and † Clinical Neurophysiology, Glostrup Hospital, Denmark

In the present study we have investigated patients with various well-defined types of epilepsy (juvenile myoclonic epilepsy, psychomotor epilepsy, and cryptogenic grand mal epilepsy) in regard to personality traits by use of an inventory based on Sjöbring's (1973) neurophysiological model of personality.

PATIENTS AND METHODS

Subjects

The subjects were patients selected from the Epilepsy Out-Patients' Clinic, Department of Neurology, Glostrup Hospital. The great majority had previously been admitted to the department and subjected to routine neurological, ophthalmological, otological, and electroencephalographic investigations as well as X-ray examination of the skull. When indicated, isotope brain scan and diagnostic PEG or cerebral angiography was performed. Tumors and gross pathological lesions were excluded. A few patients with slight-to-moderate focal or diffuse cerebral atrophy were included.

The following three groups participated in the investigation.

1. Juvenile myoclonic epilepsy. Impulsive petit mal (Janz, 1969) defined as cryptogenic epilepsy with onset between 10 and 20 years of age, characterized by bilateral myoclonic jerks as the typical seizure type, but very often exhibiting grand mal and petit mal, and occasionally also akinetic (astatic) seizures. The admission criterion was the presence of bilateral myoclonic jerks.

2. Psychomotor epilepsy. Complex partial seizures, often associated with grand mal. The admission criterion was presence of psychomotor epilepsy for at least 1 year, and a frequency of seizures of at least one per month. Patients with identified tumor and patients with temporal lobe resection were excluded.

3. Grand mal epilepsy with or without petit mal. Only patients in whom no focal cerebral pathology had been found were included.

The patient group with juvenile myoclonic epilepsy represented the total number of patients with this form of epilepsy attending our outpatients' clinic. The other two epilepsy groups were selected from our clinic to match with juvenile myoclonic epilepsy according to age, sex, and duration of disease. On the test day, four patients (two with juvenile myoclonic epilepsy, one with psychomotor epilepsy, and one with grand mal epilepsy) refused to cooperate; thus a total number of 89 patients took part in the study. In the juvenile myoclonic epilepsy group there were 12 males and 18 females, aged 15 to 63 years (median 30 years); in the psychomotor epilepsy group there were 13 males and 16 females, aged 15 to 55 years (median 37 years); and in the grand mal epilepsy group there were 16 males and 14 females, aged 18 to 53 years (median 29 years).

Patients suffering from Menière's disease served as a control group. These patients (11 males and 11 females) participated in a double-blind crossover trial to test the effect of lithium against placebo (Thomsen et al., 1976). The test periods were 6 months, and the results shown here are collected in the placebo period. The patients matched with the epilepsy group in regard to sex, duration of disease, and social level, whereas the age was statistically significantly higher, median 54.5 and range 36 to 71 years.

Methods and Procedure

The investigation took place in the autumn of 1974. The patients' records were reviewed for evaluation of electroencephalographic findings and social data.

EEG Findings

The EEG findings were classified according to the dominating features into groups including:

1. bilateral synchronous polyspike and wave paroxysms;
2. bilateral synchronous paroxysms without polyspike and wave paroxysms;
3. temporal focus of spikes or sharp waves and/or slow waves;
4. bitemporal abnormalities;
5. pathological traits, but excluding 1 through 4;
6. no abnormalities.

Social Evaluation

The social evaluation was made according to the principles of social stratification given by Svalastoga (1959) dividing patients and controls into five social groups: (1) upper classes and higher middle class, (2) middle class, (3) lower middle class, (4) higher working class, and (5) lower working class.

Rating Scales

The procedure also included a rating scale, on which the patients estimated retrospectively the frequency of seizures during the 4 weeks preceding the test day. Finally, a questionnaire, the Marke-Nyman inventory, was used as a measure of personality traits (Nyman and Marke, 1962; Perris, 1966; Coppen, 1966; Bech et al., 1976, *a,b,c*).

The questionnaire is based on Sjöbring's (1973) theory of personality structure including the three variables validity, stability, and solidity. Validity is a measure of available and effective energy; stability is a measure of emotional control; and solidity is a measure of maturity. Accordingly, subvalidity, substability, and subsolidity largely correspond to psychoasthenia, syntony, and hysteroidy, respectively. The item score on this scale was analyzed both according to Marke-Nyman and according to Perris (1966). In the original study (Marke and Nyman) the total of 60 items is made up of 20 items for each of the three variables. In accordance with this, the item scores are added for all 20 items for each variable, so that the scores range from 0 (the highest minus variant) to 40 (highest plus variant). Perris (1966) selected 10 items for each variable. The items were added for the 10 selected items for each variable, and the total score on this subscale ranged from 0 to 20. Only the subscale data will be mentioned here; for further data see Bech et al. (1976*b*).

Treatment

All patients regularly attended our clinic, and each control included interview, clinical examination, and determination of serum concentration of the anticonvulsant given. Hydantoins (diphenylhydantoin and ethotoin) dominated among the anticonvulsants. In general, there was no marked difference in the antiepileptic treatment among the diagnostic groups.

Statistical Analysis

Nonparametric statistics were used throughout the study. When the level of measurement was nominal, the X^2 test for independent samples was used. When the level of measurement was ordinal, the Mann-Whitney test was used for independent two-sample cases and the Kruskal-Wallis test for independent three-sample cases. As a measure of correlation, the Spearman test was used (Siegel, 1956). Throughout the study the median was used to express the central tendency, and the 10 through 90 percentiles to express the dispersion.

RESULTS

Social Data

There was no statistically significant difference between the epileptic groups and the Menière group, neither were there any significant differences within the epileptic groups. When the epileptic groups were analyzed according to the EEG findings, no statistically significant differences were obtained.

Frequency of Seizures

The patients' self-ratings of the frequency of all kinds of seizures during the 4 weeks before the test day showed that whereas only one grand mal epilepsy patient had seizures, 12 juvenile myoclonic epilepsy and 12 psychomotor epilepsy patients reported to have had seizures in the test period.

Marke-Nyman Scale

Neither in the epilepsy group nor in the Menière group was there any correlation between the three variables on the Marke-Nyman scale and the age of the patients.

Validity

When the epilepsy groups were analyzed in total, there was no statistically significant difference in validity between the epilepsy group and the Menière group, as shown in Table 1. In the epileptic groups, those with juvenile myoclonic epilepsy scored less valid than did those with grand mal epilepsy ($p < 0.05$). The score in the psychomotor epilepsy group was intermediate between that in the juvenile myoclonic epilepsy and grand mal epilepsy groups, and the difference among the three epileptic groups reached statistical significance only at $p < 0.10$.

The subgroup of patients in the juvenile myoclonic epilepsy group ($N = 25$) and in the grand mal epilepsy group ($N = 9$) with electroencephalographic polyspike and wave paroxysms had a score pattern similar to the results within and between the groups, respectively, as shown in Table 1. In the psychomotor epilepsy group, however, patients with a unilateral temporal focus in the EEG ($N = 10$) scored significantly lower in validity than did those patients without such a focus but with bitemporal abnormalities ($N = 14$).

There was no statistically significant difference between males and females when the epilepsy groups were analyzed in total.

Neither in the control group was there any statistically significant difference

TABLE 1. *The Marke-Nyman subscale (median and 10–90 percentiles).*

Diagnostic group	Marke-Nyman scale (median and 10–90 percentiles)		
	Validity	Stability	Solidity
Juvenile myoclonic epilepsy ($N = 30$)	7 (2–14)	6 (0–14)	8 (2.2–13.7)
Psychomotor epilepsy ($N = 29$)	8 (2–16)	8 (2–10)	10 (2–18)
Grand mal epilepsy ($N = 30$)	10 (4–18)	5.4 (2–14)	10.6 (6–16)
	< 0.10	ns	ns
All 3 epileptic groups ($N = 89$)	8 (2–16)	6 (2–14)	10 (4–16)
Menière ($N = 22$)	8 (2–16)	8 (2.0–17.3)	11 (8–16)
	ns	< 0.05	< 0.05

between females and males. When the results were analyzed for females and males separately, the scored pattern was similar to the results shown in the table.

Stability

When the three epileptic groups were analyzed in total, the epilepsy group scored statistically significantly less stable than did the control group ($p < 0.05$). Within the three epileptic groups there was no statistically significant difference in stability. Females scored less stable than did males in the epilepsy group ($p < 0.05$), whereas there was no statistically significant difference between the two sexes in the control group. When the results were analyzed for females and males separately, it was found that the difference between the epilepsy group and the control group reached statistical significance only for females ($p < 0.01$).

Solidity

As shown in Table 1, the epilepsy group scored normosolid but less solid than did the Menière group ($p < 0.05$). Within the epileptic groups there was no statistically significant difference in solidity, although juvenile myoclonic epilepsy patients had a tendency to lower scores. This tendency to subsolidity in the juvenile myoclonic epilepsy group was also found when juvenile myoclonic epilepsy and grand mal epilepsy patients with polyspike and wave paroxysms were compared, but it never reached statistical significance. Psychomotor epilepsy patients with temporal lobe focus on the EEG scored less solid than patients without a focus, and the difference was statistically significant. When psychomotor epilepsy patients with temporal lobe focus were compared with grand mal epilepsy patients, the difference in solidity was statistically insignificant.

Neither in the epilepsy group analyzed in total nor in the control group was there any statistically significant difference between females and males. When the results were analyzed for females and males separately, the scored pattern was similar to the results shown in the table.

Comparison Between Patients With and Without Seizures in the Test Period

Neither in the juvenile myoclonic epilepsy group nor in the psychomotor epilepsy group was there any difference between patients with and without seizures during the 4 weeks before the test day concerning the three variables on the Marke-Nyman scale.

DISCUSSION

Although the epileptic subgroups matched according to sex, age, duration of disease, treatment, and social level, we used as a control group patients with Menière's disease to take into account the effect of a comparable disease characterized by repeated attacks. Our results showed that there was no difference between epileptic patients with and without seizures up to the test day indicating that our findings could not be ascribed to the effect of recent seizures.

Our results showed that the epilepsy group compared with the Menière group had low stability, this being especially due to a low score in the females. The difference in solidity showed the Menière group to be supersolid and the epilepsy group mainly normosolid. Within the epileptic groups the low stability was associated with a low validity in the juvenile myoclonic epilepsy group irrespective of electroencephalographic findings, whereas the grand mal epilepsy group was normovalid, and the psychomotor epilepsy group scored between the two groups on validity. However, when the psychomotor epilepsy group was divided according to the electroencephalographic findings, patients with temporal lobe focus were statistically significantly subvalid. The combination of low validity and low stability was not reflected in the social findings, but in this study we have focused on the character and not on intellectual capacity. A report of the juvenile myoclonic epilepsy group describing social level and mental capacity is published elsewhere (Lund et al., 1975).

In contrast to the Rorschach test and the Minnesota Multiphasic Personality Inventory, which so far have been found relatively inadequate to evaluate epileptic patients (Reitan, 1974; Stevens, 1975), the Marke-Nyman inventory is based on a personality theory, and the three variables validity, stability, and solidity on that scale have been verified by use of factor analysis (Barret, 1972).

The conclusion which can be drawn from the results here reported is that our patients with epilepsy, irrespective of type of seizure, were substable, whereas the validity dimension varied from normovalidity to subvalidity. Low validity was found in patients with juvenile myoclonic epilepsy and in patients with psychomotor epilepsy in whom there was electroencephalographic evidence of temporal lobe focus. In those latter groups of epilepsy a tendency to subsolidity was also seen. In Sjöbring's frame of reference, substable patients of low validity have a psychological vulnerability, being unable to overcome the small concrete adversities of life. Being unable to solve problems, they tend to react in a mood of discontent or in maladjustment. Our findings support the observations by Janz (1969) on juvenile myoclonic epilepsy and by Peters (1969) on psychomotor epilepsy, in that a high proportion of those patients show character traits of psychoasthenia, emotional instability, and self-centeredness.

ACKNOWLEDGMENTS

This study was supported in part by a grant from Dansk Esso Fund. The authors are indebted to the patients for their cooperation in this study.

REFERENCES

Barret, J. E. (1972): Use of the M-N-T inventory (Sjöbring's personality dimensions) on an American population. *Acta Psychiatr. Scand.,* 48:501–509.

Bech, P., Vendsborg, P. B., and Rafaelsen, O. J. (1976a): Lithium maintenance treatment of manic-melancholic patients: Its role in the daily routine. *Acta Psychiatr. Scand.,* 53:70–81.

Bech, P., Kjaersgård Pedersen, K., Simonsen, N., and Lund, M. (1976b): Personality in epilepsy. *Acta Neurol. Scand.* 54:348–358.

Bech, P., Thomsen, J., and Rafaelsen, O. J. (1977b): Long-term lithium treatment: Effect on simulated car driving and other psychological tests. *Eur. J. Clin. Pharmacol.* 10:331–335.

Coppen, A. (1966): The Marke-Nyman temperament scale: An English translation. *Br. J. Med. Psychol.,* 39:55–59.

Janz, D. (1969): *Die Epilepsien.* G. Thieme, Stuttgart.

Lund, M., Reintoft, H., and Simonsen, N. (1975): En kontrolleret social og psykologisk undersøgelse af patienter med juvenil myoklon epilepsi. *Ugeskr.* Laeger, 137:2415–2418.

Nyman, G. E., and Marke, S. (1962): *Sjöbring's differentiella psykologi* (The Differential Psychology of Sjöbring). Gleerups, Lund.

Perris, C. (1966): A study of bipolar (manic-depressive) and unipolar recurrent depressive psychoses. IV. A multidimensional study of personality traits. *Acta Psychiatr. Scand. [Suppl.],* 194:68–82.

Peters, U. H. (1969): Das pseudopsychopatische Affektsyndrom der Temporallappenepileptiker. *Nervenarzt,* 40:75–82.

Reitan, R. M. (1974): Psychological testing of epileptic patients. In: *Handbook of Clinical Neurology,* edited by P. J. Vinken and C. W. Bruyn, pp. 559–575. North-Holland Publishing Company, Amsterdam.

Siegel, S. (1956): *Non-parametric Statistics.* McGraw-Hill, New York.

Sjöbring, H. (1973): Personality structure and development. *Acta Psychiatr. Scand. [Suppl.],* 244: 113–157.

Stevens, J. R. (1975): Interictal clinical manifestations of complex partial seizures. In: *Complex Partial Seizures and Their Treatment, Advances in Neurology, Vol. 2,* edited by J. K. Penry and D. D. Daly, pp. 85–112. Raven Press, New York.

Svalastoga, K. (1959): *Prestige, Class and Mobility.* Scandinavian University Books, Gyldendal, Copenhagen.

Thomsen, J., Bech, P., Geisler, A., Prytz, S., Rafaelsen, O. J., Vendsborg, P. B., and Zilstorff, K. (1976): Lithium treatment of Menière's disease. *Acta Otolaryngol.* 82:294–296.

Epilepsy, The Eighth International Symposium,
edited by J. K. Penry. Raven Press, New York
© 1977.

The Concept of Preventive Rehabilitation in Childhood Epilepsy: A Plea Against Overprotection and Overindulgence

P. Lerman

Epileptic Clinic and EEG Laboratory, Beilinson Medical Center, Petah Tikva, Israel

An epileptic is successfully rehabilitated if he is able to obtain and keep a job, thus achieving financial security and a satisfactory social status. Many conditions must be fulfilled to attain this goal, including adequate seizure control, good working habits and social adjustment on the part of the employee, and an enlightened attitude toward epilepsy on the part of the employer and the patient's co-workers.

I would like to focus attention on a common psychosocial problem which creates great difficulties in rehabilitation and which, I believe, is preventable. Many seizure-free epileptics are almost unemployable not because of the cerebral dysrhythmia or feeble-mindedness, but because of a personality problem. Apart from the personality disturbances due to organic brain disease and/or seizures, the epileptic is often afflicted with maladjustment problems, including lack of emotional maturity, dependability, and motivation to work, which are purely psychogenic and not produced by the epilepsy *per se.*

I claim that a major factor in the genesis of these psychosocial problems, obviating employability, is faulty upbringing, namely, a wrong parental attitude toward the epileptic child, often encouraged by the medical and educational professions.

Epileptologists and particularly social workers are certainly familiar with the type of problematic youngster suffering from epilepsy from childhood. He tends to be irritable and even belligerent, has a low frustration threshold, and makes unrealistic demands. He fails at work because he has learned no skills, lacks suitable preparation, and, most important, has no motivation. He takes it for granted that he should be supported by social welfare agencies, considering himself a handicapped person unable to work. In our opinion he is merely a mental cripple who is the product of his environment—the result of parental overprotection and overindulgence.

Surprisingly, there is little reference to this problem in the literature dealing with the psychosocial aspects of epilepsy. In the extensive review of "social aspects of epilepsy in childhood" by Lorentz de Haas (1962) as well as that of Jüül-Jensen (1974), only a few sketchy remarks on this problem are to be found, such as the quotation from Kanner (1960) that "overprotection may result in spoilt behavior and retardation of mental and social maturation." Tylor Fox (1947) justly holds that "physical danger likely to accrue from underprotection is really less than the mental damage resulting from overprotection." Kaye (1951), investigating psychosocial maladjustment in children with petit mal, found an impaired parent-child relationship as a cause. In all cases there was parental rejection leading to hostility or compensatory overprotection. Finally, Pond and Bidwell (1954) found that 40% of the patients in their large series had difficulties in social adjustment due to behavior problems.

In a pilot study of 20 families of epileptic children performed by us, the parents were questioned regarding a possible change in their attitude toward the affected child after the diagnosis of epilepsy had been disclosed to them. Fully 80% admitted that they had consequently become more indulgent and permissive.

In a review of 100 children suffering from benign focal epilepsy of childhood (Lerman and Kivity, 1975), we had the unique opportunity to compare two groups—one retrospective and the other prospective—which were similar clinically but differed in the way in which they had been brought up due to dissimilar attitudes on the part of the treating physicians and the parents. In the older (retrospective) group a guarded prognosis had been pronounced and excessive restrictions had been imposed, resulting in anxiety, overprotection, and overindulgence in most cases. In the prospective group, the favorable prognosis was stressed, the parents were told that full recovery would ensue within several years, and they were warned against overprotection and overpermissiveness. In the former group, emotional difficulties, behavior problems, and social maladjustment were much more prominent. Thus we have the same kind of epilepsy but different psychosocial consequences, clearly due to environmental factors.

Interestingly, we had the chance to observe an 18-year-old who was not an epileptic but had been brought up as one because of an erroneous diagnosis. When he was called for military service his father appealed to the authorities, explaining that the youngster was not fit to be a soldier because of behavior problems. He wrote, "We gave up all principles of education because of his ailment and consequently he has grown up to be completely spoiled."

Now let us analyze the psychodynamics of this problem. In most cases, at least in our culture, parents react to the diagnosis of epilepsy with a mixture of extreme feelings—apprehension, shame, anxiety, frustration, and helplessness. This leads to an oppressive atmosphere of secrecy and despair which affects the child adversely, as so aptly described by Lennox (1960). The child has no one to talk to about his condition and he is convinced that it is something utterly terrible. Add to this the rejection on the part of schoolmates, friends, and neighbors. In most cases the epileptic child becomes confined to his home, lacking playmates and friends. He has no chance to develop the intricate skills of social interrelationships. This social isolation takes a heavy toll on him when he grows up unprepared for life because he has had no normal social contacts, so essential to the healthy youngster in becoming a functioning member of society. He remains insecure, overdependent, emotionally immature, and is inept when he reaches adulthood.

The parents develop emotions of guilt and anger. Most of them come to believe that they are responsible for their child's plight. They often regard it as a retribution for some sin committed in the past. This guilt complex, which is often a corollary of rejection and hidden anger, leads to an excessive desire to protect the child. Sometimes this becomes an irrational obsession. We encounter mothers who keep their epileptic child under constant surveillance. To quote Lennox (1960): "Many parents believe it their duty to keep the child always in sight and forbid all activities which involve any danger."

Extreme overprotection is illustrated in the case of a 23-year-old patient who has never had a job. During his childhood he had numerous petit mal absences subsequently followed by rare grand mal seizures. All through high school his mother escorted him to school in the morning and home in the afternoon. When the boy was 17 his father shaved him every morning since he "couldn't be trusted with a razor."

Another factor is the imposition of excessive and often unnecessary restrictions on the epileptic child: he must not stay out in the sun and should refrain from swimming, other sports, and physical exercise. Unfortunately, these harmful recommendations are usually made by the good doctor with the best intentions. Most school physicians automatically bar the epileptic child from almost all school activities. But isn't the risk of a broken leg by far preferable to that of a broken heart?

The most disastrous advice, often given by those involved in the care and treatment of these children, is that they should not be angered, aggravated, or opposed lest they have a fit—which is equally true concerning children suffering from congenital heart disease, bronchial asthma, breath holding spells, and other disorders. This absurd attitude inevitably results in the parents' becoming overpermissive and overindulgent and in the child's becoming pampered and spoiled. He quickly learns that the parents are there to serve him and that he can get away with anything. He becomes more and more demanding, capricious, and self-centered. He is taught to take but not to give. His personality becomes distorted. He is brought up to believe that society has to provide for him in the same way that his parents have always supplied all his needs and answered all his whims. Thus is the mental cripple engendered.

Shalom Aleichem, often called the Jewish Mark Twain, has an instructive story about Motel, who found how delightful it was to be an orphan, spoiled by the family and soft-hearted neighbors. The story is entitled "Happy I Am, Being an Orphan." One might paraphrase this to "Happy I Am, Being an Epileptic Child," spoiled by compassionate parents.

I believe that this unfortunate situation is largely preventable if strict prophylactic measures are taken. Since in the great majority of cases epilepsy starts in childhood, this problem is of paramount importance and magnitude. It should be recognized and treated vigorously as early as possible. All those concerned with the treatment of the epileptic child—doctors, nurses, psychologists, social workers, and teachers—should warn parents against overindulgence, permissiveness, and overprotection. They should insist that the epileptic child be brought up essentially as a healthy child, with the same privileges accorded and the same duties demanded. Group therapy for the parents and guidance for the child are very helpful. The young epileptic should be helped to face the misconceptions concerning epilepsy and the prejudice against epileptics in society.

Let me conclude with the words of Lennox (1960): The disability of epilepsy is more social than physical.

SUMMARY

From the experience gained in the care and observation of a large number of epileptic children throughout the years in the EEG Laboratory and Neuropediatric Service of Beilinson Medical Center, it was concluded that the main factors engendering psychosocial problems in young epileptics are as follows: (1) the atmosphere of secrecy and shame at home, leading to a distorted self-image and low esteem of the patient; (2) parental overprotection and nonacceptance by peers, leading to poor development of social interrelationships; and (3) overindulgence and overpermissive parental attitude, leading to "spoiled-bratism" and an irreversible malformation of the child's personality, obviating employability.

REFERENCES

Jüül-Jensen, P. (1974): Social prognosis in epilepsy. In: *Handbook of Clinical Neurology, Vol. 15,* pp. 800–814 North-Holland Publishing Corp., Amsterdam.
Kanner, L. (1960): *Child Psychiatry,* pp. 129–131. Charles C Thomas, Springfield, Ill.
Kaye, I. (1951): What are the evidences of social and psychological maladjustment revealed in a study of 17 children who have idiopathic petit-mal epilepsy? *J. Child Psychiatry,* 2:115–160.
Lennox, W. G. (1960): *Epilepsy and Related Disorders,* p. 932. Little, Brown and Co., Boston.
Lerman, P., and Kivity, S. (1975): Benign focal epilepsy of childhood. *Arch. Neurol.,* 32:261–264.
Lorentz de Haas, H. M. (1962): Social aspects of epilepsy in childhood. *Epilepsia,* 3:44–55.
Pond, D. A., and Bidwell, B. H. (1954): Management of behaviour disorders in epileptic children. *Br. Med. J.,* 11:1520.
Tylor Fox, J. (1947): The epileptic child. *Public Health,* 61:149–150.

Epilepsy, The Eighth International Symposium,
edited by J. K. Penry. Raven Press, New York
© 1977.

How Doctors "Manage" Epilepsy

Anthony Hopkins and Graham Scambler

Department of Neurological Sciences, St. Bartholomew's Hospital, London, EC1A 7BE

There seems to be a generally accepted view of how epilepsy "ought" to be "managed." The Reid Report (H.M.S.O., 1969) states, "The family doctor will undoubtedly wish to refer the majority of his patients [with epilepsy] for consultant advice, as an epileptic fit is a symptom, rather than a disease, and prolonged investigation may be necessary before a firm diagnosis can be reached." We were interested to see, firstly, what doctors actually did for their patients with epilepsy in a developed country today, where there is free and easy access to specialist care, and, secondly, whether such medical intervention and specialist referral were beneficial. This forms part of a wider study in the sociology of epilepsy to be published in monograph form (G. Scambler and A. Hopkins, *in preparation*).

METHODS

We identified all those subjects who, on prevalence day, (1) were aged 16 or over, (2) had had more than one nonfebrile seizure of any type, (3) had had at least one seizure in the preceding 2 years and/or had been on continuing anticonvulsants for more than one nonfebrile seizure in the past, (4) were not in long-term institutional care, and (5) were present in a population of 42,339 registered with 17 Health Service Practitioners in suburban London. Of this population 32,000 were aged 16 or over. We identified 108 subjects who met our restrictive criteria, giving a prevalence of 340/100,000. General practitioner records and correspondence from specialist units were available on these subjects; in addition, 94 of them (87%) consented to domiciliary visits by the neurologist (A.P.H.) and sociologist (G.S.).

The sociologist collected his information using tape-recorded nonstructured interviews and analyzed the tapes with rating scales developed for this study. Eighty-nine of the 94 subjects (95%) had been referred to a hospital clinic because of their epilepsy and at least one set of hospital notes could be inspected for 84 of these 89. Information available on those subjects who did not wish to be interviewed indicated that they did not differ from the interviewed subjects in terms of age, sex, social class, seizure type, or seizure frequency. We therefore believe our sample to be representative of (diagnosed) epilepsy "as it really is" in metropolitan society today.

RESULTS

The distribution of seizure types and seizure frequency in the population has already been published elsewhere (Hopkins and Scambler, 1976).

We were interested in patients' actions at the onset of their epilepsy. For this purpose we studied those 34 subjects in whom only generalized seizures had occurred. In 24 of the 29 respondents in this group medical advice was sought in close relation to the first attack, in 10 of them in immediate relation to the attack, often in an Emergency Department of a Hospital. In spite of seeking early advice, only one-third of the respondents who had had only generalized seizures anticipated the diagnosis of an epileptic seizure before they were informed of this. In the whole sample this proportion was only 20%.

If the patient is not successful at diagnosing his own illness, who is? In order to answer this question, we studied the notes from the hospital to which the subject had been first referred for his epilepsy. We retrieved 64 such records and studied the general practitioner's letter from all the records in which it was available (44 letters). In 80% of these cases the correct diagnosis of epilepsy had been made by the general practitioner, and in a further 11% epilepsy was mentioned by him as a possible diagnosis. In spite of this early correct diagnosis, 18% of respondents in the whole sample indicated in their tape-recorded interviews that they were either unaware of or did not accept the diagnosis of epilepsy. The probability of failure of communication was inversely related to the educational attainment of the subject. More of the respondents who understood that they had epilepsy, and who had been told by a doctor, had been informed of the diagnosis by a specialist (30) than by the general practitioner (23).

It is not possible here to indicate all the investigations undertaken by the neurologists to whom these subjects were referred, but we have some interesting information about electroencephalography. Of the 89 subjects, 77 (86%) referred to hospital had EEGs, and at least one record or report was available for review for 72 subjects (Table 1). If more than one record or report was available, the most abnormal has been included in the table. For 15 subjects the records were entirely normal, and a further 23 reports contained statements such as "virtually normal," "trivial abnormality," or "probably normal." If these are included with those reported as entirely normal, more than half the subjects (38 of 72, or 53%) had records that were normal. This figure includes 9 of 23 subjects with physical signs.

Six patients had 3-Hz spike-and-wave discharges, three a major excess of theta rhythms symmetrically, and six a major excess of theta rhythms asymmetrically. Spikes confined to one site were found in six subjects and multiple spikes in thirteen.

An attempt was made to correlate this broad classification with present seizure frequency (Table 1). Attention is drawn in particular to two groups. Five of the twelve patients having generalized seizures, other than petit mal, monthly or more frequently had never had an abnormal EEG. Nine of the thirteen patients

TABLE 1. Review of records or reports on EEGs obtained from a sample of people with epilepsy in the community, and present seizure frequency.

EEG	Petit mal		Partial seizures		Generalized seizures		Total
	Monthly or more frequently	Less than monthly	Monthly or more frequently	Less than monthly	Monthly or more frequently	Less than monthly	
Normal, or minor theta abnormalities only			9	11	5	30	39
Symmetrical excess of theta activity				2		2	3
Asymmetrical excess of theta activity			3			5	5
3-Hz spike and wave	1	3				6	6
Multiple spikes			6	6	4	9	13
Spike at one site			4		1	5	6
Record unavailable			3	1	2	3	5
No record made	2	1	2	6		17	17
Total	3	4	27	26	12	77	94

with multiple sites of epileptic discharges had seizures less frequently than monthly.

We reviewed the hospital records of those in our sample with progressive neurological disease to see if the EEG had in any way aided management. Two of the ninety-four subjects had astrocytoma, one a meningioma, one a gumma, and one an angioma (see Hopkins and Scambler, 1976). We reviewed the medical records to see if the decision to investigate these patients further had hinged on an abnormal EEG or some other finding. In no case was the EEG an important factor. Plain skull films showed sclerosis of the planum sphenoidale in the subject with the meningioma and intracranial calcification in one of the subjects with an astrocytoma. The other subject with an astrocytoma had papilledema and a left hemiplegia. The subject with an angioma had proptosis and an orbital bruit.

We also attempted to assess how realistically anticonvulsants were prescribed. Five of the ninety-four subjects were taking no medication at all, and a sixth was taking only oral diazepam. Five of these subjects had had generalized seizures (other than petit mal) within the last 2 years, and three of those had had partial seizures (weekly in two cases, every 2 to 3 months in the third). The sixth subject had not had a generalized seizure for nearly 30 years but continued to have monthly partial seizures.

By far the most frequently used drugs were phenobarbital and phenytoin—86 of the 89 people on medication took one or both drugs. Of these, 24 took phenobarbital without phenytoin, 19 took phenytoin without phenobarbital, and 43 took both. Two subjects were on primidone alone, and one on diazepam alone. Other drugs were used in combination with phenobarbital and phenytoin. Primidone, the most popular, was used by sixteen subjects, ethosuximide by three, sulthiame by two, pheneturide by two, and troxidone, carbamazepine, and acetazolamide each by one subject. Diazepam was used by six subjects and nitrazepam was used by five subjects, but in each case it appeared that these drugs were used for their sedative or hypnotic effect rather than for any belief in their anticonvulsant action.

Drug dosage in the population studied was extremely conservative, the mean dose of phenobarbital being 86 mg, of phenytoin 218 mg, and of primidone 680 mg. In an attempt to express the range of anticonvulsant dosage in the population, we have used, with modifications, the system of Richens (1970). He expressed the dose of the major anticonvulsants in units so that the dosages of the commonly prescribed drugs could be equated. He allowed one unit for every 50 mg of phenytoin or 30 mg of phenobarbital, and 1.5 units for every 250 mg of primidone or 200 mg pheneturide. We have used this scale, allocating also 1.5 units to every 200 mg of carbamazepine, sulthiame, and troxidone and to every 250 mg of ethosuximide. One unit has also been allocated to every 10 mg of diazepam and nitrazepam. A subject on phenobarbital 30 mg three times a day and phenytoin 100 mg three times a day is therefore on 9 units of anticonvulsants on this scale. We found that 35 subjects were on less than 4.9 units per day, 41 on 5.0 to 9.9 units, 15 on 10.0 to 15.0, and only 3 on more than 15.0 units per day.

There was no correlation between the weight of the subject and the dose of drugs. Furthermore, there was in many cases little attempt to control frequent seizures with an adequate dose of medication. Half those with frequent generalized seizures (other than petit mal) were probably undertreated. Of the 12 subjects having such seizures monthly or more frequently, 1 was having no medication, 1 less than 4.9 units, and 4 between 5.0 and 9.9 units. Of the 29 subjects having partial seizures monthly or more frequently, 2 had no medication, 5 less than 4.9 units, and 10 between 5.0 and 9.9 units.

In an attempt to assess the activity of medical supervision, we asked 74 of the subjects when they had last seen their general practitioner. Twenty-four of these (32%) had seen him within the last month, 49% within the last 2 months, 65% within the last 6 months, and 85% within the last year. Three subjects (4%) had not seen their doctor for 2 years or more.

Supervision of those with the worst epilepsy is not as good as it might be. Three subjects were having generalized seizures daily or more frequently; one had not seen his general practitioner for 2 to 4 months, and one for 6 to 12 months.

Only 10 subjects in the whole sample were under current outpatient supervision for their epilepsy, and in half of these such supervision seemed rather unnecessary—5 subjects had generalized seizures other than petit mal yearly or less frequently. Conversely, three subjects were discharged from hospital supervision when the frequency of attacks was weekly or more frequently.

At one stage we began to review the pattern of patient care within outpatient clinics. The quality of the notes did not allow a useful conclusion to be drawn, apart from the observation that in small units the patient could usually expect to see the consultant, whereas in large units he stood little chance of so doing. For example, for 22 visits made by one subject to one hospital, 16 different signatures were present in the notes, and there was no record of a consultant seeing him. Ross (1975) found that "the number of different doctors seen [by children with epilepsy] appeared to be almost directly proportional to the number of visits paid to the hospital."

DISCUSSION

Those aspects of medical "management" that we have chosen to accent reveal the following pattern of events and care. People with epilepsy generally do not anticipate the diagnosis of epilepsy, but those who seek help usually do so after the first episode. Nearly all are referred for specialist advice, even though the correct diagnosis of epilepsy is nearly always made by the general practitioner. The hospital doctor, however, usually tells the patient the diagnosis, although in a significant minority (18%) communication of the diagnosis fails to take place. Failure of communication is more likely to occur in the poorly educated.

Of those who are referred to hospital, 86% have one or more EEGs, but more than half of these are normal, and in no way do these contribute to management. Only normal traces had been recorded in 5 of 12 subjects having generalized seizures monthly or more frequently at the time of interview; conversely, highly abnormal records with multiple sites of epileptic discharges occurred in 4 out of 13 having at the time of interview occasional seizures only. We fully accept that intensive EEG monitoring as described by Penry and by Wolf *(this volume)* will increase the yield of recorded abnormal discharges, but it is remarkable how routine records have been carried out for nearly 40 years with so little benefit to doctor or patient (Matthews, 1973). A biochemical test with so many false negatives would never have entered clinical practice. Our study has also shown that anticonvulsant treatment is extremely conservative in both choice and quantity of drug, and half those having generalized seizures monthly or more frequently are probably undertreated. Continuing medical supervision seems fairly random—half of the few still attending hospital clinics have rare seizures, whereas some of those with frequent seizures do not see even their general practitioner for some months.

This irregular pattern of medical care contrasts with the precepts of the Reid Report (H.M.S.O., 1969) quoted in the first paragraph of this chapter: "The family doctor will undoubtedly wish to refer the majority of his patients [with epilepsy] for consultant advice, as an epileptic fit is a symptom, rather than a disease, and prolonged investigation may be necessary before a firm diagnosis can be reached."

Our view is the converse, and we believe that the great majority of people with epilepsy would benefit from a less ritualistic management of their condition. Although general practitioners have shown themselves, from their referral letters, to be perfectly capable of making the diagnosis of epilepsy and instituting anticonvulsant treatment, referral to a specialist has become a ritual necessity. We suggest that the reason for hospital referral of people with epilepsy is that the illness "epilepsy" can be legitimized, in sociological terms, only by a specialist, even if diagnosed by the general practitioner.

The specialist often reveals the diagnosis. But the specialist has his rituals too. Legitimization of his diagnosis by the EEG is his ritual, although our own material and many other studies (reviewed by Matthews, 1973) have shown the result to be of no value in predicting outcome or in diagnosing the underlying cause. There are further ritual aspects of management. We draw attention particularly to the customs of altering anticonvulsant regimens with no adequate statistical method of comparing intervals between seizures and adjusting dosage without, in the great majority of subjects, assessment of blood levels. The inadequate regimens prescribed for many of our subjects with continuing seizures suggest that a physician's honor is satisfied as long as *some* tablets are taken. The finding that some with rare generalized seizures still attend hospital clinics whereas other patients with daily or weekly generalized seizures—other than petit mal—have not seen their general practitioner for some months suggests that medical supervision is not related to patient need.

ACKNOWLEDGMENTS

This work was supported by the Epilepsy Research Fund of the British Epilepsy Association. We are grateful to those general practitioners who allowed us access to their records and to the people who told us about their epilepsy.

REFERENCES

H.M.S.O. (1969): *The Reid Report: People with Epilepsy.* Her Majesty's Stationery Office, London.
Hopkins, A., and Scambler, G. (1976): The social implications of epilepsy. *Adv. Med.,* 12:100–105.
Matthews, W. B. (1973): The clinical value of routine electroencephalography. *J. R. Coll. Physicians London,* 7:207–212.
Richens, A. (1970): Disturbance of calcium metabolism by anticonvulsant drugs. *Br. Med. J.,* 4:73–76.
Ross, E. M. (1975): A Bristol study of secondary school children with epilepsy. M.D. thesis, University of Bristol.

Epilepsy, The Eighth International Symposium,
edited by J. K. Penry. Raven Press, New York
© 1977.

Pilot Study on Theme-Centered Interaction Groups with Epileptic Patients

*Brunhilde Mayer and **Leopold Gutjahr

*Medical Psychology Division and **Clinical Neurophysiology and Experimental Neurology Division, Medical School Hannover, 61, Germany*

Epileptic patients as a group are characterized by their specific illness profile and the sociocultural effect thereof. In their seizure-free periods there is no difference between them and their healthy social partners within the family and their professions. They have analogous abilities for dealing with reality, taking into account their scholastic and professional development and their social class. Their illness is not visible and the so-called epileptic character changes are often changes more of social etiquette than real changes in intellectual or personal characteristics. Similar signs can also be seen in healthy individuals.

Persons with epilepsy, however, form a special group because of the particular pressures on them as the result of their illness. Certain civil rights are denied them, such as the freedom of choice in a place of work and the right to drive a motorized vehicle. The consumption of alcohol is forbidden, partaking in sports is possible only to a limited extent, and so on. They have the same chances within their social strata only until their first seizure, that is, until others have experienced them and their illness. Epileptic patients cannot acquire their own picture of their illness and so have to rely on the descriptions given by those in their immediate environment. Thus, they cannot themselves experience an important part of their social picture. Throughout their seizures they are completely at the mercy of the reaction of their environment, a reaction that they are unable to experience. With each new adaptation or change of medication resulting in a seizure-free period comes the hope of being completely seizure-free, until the next attack destroys these hopes. Depending on seizure frequency, the feelings of oppression may take different levels, but they have no principal differences.

The special form of the disease leads to the effect that epileptic patients are at least in part dominated by some members of their social group. Since they are dependent on help and assistance, their social role is generally that of dependence. From morning to evening, what they do and do not do is controlled. The temporary condition of unconsciousness is expanded by their environment to a reduction in their social responsibility. The patient experiences in his illness and social situation a feeling of helplessness and comes against an apparently unbreakable social chain that forces on him a feeling of dependence.

Although the causal mechanisms of the central nervous system which lead to seizures are not yet sufficiently understood, the correlation to corporeal and stress situations has been extensively proven. Treatment of epileptic patients must provide support in the psychosocial area, in addition to the medicative treatment, so that the patient may be in a position to consider objectively his real possibilities. These patients must learn to be specific about their own needs and desires and to adapt these to their potential and illness-specific limitations in order to achieve conditions for self-realization that have been worked out in cooperation with their social partners. How such treatment could be carried out with a group of outpatients is demonstrated by means of the group therapy we performed and the results on the life style of our patients. The aim of this work is to provide suggestions, not to set up directives.

DISCUSSION OF THE LITERATURE

In spite of repeated demands for new psychiatric, psychological, and psychotherapeutic methods in research and therapy by, among others, the Federal Research Council of Germany in *Memorandum Epilepsy,* the pertinent literature reports, if at all, only on general concepts of rehabilitation. Van Wessem (1976), for example, was critical at last year's congress of the medicosomatic understanding of the doctors and the superstitious nature of the Italian public where he estimated only 5% of the epileptics were recognized as such. He considered a lay organization that he had set up to be a relatively optimal form of self-assistance. At the same time, Burden (1976) demonstrated the social problems of such lay organizations, whose endeavors at social integration of the patients are doomed to failure through lack of institutional support and often result in deeper isolation instead of the desired integration. Brullemann (1972) reported on the only group therapeutic attempt that we are aware of. He used Rogers' client-centered method and emphasized that a direct approach is sometimes suitable if one is to achieve in the patient an effective adaptation to reality and awareness of his problems. He further emphasized that the basis of group therapy must remain the interaction among the group members.

As in all psychotherapeutic methods, there is a dependence on the selection of the patients who should be, in the opinion of the doctor in charge, capable of rehabilitation, but are also limited in their communicative ability as a result of their social isolation. In such cases, the group provides significant possibilities for communicative and self-confidence training, possibilities that could not be provided by a doctor only.

Hakkarainen (1976) estimates that 8% of patients with epilepsy can be rehabilitated through employment. About 10% of the patients in the epilepsy outpatient department of the Medical School Hannover fall into this category. We selected the patients to participate in group therapy from 280 regularly treated patients.

We finally asked 15 patients, of whom 8 partook more or less regularly in the group meeting.

DESCRIPTION OF THE PATIENT POPULATION

Table 1 shows that five of the eight patients had left school, one was undergoing job training, and three had completed their apprenticeship. Three patients were out of work, the patient in training being considered as having the same status as those in work. Most of the patients lived at home, although the only well-qualified professional of our patients had been in the hospital for 1 year due to chronic alcoholism. Only one of the patients was professionally and socially fully integrated and had private contacts outside of his immediate family. None of the patients had a relationship with a definite partner, two being widowed after ruined marriages. With regard to their family relationships, we noted that our two youngest patients lived in a pleasant home atmosphere and felt secure therein. All others considered their situation somewhat conflicting and ambivalent. The biggest problem was that of patient No. 5, who was rejected by his extremely domineering mother and who needed the immediate active support of the therapist before he would provide even a minimum of information, such as the amount of state-provided financial assistance that was being withheld from him by his mother. The parents of patient No. 3, who was herself the mother of two children, attempted to forbid her to take part in the group therapy, which she had described as being "tuition."

Table 2 summarizes data regarding seizure type, EEG findings, and psychiatric

TABLE 1. *Social situation during group therapy*

	Before therapy	After therapy
Education		
Elementary school completed	5	5
Job training	1	2
Job training completed	3	3
Financial support		
Disability pension	1	1
Employed	4	6
Unemployed	3	1
Place of living		
Family	5	4
Alone	2	2
Commune	0	1
At a sheltered workplace	0	1
Hospital	1	0
Private contacts outside the family		
Normal	1	2
Occasional	5	4
None	2	2

TABLE 2. Medical data of patients joining theme-centered group therapy

Patient	Age	Sex	Family attitudes			Seizures				EEG			Psychiatric symptoms			
			Pro-tective	Over pro-tective	Oppres-sive	Grand mal	Psycho motor	Absences	Other	Seizure dis-charges	Focus	Dysrhyth-mia	Psycho-motor retarda-ation	Disturb-ance of atten-tiveness	Marked Intel-lectual reduction	Depression
1	16	F	+			+	+	+	–	+	–	+	–	+	+	+
2	30	F		+		+	+	–	–	–	+	+	+	–	+	–
3	37	F		+		+	–	–	–	+	+	+	–	+	+	–
4	21	M			+	+	–	–	+	+	–	–	–	–	–	+
5	28	M			+	+	–	+	–	–	–	+	–	–	–	+
6	24	M	+			+	+	+	–	–	+	+	+	–	Unknown	–
7	38	M	+ (mother)			+	+	–	–	–	–	+	–	–	–	–
8	34	M			+	+	+	–	–	–	–	–	–	–	–	–
Total			3	2	3	8	5	2	1	3	3	6	2	2	2	3

symptoms. The patients showed vast differences with regard to the frequency of their attacks; however, each of them had suffered from epilepsy for a number of years.

Therapeutic Method

The group met one evening a week for 1½ hr over a period of 3 months and then, after the summer break, for another 4 months. The conversations were recorded on videotape and used in exemplary cases as a feedback on the patients' behavior. At the beginning of each session, the patients reported on the latest happenings of the week. Then followed the discussion of a topic agreed on in the previous week. The topics discussed included, for example: "We want to live— alone or with other people—in small or large groups;" "Fear of an attack and how to live with it;" "Everyone should bring something he thinks will cheer up the others and say why he is of this opinion." Further points of discussion were the patients' attitudes to the family, to children, to partnerhood, and to religion. The so-called controlled dialogue method was used upon consideration of the topic "talking and listening to one another, and understanding each other," whereupon we noticed that the individual's ability to concentrate was drastically reduced when he or she was no longer the focal point of the group's activities. It was noticeable that the patients' egocentricity contributed to a large extent to their isolation and that they should learn to expand their areas of interest to topics that did not have primary interest to them. The initial topic, "problems of epilepsy," took on lesser and lesser importance. Problems of adaptation to their immediate environment were of vital interest to all, and one could see the effects of being able to provide mutual support and useful assistance. Because of the interactions within the group and the necessity of being able to specify their intrafamiliar dependency, this dependency was recognized and ways of dealing with such conflicts were specifically discussed. The patients were actively supported by the group members with regard to the resultant conflicts with their families, and they received a very critical feedback on their behavior and the consequences thereof. They received in some cases such active support for their attempts in emancipation that we as therapists were forced to restrictiveness so that they did not lose sight of their actual dependency.

The respective sociological and medical data show in some cases a definite improvement in the social and medical condition, something that we had not hoped for.

Social Situation

Three patients found employment. The position held by patient No. 2 could not, however, be continued after its predefined termination date. Patient No. 4 was accepted for training as a nurse's assistant. The living conditions improved for patients No. 5 and No. 8, patient No. 8 attaining a definite partner relationship for the first time in his life. However, patient No. 1, after completion of her scholastic education, was confronted with the strong social rejection resulting from her illness. Because she could not get accepted for an apprenticeship, she had to go to a school catering for job training that was governed by retired schoolteachers. The lack of understanding there deepened her feelings of social isolation. The group was also of little help for the next youngest patient (patient No. 6), who felt no necessity for leaving his parents' home. He followed the group's suggestion for making extrafamiliar contacts but was unable to break out of isolation. Anyhow, it was not possible for most of the patients to achieve an increase in their extrafamiliar contacts in such a short time.

Medical Data

After a manifest improvement in certain patients throughout the group therapy, the deterioration in the condition of some of our patients after its conclusion came as a shock to us. We have useful data regarding the seizure rate of four of our eight patients (Fig. 1). These data have been analyzed with respect to the sequential test method of Johnson et al. (1959) that we presented last year (Gutjahr et al., 1976).

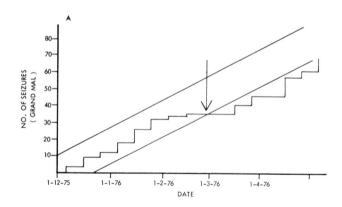

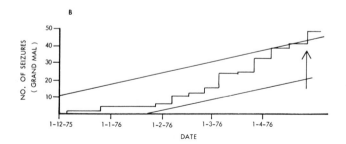

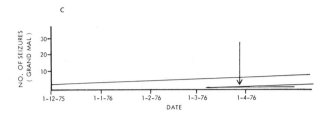

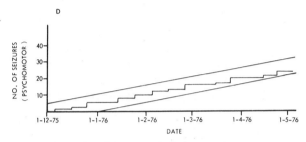

FIG. 1. Graphic monitoring of the absolute frequencies of seizures summarized over 10-day periods. The significant changes were tested by sequential analysis. The crossing of the confidence boundaries shows a change in seizure incidence at the 5% significance level. The pretest period commenced 120 days before the start of group therapy, and follow-up studies were done for 2 months after the end of therapy. **A:** Patient No. 3. Seizures in pretest period: 0.72/day; significant reduction of 25% of attacks at the end of group therapy, with obvious increase afterwards. **B:** Patient No. 2. Seizures in pretest period: 0.24/day; strong trend toward seizure reduction during therapy, with a significant increase 2 months after the end of group therapy. **C:** Patient No. 5. Seizures in pretest period: 0.08/day; significant reduction of 75%; because of minimal seizure frequency, a significant reduction occurred after the end of group therapy, although no attack occurred during the therapy period. **D:** Patient No. 6. Seizures in pretest period: 0.13/day; no significant change during or after group therapy.

A significant reduction in the seizure rate within the therapy period can be seen for patients No. 3 and No. 5 from the crossing of the lower tolerance boundary in their seizure profile. A direct improvement could not be read from the other two profiles. On the other hand, a significant increase in seizure rate after the breakup of the group could be seen in the profile of patient No. 2.

CONCLUSION

In spite of our small patient population and our conscious abandonment of experimental procedures and thereby the possibility of a scientific control, we have reported here on our pilot studies.

The meaning of group therapy to the patients was: the major function of the group for all patients who took part was the possibility of interaction with others. It was the only weekly event that was, perhaps because of the long journey to the big city of Hannover, an adventure. They all emphasized the importance of knowing that someone would be there who would listen, who would give of his time, whom they could talk to, and who needed them. This alone would in our opinion justify the time and effort involved. Apart from this, we as therapists saw that we were able to obtain data that proved our influence on the course of the illness in half of the cases. One could possibly achieve by means of group therapy a psychic stabilization and improved tolerance of affects that have until now been merely attempted in vain by chemotherapy.

We make our appeal in the small hope that some workers may be in charge of improved research and working environments and will have the financial capabilities of furthering the psychosocial approach we have mentioned in order to achieve a modern understanding of epileptic patients and to offer concrete assistance to such patients. We consider outpatient care in real-life situations, with its possibilities for the reduction of a conflict situation, to be at least as sensible and perhaps less costly than short-term confinement of the patients in rehabilitation centers, which build up hopes that are quickly shattered in the reality and lack of understanding of society, forcing the patients back into their loneliness.

REFERENCES

Brullemann, L. H. (1972): Group therapy with epileptic patients at the Instituut voor Epilepsiebestrijding. *Epilepsia,* 13:225–231.
Burden, G. (1976): The role of lay organizations in the treatment of people with epilepsy. In: *Epileptology,* Proceedings of the Seventh International Symposium on Epilepsy, Berlin (West), June 1975, edited by D. Janz. Thieme/PSG, Stuttgart.
Gutjahr, L., Kunkel, H., and Starck, R. (1976): The usefulness of modern documentation methods in treating outpatients with epileptic seizures. In: *Epileptology,* Proceedings of the Seventh International Symposium on Epilepsy, Berlin (West), June 1975, edited by D. Janz. Thieme/PSG, Stuttgart.
Hakkarainen, H. (1976): Criteria of assessment in rehabilitation of patients with epilepsy. In: *Epileptology,* Proceedings of the Seventh International Symposium on Epilepsy, Berlin (West), June 1975, edited by D. Janz. Thieme/PSG, Stuttgart.
Janz, D. (1975): *Memorandum Epilepsy.* Harald Boldt Verlag, Boppard.
Johnson, E., Haus, E., Halberg, F., and Wadsworth, G. L. (1959): Graphic monitoring of seizure incidence changes in epileptic patients. *Minn. Med.,* 42:1250–1257.
van Wessem, G. C. (1976): Certain aspects of lay organizations with special emphasis on the situation in Italy. In: *Epileptology,* Proceedings of the Seventh International Symposium on Epilepsy, Berlin (West), June 1975, edited by D. Janz. Thieme/PSG, Stuttgart.

Epilepsy, The Eighth International Symposium,
edited by J. K. Penry. Raven Press, New York
© 1977.

Operant Conditioning for Behavior Modification in Institutionalized Retarded Children

Ulrike Zöllner-Breusch

Swiss Institute for Epilepsy, Zurich, Switzerland

The rehabilitation of patients suffering from epileptic reactions is interdependent not only with the medical control of the fits but also with the socialization of the accompanying psychic symptoms (in particular, the lability of affective structures with tendency to egocentric, explosive reactions). These symptoms are considered to be due partly to a cerebral dysfunction, partly to an alteration of the patient's relationship with his social environment.

The majority of patients who need to be hospitalized will benefit little from psychotherapeutic treatment because their intellectual abilities are reduced; they have trouble exercising self-criticism, lack objectivity toward themselves, and cannot control themselves sufficiently. The therapy must therefore have an extrapsychic basis.

The operant techniques used in behavior therapy allow the modification of psychic disorders by influencing the external social situation of the patient. It is then possible, by controlling the external frame of the patient's behavior and by using contingent sanctions, to correct the behavioral disorders. The aim of the therapy is the modification of the individual's disturbed learning process.

Operant techniques have been used successfully for 10 years with psychiatric patients suffering from maladjustment and with mentally retarded patients. There is a complete description in the literature of the problems encountered and the results obtained with these patients by using behavior therapy (Gottwald and Redlin, 1972; Aitchison and Green, 1974). In the field of epilepsy the use of behavior therapy has so far been limited for the most to classic conditioning. Efron (1956) describes a case of psychomotor epilepsy in which he succeeded in interrupting the aura by applying a conditioned stimulus. Recently biofeedback experiments have shown possible interesting applications of the classic conditioning methods (Sterman, 1973). So far only Buddeberg (1975) has reported on using operant conditioning with a hospitalized epileptic patient suffering from a severe personality change. Buddeberg stresses the significance of behavior therapy with epileptic patients who present psychopathological symptoms consisting mainly of behavior and adaptation disorders.

We are reporting on our experiences in the use of operant techniques for the rehabilitation of epileptic patients on the basis of two case studies.

CASE STUDIES

Eating Training with a Mentally Retarded Child

At the beginning of therapy the girl was 3 years and 7 months old. The following diagnosis was made: (1) epileptic reactions from the first year of life, first salaam fits, later myoclonic-astatic fits (Lennox syndrome); and (2) severe psychomotor retardation corresponding to an idiocy following early brain damage.

In the course of the antiepileptic treatment the girl developed a loss of appetite which required her to be fed through a nasogastric tube, at first intermittently, and later permanently. After her general condition had improved, the child refused to eat in a normal way and reacted with crying and screaming to the presentation of food or a spoon.

We decided that three factors were responsible for the patient's disturbed behavior:

1. Classic conditioning processes, i.e., while eating the patient had experienced negative intra- or extrapsychic stimuli which had led her to react with aversion;
2. Momentary worsening of the patient's physical condition leading to a regression, to apathy, and to sleepiness;
3. Fixation and stereotyping of the faulty behavior based on 1 and 2.

The therapeutic aims were therefore reduction of the aversion by gradually bringing food and spoon closer to the patient, and progressive building of normal eating behavior supported by positive and negative reinforcement.

The design of the therapy program was as follows:

Stage 1
  Aim: Acceptance of the spoon without food
Stage 2
  Aim: Acceptance of the spoon in the mouth without food
Stage 3
  Aim: Acceptance of the spoon with food
Stage 4
  Aim: Acceptance of the food in the mouth
Stage 5
  Aim: The food to be chewed and swallowed

Contingent positive and negative reinforcement was used in each stage. Positive reinforcement was used whenever the behavior aimed at in each phase was elicited. For positive reinforcers, we used a light (the child reacted promptly only to a red flashlight) or verbal reinforcement with the words "nice" and "good" connected with caressing. Negative reinforcers were used whenever defense mechanisms appeared, and they included turning off the light, punishment, i.e., time-out (the child's head was held down for a short period of time, which implied

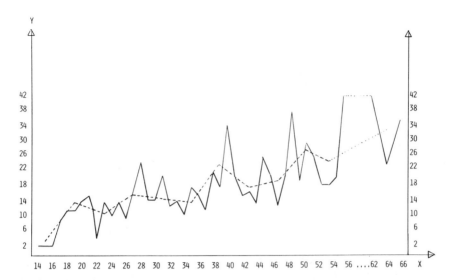

FIG. 1. Results from stage 5 of the therapy program. X, days in training stage 5; Y, number of spoonfuls eaten; ————, average in 1 day; – – – –, average in 4 days.

a lack of social reinforcement by the environment), and verbal punishment using the word "no" in conjunction with a short shaking of the child. A similar approach is described by Gutezeit et al. (1976).

During training stages 1 through 3, the therapeutic aims were reached very quickly. After a few sessions the child no longer reacted defensively to the spoon and opened her mouth spontaneously. But for a long time this spontaneous behavior was unstable, that is, during stage 4 of the training the child held her mouth closely shut as soon as food was presented. We encountered another problem during stage 5 which could be overcome only after a long training period: the child accepted the food willingly but did not chew or swallow it. In this case punishment with the word "no" and shaking proved very effective.

A few results from stage 5 are summarized graphically in Fig. 1. The number of training stages on the abscissa shows that progress was very slow. It was possible to keep the eating frequency reached at the end of the curve on a constant level until the child was sent home.

We followed the program for 1½ months in sessions of 30 min three times a day. Later it was carried out under supervision by the nursing staff for 2½ months until the child was able to eat normally for her age. The catamnesis confirms the success of the therapy. Ten months later the patient's eating behavior is still normal.

Group Management Based on the Principles of Behavior Therapy

We used techniques of behavior therapy with a group of nine male epileptic adolescents with a normal to imbecile level of intelligence and an average age of 16 years and 8 months. These techniques have been used so far for 1 year successfully as a basis of group management, with two purposes in the rehabilitation program in view: socialization (training adaptability and conflict management) and work training (practicing simple activities at the protected workshop level, training positive work orientation).

The contingent reinforcement of the defined behavior is done through a token rewarding system. The behavior to be rewarded is defined uniformly for all members of the group, except for individual differences with regard to the kind and quantity of work. The behavior to be corrected through punishment (taking back of tokens) is also defined uniformly. The exchange value of the tokens is adjusted to the boy's individual needs and interests (e.g., acquisition of food or records, movie going, taking care of the institute's animals). We also made good experiences in offering to exchange tokens for a certain amount of our time (e.g., 30-min discussions). These opportunities for discussion are useful on one hand in promoting the patient's need of relationship and transference, on the other hand in taking away some of the pressures put on the patient in the course of the program. They also help us correct therapeutically the patient's exaggerated need for negation. Also, the nurses find it useful to be able to tell patients, when they tend to become too talkative or too invading, to wait until the evening discussion.

We are supporting the token system successfully by a special evaluation of the work done in the workshop. We fix a basic salary according to the individual average; if the patient works well, we add a certain amount to it, if his work is unsatisfactory, we subtract from it. The day's salary is written down every evening in the patient's salary book. At the same time we discuss with him the day's events, warn him, or motivate him. At the end of the week the sum that the patient has earned by working especially well is doubled and given to him as pocket money, which works as an added motivation.

When working with groups on the basis of behavior therapy, it is possible to use social competition to promote social values. The tendency to compete within the group works in a regulatory manner on the patient's egocentric behavior. We try to teach the patients social criticism and to build their self-control by having them meet every evening for a group discussion during which they give each other the points earned during the day. A big board hangs on the wall of the group room, with columns for the whole week. The points are marked on this board, which allows a judgment of the individual's efforts and a comparison with the other members of the group; this works as a supplementary inducement.[1]

Most important for group management is the fact that the behavior modification programs allow continuous and congruent care of the patients even when the nursing staff changes. Also, these programs give us a chance to include difficult cases in a resocialization process, in particular adolescents who, because of their aggressive behavior, have been put in a closed ward.

---

[1] An introduction to the possibilities of the token system is given by Ayllon and Azrin (1968).

FURTHER PROBLEMS

The elaboration of a behavior therapy program should have two aims: (1) the guiding principles must be transferable (so that continuity is provided when the nursing staff changes), and (2) autonomy of the nursing staff working on the program must be possible.

The following points have proven to be relevant to the elaboration of a program:

1. Patient's description (epileptic fits, short anamnesis, present clinical status)
2. Results of the neuropsychological investigation (intelligence and personality, extent of mental retardation, individual handicaps, points relevant to the training)
3. Description of the behavior disorders (defined at an operational level—base line of behavior)
4. Aims of therapy
5. Description of the therapeutic methods (e.g., primary reinforcement, token reinforcement)
6. Reinforcement schedule (e.g., fixed ratio reinforcement, contingent reinforcement)
7. Description of the behavior to be rewarded (defined at an operational level)
8. Description of the behavior to be punished (defined at an operational level)
9. Exchange of reinforcers
10. Additional indications for education and management

After similar coaching, the nursing staff can normally work on its own under loose supervision. Regular discussions of critical situations are used mainly to train the staff to think in terms of behavior therapy. The problems encountered with the nursing staff are related mainly to the fact that they consider behavior modification to be an inhuman technology. Concretely these resistances diminish rapidly when the staff realize that the coaching they have received is helpful and gives them a feeling of safety. Also, the rapid success of the therapy helps to engender a more positive attitude toward patients who previously had been feared and rejected.

It is important to modify the program continuously (in particular the rewards) and to give the nursing staff full support if, after the well-known initial success, some setbacks appear. If severe, nonreactive episodes of irritability and psychotic disturbances occur, it makes sense to withdraw the patient immediately from the group and to fade out the program until the trouble disappears. This prevents a violation of the therapeutic principles by the patient's lack of interest and his diminished sense of reality.

In our experience the frequency of epileptic seizures cannot be influenced by such a program. In a few cases of severe psychogenic reactions it is possible to punish hysterical fits within the program framework. This is rarely useful because both the patient and the other members of the group tend to perceive it as a lack of insight and can react with behavioral problems. It is useful, though, to ignore consequently or to reinforce the attitudes that are not compatible.

The side effects of medication can modify the therapeutic aims to a large extent. It is therefore essential to keep adapting the program to the patient's achievement level. In extreme cases sedation can hinder the therapeutic effort because the patient is not able to react sufficiently to the demands of the program. This is why we try to use drugs carefully and, if possible, in small dosages.

REFERENCES

Aitchison, R. A., and Green, D. R. (1974): A token reinforcement system for large wards of institutionalized adolescents. *Behav. Res. Ther.,* 12:181–190.

Ayllon, T., and Azrin, N. H. (1968): *Token Economy: A Motivational System for Therapy and Rehabilitation.* Appleton-Century-Crofts, New York.

Buddeberg, C. (1975): Möglichkeiten und Grenzen der Verhaltenstherapie in der Behandlung schwer wesensgeänderter Epileptiker. *Nervenarzt,* 46:447–452.

Efron, R. (1956): Effect of olfactory stimuli in arresting uncinate fits. *Brain,* 79:267–281.

Gottwald, P., and Redlin, W. (1972): Verhaltenstherapie bei geistig behinderten Kindern. Göttingen.

Gutezeit, G., Delfs-Heuer, F., and Grosse, R. (1976): Zur Behandlung einer schweren Esstörung bei einem 7-jährigen retardierten Mädchen. *Prax. Kinderpsychol. Kinderpsychiatr.,* 25(5):161–173.

Sterman, M. B. (1973): Neurophysiological and clinical studies of sensorimotor EEG biofeedback training: Some effects on epilepsy. *Semin. Psychiatry,* 5:507–525.

Epilepsy, The Eighth International Symposium,
edited by J. K. Penry. Raven Press, New York
© 1977.

A Study of Intellectual Function in Children with Epilepsy Attending Ordinary Schools

* D. H. Mellor and ** I. Lowit

** City Hospital, Hucknall Road, Nottingham, England; and ** Royal Aberdeen
Children's Hospital, Cornhill Road, Aberdeen, Scotland*

Until recently most studies, as reviewed by Keating (1960), have shown a high incidence of intellectual impairment among epileptic children. However, many of these studies did not differentiate between children with symptomatic and those with idiopathic epilepsy. Often highly selected and even institutionalized epileptic children were studied, and carefully matched control groups were rarely used. Of recent studies, that of Rutter, Graham, and Yule (1970a) is particularly valuable. They identified 86 epileptic children aged 5 to 14 years on the Isle of Wight among a total school population of 11,865, a prevalence of 7.2 per 1,000. In 22 of the children the fits were associated with cerebral palsy or other brain disorder, and, not surprisingly, many of these children were found to be of low intelligence. The remaining 64 children had uncomplicated epilepsy and were found to have a normal distribution of full-scale IQ scores on the Wechsler Intelligence Scale for Children (WISC) with a mean score of 102. Stores (1971) has made a plea for more careful studies of cognitive function in well-defined subgroups of children with epilepsy.

PATIENTS AND METHODS

A group of 285 children was identified through hospital and other records, who were aged 7 to 15 years, had been diagnosed as having epilepsy, and were attending ordinary schools in the northeast (Grampian) region of Scotland. This represents a prevalence rate of 5.87 per 1,000, which is similar to the prevalence rates found in other surveys of childhood epilepsy (Pond et al., 1960; Brewis et al., 1966; Rutter et al., 1970b). Each epileptic schoolchild was matched with the classmate nearest in age and of the same sex. In this way a matched control group of children was formed.

Children attending ordinary schools in the northeast region of Scotland routinely receive the Moray House Test at 9 or 11 years of age. This test is one of reasoning ability and yields a reasoning quotient which is comparable to a ratio IQ with a mean value of 100 and a standard deviation of 15 for the normal population (University of Edinburgh Department of Education, 1961, 1968).

Results of this test were available for 221 of the epileptic children, 224 of the control children, and 216 matched pairs of epileptic and control children.

The child's father's occupation was used to determine the family's social class group as described by Birch et al. (1970). With this scheme social classes I through IIIB comprise nonmanual and artisan occupations and IIIC through V are manual occupations. Information was available to classify 209 of the epileptic children with Moray House scores in this way.

To assess behavior, we used the questionnaire for completion by the child's teacher devised by Rutter (1967). The higher the score on this questionnaire, the less desirable is the child's behavior. Also, a correlation has been found between behavior disorder as judged by traditional psychiatric assessment and a score of more than 8 on the questionnaire. Questionnaires were returned for 212 of our epileptic children with Moray House scores.

Prospectively coded perinatal information was available for 133 of the epileptic children with Moray House scores from data recorded as part of a Medical Research Council Obstetric study in Aberdeen. An adverse perinatal factor score was devised which was composed of those events known to be related to increased perinatal mortality (Butler and Bonham, 1963).

RESULTS

Table 1 summarizes the results. Comparison of the epileptic children with their matched controls on the results of the Moray House scores showed significantly more epileptic children with low scores. Exclusion of 6 children with evidence of symptomatic epilepsy did not alter this finding. Epileptic children from families of social classes IIIC through V had significantly lower scores than those from social classes I through IIIB. This was also the case in the control group, but there was no significant difference in social class distribution between the epileptic and control children. Lower Moray House scores in both epileptic and control children were significantly associated with high scores on the behavior questionnaire and therefore with behavior disorder. When compared with their matched controls, the epileptic boys showed significantly lower Moray House scores, but the epileptic girls' scores were not significantly different from those of their matched controls. There was a tendency for low Moray House scores to be associated with a high incidence of adverse perinatal factors, onset of epilepsy in the first year of life, a negative family history of epilepsy, and a mixed seizure type, but none of these differences reached statistical significance.

DISCUSSION

Reviewing the literature on the relationship between intelligence and epilepsy, Rodin (1968) concludes that children with "non-organic" epilepsy usually have intellectual abilities within the normal range, but there is a tendency for the lower end of the normal range to be overrepresented. Our results strongly support this conclusion and are somewhat at variance with those of Rutter, Graham, and Yule

TABLE 1. *Comparisons between the various identified groups on the basis of Moray House scores*

Groups compared	Moray House scores
Epileptic children/matched controls	Lower scores in epileptic children ($p < 0.001$)
Children with idiopathic epilepsy/ matched controls	Lower scores in epileptic children ($p < 0.001$)
Epileptic children from social class I–IIIB families/epileptic children from social class IIIC–V families	Lower scores in epileptic children from social class IIIC–V families ($p < 0.02$)
Epileptic children with behavior disorder/epileptic children without behavior disorder	Lower scores in epileptic children with behavior disorder ($p < 0.001$)
Epileptic boys/matched control boys	Lower scores in epileptic boys ($p < 0.01$)
Epileptic girls/matched control girls	No significant difference (trend for lower scores in epileptic girls)
Epileptic children with adverse perinatal factors/epileptic children without adverse perinatal factors	No significant difference (trend for lower scores in epileptic children with adverse perinatal factors)
Epileptic children with onset in early childhood/epileptic children with onset in later childhood	No significant difference (trend for lower scores in epileptic children with onset in early childhood)
Epileptic children with positive family history/epileptic children with negative family history	No significant difference (trend for lower scores in epileptic children with negative family history)
Epileptic children with single seizure type/epileptic children with mixed seizure type	No significant difference (trend for lower scores in epileptic children with mixed seizure type)

(1970*a*) who found a normal distribution of full-scale WISC scores among children on the Isle of Wight with uncomplicated epilepsy. However, they did show a higher than expected frequency of discrepancies between the WISC verbal and performance subscales, and 18% of the children had significant reading retardation on the Neale Analysis of Reading Ability, suggesting a high incidence of more subtle cognitive disabilities.

In the general childhood population, milder degrees of intellectual impairment are commoner in the lower socioeconomic groups (Birch et al., 1970). Our finding of lower Moray House scores in the epileptic children of manual workers is therefore not unexpected and suggests that social class has a role in determining intellectual ability in epileptic children similar to that in other children.

Lower IQ scores have been shown to be associated with a higher rate of psychiatric disability within the general childhood population (Rutter et al., 1970*b*). Our study shows that this is also true for epileptic children attending ordinary schools. Stores (1971) has suggested that cognitive deficits in epileptic children may interfere with the normal process of social learning and so generate disturbed behavior.

The poorer intellectual showing of the epileptic boys is of interest as most previous studies of uncomplicated epilepsy have not shown any sex differences in overall cognitive function.

Failure to find a significant relationship between perinatal events and intellectual ability in this study may be because it was limited to children attending ordinary schools. Pasamanick and Lilienfeld (1955) were able to show an association between adverse perinatal events and mental handicap, but they studied a population with a wider range of intellectual ability.

Several previous studies have shown that epilepsy commencing in infancy carries a poorer prognosis for intellectual ability than when it starts later in childhood (Zimmerman et al., 1951; Halstead, 1957; Rodin, 1968). Halstead (1957) was also able to show that lower scores on the Stanford-Binet test were more common in the absence of a family history of epilepsy and in children with a mixed seizure pattern. That the present study was able to show similar trends without their reaching statistical significance is probably because the study was limited to children attending ordinary schools so that mentally handicapped children were excluded.

REFERENCES

Birch, H. G., Richardson, S. A., Baird, D., Horobin, G., and Illsley, R. (1970): *Mental Subnormality in the Community*. Williams & Wilkins, Baltimore.

Brewis, M., Poskaner, D. C., Rolland, C., and Miller, H. (1966): Neurological disease in an English City. *Acta Neurol. Scand.* [Suppl.] 24:42.

Butler, N. R., and Bonham, D. G. (1963): *Perinatal Mortality*. Livingstone, Edinburgh.

Halstead, H. (1957): Abilities and behaviour of epileptic children. *J. Ment. Sci.,* 102:28.

Keating, L. E. (1960): A review of the literature on the relationship of epilepsy and intelligence in schoolchildren. *J. Ment. Sci.,* 106:1042.

Pasamanick, B., and Lilienfeld, A. M. (1955): Association of maternal and fetal factors with development of mental deficiency. *J.A.M.A.,* 159:155.

Pond, D. A., Bidwell, B. H., and Stein, L. (1960): A survey of epilepsy in fourteen general practices. I. Demographic and medical data. *Psychiatr. Neurol. Neurochir. (Amst.),* 63:217.

Rodin, E. A. (1968): *The Prognosis of Patients with Epilepsy*. Charles C Thomas, Springfield, Ill.

Rutter, M. (1967): Children's behaviour questionnaire for completion by teachers. Preliminary findings. *J. Child Psychol. Psychiatry,* 8:1.

Rutter, M., Graham, P., and Yule, W. (1970a): *A Neuropsychiatric Study in Childhood*. Spastics International Medical Publications, London.

Rutter, M., Tizard, J., and Whitmore, K. (1970b): *Education, Health and Behavior*. Longmans, London.

Stores, G. (1971): Cognitive function in children with epilepsy. *Dev. Med. Child Neurol.,* 13:390.

University of Edinburgh Department of Education (1961): *Manual of Instructions for the Moray House Junior Reasoning Test 2*. University of London Press, London.

University of Edinburgh Department of Education (1968): *Manual of Instructions for the Moray House Verbal Reasoning Test 81*. University of London Press, London.

Zimmerman, F. T., Burgemeister, B. B., and Putnam, T. J. (1951): Intellectual and emotional make-up of the epileptic. *Arch. Neurol. Psychiatry,* 65:545.

Epilepsy, The Eighth International Symposium,
edited by J. K. Penry. Raven Press, New York
© 1977.

Progressive Aphasia and Epilepsy with a Self-Limited Course

Hans C. Lou, Sven Brandt and * Peter Bruhn

*Department of Pediatrics TG, and * Department of Neurology, Rigshospitalet,
Copenhagen, Denmark*

The present chapter concerns four young patients with normal or nearly normal development in every respect until the ages of 4 to 5 years. At that time, a rapid deterioration of spoken language and comprehension took place. In all cases the EEGs were found to be severely abnormal with bilateral spikes and spike waves, especially in the temporal regions, and in three cases epileptic seizures occurred. The onset of the disorder was insidious and was not accompanied by any overt sign of acute illness, except in the youngest patient (P.D.T.). The aphasia persisted for years in three cases, as did the EEG changes. The seizures were quite easily controlled with medication. At the time of EEG normalization, the antiepileptic medication could be discontinued. The EEGs of patient J. A. at the ages of 5, 6, and 15 years are shown in Fig. 1. The condition showed a

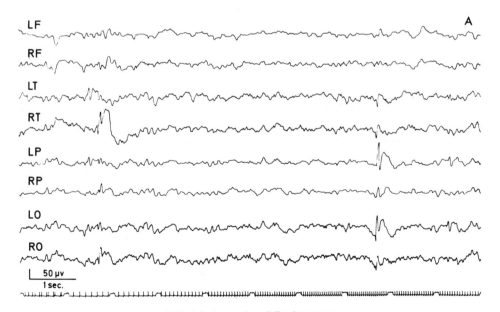

FIG. 1.A. Legend on following page.

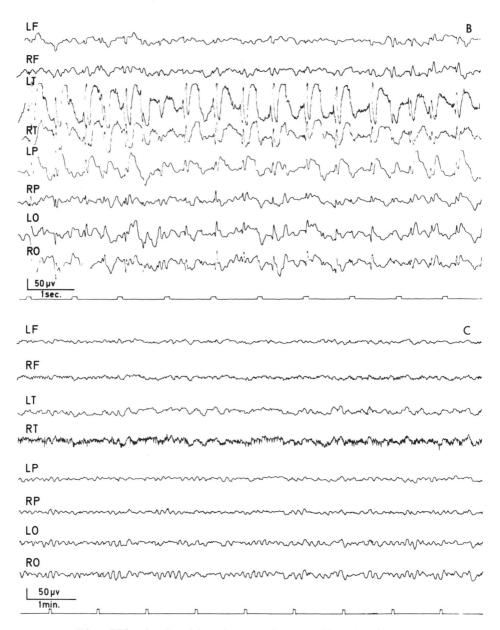

FIG. 1. EEGs of patient J.A. at the ages of 5 **(A)**, 6 **(B)**, and 15 **(C)** years.

fluctuating course with tendency to stepwise aggravation until it gradually improved. A severe aphasia persisted in only one patient.

   In 1957 Landau and Kleffner provided the first description of this syndrome. Since then four or five reports of similar cases have appeared (Worster-Drought,

1971; Gascon et al., 1973; Shoumaker et al., 1974; Deonna et al., 1975). In all cases, aphasia developed at ages 4 to 8, and in most cases myoclonic fits of the facial muscles or upper extremities, akinetic seizures, or psychomotor seizures preceded or accompanied the onset of aphasia. Later in the course grand mal seizures were frequent. EEGs have shown bilateral foci in all cases and the condition has lasted for years. In many cases some degree of aphasia persisted after normalization of the other features.

OWN PATIENT GROUP

The main clinical data as well as a neuropsychological evaluation are shown in Tables 1 through 8. In most cases bilateral carotid angiograms, pneumoenceph-

TABLE 1. *Clinical history*

Age (years)	J.A. (male, born 1961) Clinical characteristics	EEG findings
4½	Spoken language becoming less intelligible.	
5	Speech limited to single words. Severe impressive difficulties also. Minor seizures with myoclonic jerks of the eyes and akinetic seizures. Hyperkinetic behavior.	Severely abnormal with independent spike and spike-wave foci in right and left temporal and parietal regions. Universal 3–4 cps activity and polyspikes accompanied by disturbed consciousness and myoclonic jerks of the eyes.
6	Increasing frequency of myoclonic seizures. Speech reduced to a few grumbling sounds. Technetium scan: increased activity in left temporal region. Explorative craniotomy: milky appearance of meninges in left temporal region. Cortical biopsy shows inflammatory changes with lymphocyte infiltration in meninges, gliosis, and loss of neurons.	Aggravation, with constant paroxysmic activity with spikes and 1½–3 cps waves, especially in temporal and parietal regions with left predominance.
7½	Begins to utter a few words. Understands simple verbal commands.	Slightly abnormal with few spikes in left temporal region.
8½	Develops difficulty in swallowing; drooling and drowsiness. CSF: protein 1,000 mg/l with augmentation of all seroproteins, especially IgG.	Aggravation with very frequent spikes with high amplitude, often followed by a slow wave. Right predominance.
10	General behavior normalized. No seizures. Still severely aphasic.	Slightly abnormal with normal alpha activity and a few 4–5 cps waves diffusely.
15	Severely aphasic, otherwise normal.	Normal.

TABLE 2. *Neuropsychological assessment: summary*

J.A., 15-year-old, right-handed male

General intelligence (Wechsler)
    Performance IQ: 101
    Verbal IQ: — (patient not able to cooperate)
Specific abilities
    Language: Practically "deaf mute"
                           Peabody vocabulary equals 2½–3 years
                           Utterances of 1–2 words only, articulation very poor
                           Primary auditory-verbal processing dysfunction seems
                              most probable
    Perception: No visual-spatial abnormalities
                           Practical performances within normal limits
    Memory: Visual memory span, learning, and retention unimpaired
    Psychomotor speed: Visuomotor reaction times slow and fluctuating
Conclusions
    Very severe verbal dysfunction and poor reaction time performance
    indicative of cerebral dysfunction; other (nonverbal) cognitive
    and motor functions within normal limits

TABLE 3. *Clinical history*

Age (years)	J.S.N. (male, born 1952) Clinical characteristics	EEG findings
4	Seizures with paleness, headache, disturbed consciousness (seconds). Akinetic seizures.	Severely abnormal with multiple diffuse spike-wave potentials.
5	Grand mal. Spoken language becoming less intelligible.	Severely abnormal with constant spike activity in left temporo-occipital region. Independent spiking focus in right parieto-occipital region.
6	Progression of impressive and expressive aphasia.	
7	Drowsy and severely aphasic. Spontaneous speech much reduced. Right supranuclear facial palsy develops during weeks.	
7–7½	Improvement of general condition and aphasia.	
7½	Sudden deterioration (weeks) with increasing aphasia and grand mal.	Severe deterioration of curve with abundant spike activity diffusely.
11	No seizures.	Spiking focus in right temporocentral region.
24	Spoken language almost normal. No impressive disturbances. Left-handed. Oral dyspraxia. Right-sided dysstereognosis and dysdiadokokinesia.	Normal.

TABLE 4. *Neuropsychological assessment: summary*

J.S.N., 24-year-old, left-handed male	

General intelligence (Wechsler)	
Verbal IQ:	119
Performance IQ:	116
Full-scale IQ:	119
Specific abilities	
Language:	Auditory-verbal memory span subnormal
	No difficulties of comprehension, object-naming, or sentence construction
	Articulation slightly impaired and difficulties of oral praxis
Perception:	No constructional apraxia
	Finger identification, fingertip number writing, and object identification impaired on right side (astereognosis)
Memory:	Verbal and spatial learning and retention unimpaired
	No disturbances of long-term memory
Psychomotor speed:	Visuomotor reaction time performance slightly impaired
Conclusions	
Normal intelligence, no generalized intellectual deterioration, but specific speech and tactile deficits indicative of localized posterior left-hemisphere dysfunction	

alograms, and computerized axial tomograms were performed with negative results. Conventional audiograms were normal in all patients, and in one (J.A.) auditory evoked potentials were evaluated and found to be normal. CSF protein and cell content were normal, except in patient J.A., in whom an increase in protein (1,000 mg/liter) was found on one occasion.

TABLE 5. *Clinical history*

	C.C.T. (female, born 1965)	
Age (years)	Clinical characteristics	EEG findings
7	School performance bad. Does not understand. Speech becomes gradually unintelligible, sounds like foreign language. Uses gestures.	Spikes and 5–7 cps activity in both temporocentral regions.
7–7½	Language functions improve somewhat.	
7½–8	Spoken language deteriorates.	Severely abnormal. Independent spike foci in right temporal and left and right centroparietal regions.
8½	Aphasia subsiding.	
10	Language almost normal. Neurological examination otherwise normal.	Awake and during hyperventilation: normal. During sleep: severely abnormal with spikes in independent centroparietal foci in both hemispheres.

TABLE 6. *Neuropsychological assessment: summary*

C.C.T., 10-year, 7-month-old, right-handed female

General intelligence (Wechsler)
  Verbal IQ: 97
  Performance IQ: 127
  Full-scale IQ: 112
Specific abilities
  Language: Slightly impaired auditory comprehension
                Auditory-verbal memory span subnormal
                Sporadic object-naming difficulties
                No disturbances of sentence construction or articulation
  Perception: Visuospatial perception and drawing ability unimpaired
  Memory: Verbal learning and retention seem appropriate
  Psychomotor speed: Visuomotor reaction times within normal limits
Conclusions
  Normal intelligence but slight verbal dysfunction; especially low receptive language functions. Spatial abilities above normal and speech unimpaired.

TABLE 7. *Clinical history*

Age (years)	P.D.T. (female, born 1971) Clinical characteristics	EEG findings
3½	Two grand mal seizures.	
4⁷⁄₁₂	Vomiting and tiredness during 1 week. Then two grand mal seizures, fever, followed by weeks of drowsiness, lingering gait. Possibly hallucinations. Monotonously repeating a few sounds. Does not speak.	
4⁸⁄₁₂	Difficulties in eating and dressing. Speech gradually improving. Still aspontaneous.	Severely abnormal. Universal 2–3 cps paroxysms with spikes. Predominantly in left frontotemporal region.
4¹⁰⁄₁₂	Computerized axial tomogram: dubious cortical atrophy.	
5	Language functions normal. Still a little aspontaneous. Neurological examination otherwise normal.	Normal.

COMMENT

Acquired aphasia of childhood has some features distinguishing it from that of adults. In a large series Alajouanine and Lhermitte (1965) found that a reduction of expressive activity was the general feature in patients with onset of aphasia in the age range 6 to 10 years due to pathology in the left hemisphere. Logorrhea,

TABLE 8. *Neuropsychological assessment: summary*

P.D.T., 5-year-old, right-handed female	
General intelligence (Wechsler)	
Verbal IQ:	130
Performance IQ:	109
Full-scale IQ:	120
Specific abilities	
Language:	All aspects unimpaired; above normal
Perception:	Perceptual subtests relatively poor
	Not very good at freehand drawing
Higher motor:	Dressing difficulties (according to mother), apraxia?
	No clumsiness in motor tests
Conclusions	
Verbal intelligence above normal, no suspicion of dementia or aphasia; slight spatial dysfunction cannot be ruled out	

verbal stereotypes, perseveration, and paraphasias were, in contrast to findings in adult aphasics, rather uncommon. The authors suggest that this is because the nervous circuits subserving language are in elaboration and less deeply established than in adults, where they provide the "automatic development of linguistic formulation." The symptoms of three of the present patients fit well with this description.

On the other hand, Alajouanine and Lhermitte (1965) demonstrated a remarkable and rapid amelioration of language in their series of children with left hemisphere pathology. They speculated that language functions in the child are readily transferred to the intact right hemisphere. This is in accordance with recent experiments with the dichotic listening technique (Kinsbourne, 1974). The present patients, in contrast, typically had an aphasia persisting for years. The explanation is near at hand: in all cases the EEGs showed a severe bilateral cerebral dysfunction.

The nature of the disease process has been a matter of speculation. Recently, theories have been forwarded suggesting deafferentiation at lower subcortical levels (Gascon et al., 1973) or "functional ablation" of primary cortical language areas by persistent discharges in these regions (Shoumaker et al., 1974). Worster-Drought (1971) has suggested a low-grade selective encephalitis. Pathoanatomical studies to elucidate the question have hitherto not been published.

The studies made on a cortical biopsy in one of the present cases are remarkable. It clearly shows inflammation of the meninges with leukocyte infiltration and thickening (Fig 2A), as well as gliosis and loss of neurons (Fig. 2B), suggesting a meningoencephalitis of the "slow virus" type. This fits well with the undulating course and stepwise aggravation seen in several patients. Rasmussen and McCann (1968) have demonstrated similar findings in adult patients with long-standing temporal seizures. The adult patients were, as a rule, not aphasic, in contrast with the children in the present group.

It is therefore suggested that the newly established language function in chil-

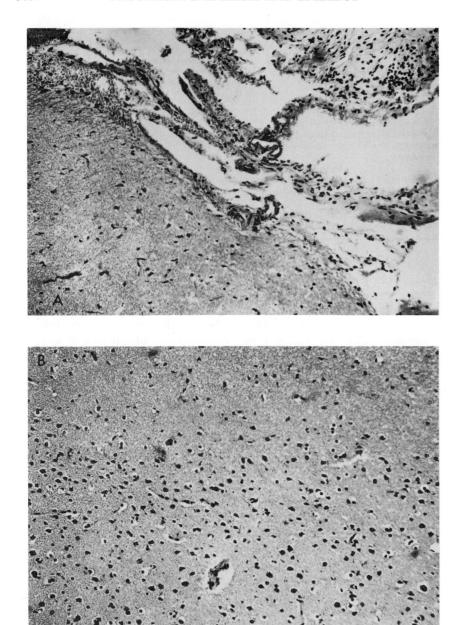

FIG. 2. Cortical biopsy of patient J.A. showing thickening of meninges with foci of lymphocyte infiltration **(A)**, as well as gliosis and loss of neurons **(B)**.

dren is particularly vulnerable to a subchronic viral encephalitis affecting both hemispheres.

ACKNOWLEDGMENTS

The authors wish to thank L. Klinken, M.D., Director of the Neuropathological Institute, University of Copenhagen, for permission to use the cortical biopsy specimen of patient J.A., and E. Reske-Nielsen, M.D., Head of Department of Neuropathology, University Hospital, Aarhus, for help with reviewing and photographing it.

REFERENCES

Alajouanine, T., and Lhermitte, F. (1965): Acquired aphasia in children. *Brain,* 88:653–662.

Deonna, T., Beaumanoir, A., Gaillard, F., and Assal, G. (1975): Syndrome of acquired aphasia in childhood with seizure disorder and EEG-abnormalities. European Group of Child Neurologists, 2nd Conference, Zurich, September 1975.

Gascon, G., Victor, D., Lombroso, C. T., and Goodglass, H. (1973): Language disorder, convulsive disorder and electroencephalographic abnormalities. *Arch. Neurol.,* 28:156–162.

Kinsbourne, M. (1974): Mechanisms of hemispheric interaction in man. In: *Hemispheric Disconnection and Cerebral Function,* edited by M. Kinsbourne and W. L. Smith. Charles C Thomas, Springfield, Ill.

Landau, W. M., and Kleffner, F. R. (1957): Syndrome of acquired aphasia with convulsive disorder in children. *Neurology (Minneap.),* 7:523–530.

Rasmussen, T., and McCann, W. (1968): Clinical studies of patients with focal epilepsy due to "chronic encephalitis." *Trans. Am. Neurol. Assoc.,* 93:89–94.

Shoumaker, R. D., Bennett, D. R., Bray, P. F., and Curless, R. G. (1974): Clinical and EEG manifestations of an unusual aphasic syndrome in children. *Neurology (Minneap.),* 24:10–16.

Worster-Drought, C. (1971): An unusual form of acquired aphasia in children. *Dev. Med. Child Neurol.,* 13:563–571.

Epilepsy, The Eighth International Symposium,
edited by J. K. Penry. Raven Press, New York
© 1977.

Aphasia and Seizure Disorders in Childhood

Christoph Foerster

University Children's Hospital Munich, Lindwurmstr. 4, Munich, Germany

Temporary aphasia is known to occur in association with idiopathic epilepsy, and especially in temporal lobe epilepsy, usually following a fit or series of fits. Such periods of aphasia regress after a variable interval but may recur after further epileptic attacks.

We are reporting on a child with a chronic language disorder and bilateral or focal spike-wave discharges in the EEG without clinical seizures.

CASE HISTORY

The girl was admitted to our hospital at the age of 7 years. The language disorder had begun at age 3 when she had the first episode of progressive loss of comprehension. An EEG showed bilateral spike-wave discharges. However, clinical seizures could not be observed. Oral administration of anticonvulsant medication caused suppression of discharges and isolated a right temporal focus. Recovery from the receptive aphasia was incomplete. Further fluctuating episodes of aphasia occurred over a period of 4 years.

The results of our neurologic examination were normal except that she exhibited dyspractic motor behavior. She was unable to follow long sentences and could answer questions only after repeating them many times. She had difficulty naming objects and made literal paraphasic errors. She showed a normal audiogram except for poor auditory direction discrimination hearing.

Intelligence and achievement testing showed her to be above average in nonverbal function, although her attention span had decreased. The EEG showed spike and slow wave discharges in right temporal and central regions. X-ray films of the skull, radioisotope brain scan, cerebrospinal fluid exam, and computerized axial transverse tomography (CT scanning) all yielded normal findings.

Anticonvulsant medication was continued. After discharge, her comprehension deteriorated so that she had to attend a school for the deaf. Some weeks later improvement of comprehension and speech occurred within 3 days.

DISCUSSION AND CONCLUSIONS

Approximately 30 cases have been reported by Landau and Kleffner (1957) and other authors in the English literature. In the German literature, the mental disturbances which may be associated with the aphasia have been stressed and the relationship with infantile psychoses emphasized.

In all cases the abrupt or slowly progressive onset of the aphasia was associated with spike and slow wave discharges or abnormalities in the EEG and/or clinical seizures. The clinical seizures which occur in the beginning or during the language disorder may be generalized, partial, or myoclonic. The degree of aphasia did parallel the EEG abnormalities only in some cases. Although our patient had paroxysmal discharges in the EEG, no clinical seizures have been observed.

The etiology of this syndrome is unknown. Landau and Kleffner (1957) suggested that the aphasia may be the result of a functional ablation of the primary cortical language areas by persistent discharges in these regions. Gascon et al. (1973) mentioned the possibility that the EEG discharges are a cortical manifestation of a lower level subcortical deafferentiating process. However, in our case as in many cases in the literature there was no dramatic improvement of language disorder when the EEG discharges were changed to focal origin or cleared. If language functions recover, they lagged behind EEG improvement in most cases. Thus medical anticonvulsant treatment controlled the fits adequately but had no obvious influence on the aphasia in most cases.

The question arises whether medical treatment is necessary in the absence of clinical seizures when only abnormalities or paroxysmal discharges in the EEG are present. We now face the problem of deciding whether or not to continue medical treatment as a prophylactic measure in our child after she has recovered completely. We know that many subnormal and brain damaged children may be at special risk of experiencing adverse effects of antiepileptic drugs on behavior and learning. Therefore, we suppose that as long as the aphasia does not appear closely related functionally to the abnormal electrical activity, anticonvulsant treatment should be recommended only if clinical seizures are present. About half of the reported cases have a self-limited course, which suggests a subacute inflammatory process. This possible etiology indicates that anticonvulsant medication and speech therapy may have only a symptomatic value without being the appropriate treatment of the suggested encephalitis.

REFERENCES

Landau, W. M., and Kleffner, F. R. (1957): Syndrome of acquired aphasia with convulsive disorder in children. *Neurology (Minneap.)*, 7:523.
Gascon, G., Victor, D., Lombroso, C. T., and Goodglass, H. (1973): Language disorder, convulsive disorder, and electroencephalographic abnormalities. Acquired syndrome in children. *Arch. Neurol.*, 28:156–162.

Epilepsy, The Eighth International Symposium,
edited by J. K. Penry. Raven Press, New York
© 1977.

Epilepsy and Driving in Israel

* Sonia Laks and Amos D. Korczyn

Institute of Criminology and Criminal Law, Faculty of Law, and Department of Physiology and Pharmacology, Sackler School of Medicine, Tel Aviv University and the Neurology Service, Soroka Medical Center, Be'er Sheba, Israel

Epilepsy is considered to hamper a motorist's driving skill and increase the risk of accidents (World Health Organization, 1956, 1975). Upon application for a driving license, the candidates in most countries are required to notify the authorities of this disease. The criteria used for issuing such licenses differ from country to country. An important consideration is that the candidate has been free from seizures for a period of 1 to 3 years. In Israel, as in most countries, a seizure-free period of 2 years is required. In addition to seizures, drugs may also affect the driving abilities of epileptic drivers by reducing alertness or coordination. Thus, relying solely or mainly on the patient's being seizure-free may not suffice. In evaluating impairment, one therefore needs more information regarding the patients. This enables definition of patients who may constitute a high risk in driving.

The extent to which epileptic patients influence road safety has been assessed in the past on the basis of statistical studies of accident rates. It has been reported that drivers suffering from epilepsy have a somewhat higher incidence of traffic accidents than controls (Hormia, 1961; Crancer and McMurray, 1968; Waller, 1973). The overall number of accidents attributed to epileptic seizures was found to be small, of the order of 1 to 3 per 10,000 accidents (Norman, 1960; Hermer et al., 1966; Grattan and Jeffcoate, 1968; Van der Lugt, 1975).

In an attempt to assess the extent to which epileptic patients drive, we have interviewed a sample population consisting of 50 patients with epilepsy. In addition, we have examined other aspects related to the application for driving licenses, problems to which only little attention was paid in the past.

Our survey differs from most previous studies in that we have approached the issue by interviewing consecutive epileptic patients attending a neurological clinic, rather than examining drivers known to be epileptic.

SUBJECTS AND METHODS

We interviewed 50 nonselected male patients, aged 18 to 58, who attended a neurological outpatient clinic. Those included consecutive subjects suffering from

---

* This is part of an M.A. thesis to be submitted by Sonia Laks to the Tel Aviv University.

various types of epilepsy but without physical, mental, or intellectual impairment.

The patients were reassured that the study was not an effort to catch them breaking the law. For each person, a questionnaire was completed, containing his personal data, details of the disease and its treatment, and information concerning driving. The attending neurologist assessed the medical condition of the patients. Information concerning the subjects was also collected from the licensing bureau and the Medical Institute of Road Safety, a government agency where problematic candidates are examined medically prior to being granted a driving license.

A control group consisting of the adult brothers of the patients was used to determine the proportion of those who owned a driving license.

RESULTS

Of the 50 patients, 16 never drove and 26 (52%) were driving at the time of the study. The drivers included only 23 (45%) license holders, as compared with 70% license holders among the controls. Only 10 of the 27 patients not possessing a driver's license were trying to receive or intended to apply for such a permit. The relatively small tendency to drive among patients was partly due to self-awareness of their impediments.

A high proportion of the drivers had not notified the licensing authority of their disease, and among those who reported, few gave false data about their condition. Only 6 of 15 patients reported the existence of epilepsy when applying for a license, and fewer did so upon renewal. Consequently, the authorities were aware of the precise neurological status in only 5 of 25 license holders. Presumably the patients concealed their epilepsy because they were afraid of being refused a license. Fourteen patients (44%) were driving their own vehicle; five (22%) owned a license to drive lorries or buses and used it (sometimes in spite of recurring seizures). Half of the licensed drivers drove 300 km/week or more, and in six the distances were 500 to 1,000 km or more. Seven were professional drivers, for whom a driving license was required to earn their living.

The interviewed subjects reported being involved in seven road traffic accidents, of which probably only one had occurred while the patient had had a fit (three accidents took place before the patients had had their first fit). In four other subjects seizures occurred while driving but an accident was prevented, in two cases by the driver's companion.

The accident rates were compared in 19 patients who drove during the period 1961 to 1974. The patients drove 2 million km during that period, and only two accidents occurred. The overall accident rate in Israel during this period was 1.6 to 2.4 per million km. Thus, the accident rate among patients seems to be lower than in controls.

Of all drivers, 18 (70%) suffered from grand mal and 8 (30%) from psychomotor seizures, 5 had nocturnal seizures, and in 5 aura preceded the attack.

The severity of the disease was determined according to the clinical manifestation—strength and frequency of attacks, loss of consciousness, and loss of self-control. Nine (35%) of all drivers or those holding licenses had a moderate form of the disease, and in only one was it severe; this patient drove without a license. Of those who did not drive, 14 (60%) suffered from moderate or severe epilepsy. Thus, nondrivers had a more severe condition than those who drove.

Twenty-two (85%) of the drivers were on anticonvulsant therapy, but only twelve took their medication regularly. In eight cases drugs had been changed during the last year, which shows that at least in a few of the cases the therapy had not been well adjusted. Of those who did not drive, all were treated medically. They showed better adherence to the drug regimen, probably due to their relatively more severe condition.

EEGs showed definite abnormalities in eight of the drivers consisting mainly of temporal foci, whereas in ten cases (seven licensed drivers) with relatively frequent seizures a normal EEG pattern was revealed. These findings show the limitations of the EEG as a tool for judging driving competence.

DISCUSSION

We found that 45% of the epileptic men examined owned valid driving licenses. This proportion was similar to that reported by Phemister (1961), Rees (1967), and Maxwell and Leyshon (1971). When these figures are compared with the proportion of license holders in the control group (70%), a striking difference emerges. This gap is partly due to the licensing procedures, preventing patients with severe forms of epilepsy from obtaining a driving permit. Indeed, we found a more severe form of the disease among nondrivers. However, in the interview it became clear that self-restriction is no less important than the formal rules, and patients with severe epilepsy have shown less inclination to drive.

In Israel driving licenses are issued only after the military medical records of the applicants are screened. Thus, we were surprised to find that 8 of 15 candidates managed to escape even this precaution, using various means. It seems that to some patients driving is a necessity, and they use all ways and means to be able to drive. Indeed, seven drivers would have been unable to continue their work if prevented from using a car, and in 70% of the drivers lack of a license would have been an impediment at work. The necessity to hold a driving license in modern society is also demonstrated by the high proportion of subjects who admitted that they drove without a valid permit (7 of 30), in several cases over long distances.

Thus it seems that epileptic patients restrict voluntarily their own driving, but those who find it essential to drive either do not disclose their medical condition to the authorities or drive without a license.

It should be stressed that the candidates had relatively good information as to the terms under which a license is issued. Thus, generally those patients who met the criteria set by the law declared their condition, whereas the "high-risk" candidates withheld the relevant data.

The question must now be answered as to whether epileptic patients do constitute a high risk on the road. According to our results, the accident rate is *lower* in epileptic patients than in the general population. This result contradicts previous studies (Hormia, 1961; Crancer and McMurray, 1968; Waller, 1973; Van der Lugt, 1975). However, these studies were obtained by analysis of official traffic records of drivers known to be epileptic. It is likely that this approach will yield higher rates because, even if patients with severe forms of epilepsy do constitute a high risk, many others with mild forms are unknown to the authorities. From our personal experience it seems that several epileptic patients drove with extra care because of their disease, and many did not drive on days when they believed that an attack might be imminent.

We conclude from our study that patients with epilepsy do not constitute a particularly high risk on the road. The limitations imposed on their driving are probably excessive. The result of the rigid approach by the authorities is that relevant information is not supplied, thus possibly increasing the accident risk. A more liberal attitude may yield better results and increase road safety.

SUMMARY

A survey was conducted concerning driving among epileptic patients. We interviewed 50 male patients, aged 18 to 58 years, suffering from various forms of epilepsy, but without physical, mental, or intellectual impairment. Among these 50 cases, 16 had never driven and 26 were presently driving. These included 23 (46%) who held driving licenses, compared with 70% of license holders among matched controls. Among licensed epileptic drivers, in 16 cases the authorities were not aware of their disease, as demanded by the law. Some of these were drivers by profession. The interviewed reported being involved in seven road traffic accidents, of which probably only one occurred while the patient had a fit (three accidents had occurred before the first attack). In four other subjects seizures occurred while driving but an accident was prevented. The accident rate was lower in patients than in the general population. Eighteen drivers suffered from grand mal and eight from psychomotor seizures. Five had nocturnal seizures only, and in five aura preceded the attack. Half of all drivers or those holding licenses had seizures at relatively short intervals (weeks or months) varying in severity. Twenty-two drivers were on anticonvulsant therapy. In eight cases drugs had been changed during the last year. EEG findings showed definite abnormalities in eight of the drivers, consisting mainly of temporal foci. The policy related to issuing driving licenses to epileptic patients is discussed.

REFERENCES

Crancer, A., and McMurray, L. (1968): Accident and violation rates of Washington's medically restricted drivers. *J.A.M.A.*, 205, 5:272–276.
Grattan, E., and Jeffcoate, G. O. (1968): Medical factors and road accidents. *Br. Med. J.*, 1:75–79.

Hermer, B., Smedbey, B., and Ysander, L. (1966): Sudden illness as a cause of motor-vehicle accidents. *Br. J. Ind. Med.*, 23:37–41.

Hormia, A. (1961): Does epilepsy mean higher susceptibility to traffic accidents? *Acta Psychiatr. Scand. [Suppl.* 150], 36:210–212.

Maxwell, R. D. H., and Leyshon, G. E. (1971): Epilepsy and driving. *Br. Med. J.,* 3:12–15.

Norman, L. G. (1960): Medical aspect of road safety. *Lancet,* 1:989–994; 1039–1042.

Phemister, J. C. (1961): Epilepsy and car-driving. *Lancet,* 1:1276–1277.

Rees, W. D. (1967): Physical and medical disabilities of 1,190 ordinary motorists. *Br. Med. J.,* 1:593–597.

Van der Lugt, P. J. M. (1975): Traffic accidents caused by epilepsy. *Epilepsia,* 16:747–751.

Waller, J. A. (1973): *Medical Impairment to Driving.* Charles C Thomas, Springfield, Ill.

World Health Organization (1956): Guiding principles in the medical examination of applicants for motor vehicle driving permits. WHO/ Accid. Prev./56.

_____ (1975): WHO/ Accid. Prev./75.

OTHER ASPECTS OF EPILEPSY

Epilepsy, The Eighth International Symposium,
edited by J. K. Penry. Raven Press, New York
© 1977.

Cerebrospinal Fluid Cyclic AMP and Epilepsy

V. V. Myllylä, E. Hokkanen, H. Nousiainen, E. R. Heikkinen,
and H. Vapaatalo

*Departments of Neurology and Pharmacology, University of Oulu; and Institute of
Biomedical Sciences, University of Tampere, Finland*

Cyclic AMP was discovered in 1957 in biological systems during investigations on the regulation of liver glycogenolysis by epinephrine and glucagon (Rall et al., 1957; Sutherland and Rall, 1957). At this moment, rapidly accumulating data verify an important role of cyclic AMP in mediating among others the actions of many hormones and drugs (Breckenridge, 1970; Major and Kilpatrick, 1972). This intracellular mediator role of cyclic AMP, the so-called second messenger theory, is based on the studies of Sutherland (1970). The specificity of the actions of many hormones is apparently based on specific receptors on outer membranes of target cells (Sutherland et al., 1968).

An important role of this nucleotide in neural function was suggested when it was found that the enzymes synthesizing and degrading it are more abundant in brain than in other tissues (Krisna et al., 1970). Although functioning as an intracellular messenger (Sutherland, 1970), cyclic AMP has also been found in extracellular fluids, for instance, cerebrospinal fluid (CSF). Changes in extracellular levels of cyclic AMP have been shown to reflect alterations in intracellular levels of the nucleotide in response to a variety of endocrinological and other manipulations (Broadus et al., 1971). In animals an increase of brain cyclic AMP content can be produced by depolarizing agents or by damaging brain cortex by freezing, resulting in epileptogenic lesions (Shimizu and Daly, 1972; Walker et al., 1973). Electroconvulsive treatment strikingly increases brain AMP levels (Goldberg et al., 1970).

The purpose of the present clinicoexperimental study was to gather information about (1) the effects of convulsions and anticonvulsive drugs on CSF cyclic AMP levels in rabbits, and (2) the possible alterations in CSF cyclic AMP concentrations in epileptic patients.

PATIENTS AND METHODS

The experimental part of this study was performed on adult rabbits. Convulsions were electrically induced under ether anesthesia to mimic epileptic attacks. Part of the animals were treated with various anticonvulsants for 1 week before electroconvulsive shock. The following dosages were used: phenobarbital 5 mg/kg (s.c.), diphenylhydantoin 10 mg/kg (s.c.), and carbamazepine 50 mg/kg (p.o.).

The CSF samples were obtained by cisternal puncture under ether anesthesia. In the clinical part of the study, CSF samples from 46 epileptics (under anticonvulsive treatment) were obtained at various times after a spontaneous attack. Proteins were precipitated from the samples by adding 55% trichloroacetic acid (final concentration 5%). The cyclic AMP concentrations were measured by the protein-binding method of Gilman (1970). The values are expressed as nanomoles per liter of CSF. Student's t-test and t-test for paired observations were used for statistical treatment of the results.

RESULTS

The CSF cyclic AMP concentrations in rabbits were increased during 6 hr following convulsions, the maximum 46.8 nmoles/liter being at 3 hr (Table 1). This value significantly differs ($p < 0.005$) from the basal level of 24.0. The basal CSF cyclic AMP concentration 17.7 ± 3.9 (SE) of the animals receiving various anticonvulsants was lower ($p < 0.01$) than that of the saline (control) group. The lowest basal value 16.9 ± 1.9 was reached in the group of animals treated by phenobarbital ($p < 0.05$ when compared with the saline group). The elevation of the CSF cyclic AMP concentration seen in the control group was to a great deal leveled off by anticonvulsive agents (Table 1). The serum concentrations of various anticonvulsants after 1 week's treatment were the following: phenobarbital 12.5 ± 2.2 (SE) $\mu g/ml$, diphenylhydantoin 1.2 ± 0.3, and carbamazepine 1.1 ± 0.3.

The CSF cyclic AMP values of epileptic patients at various times after an attack were studied in 46 patients. The cyclic AMP level 27.4 ± 2.1 of the 13 patients with a recent attack (0 to 3 days) was higher ($p < 0.02$) than the value 21.9 ± 0.6 of 22 patients free from attacks for at least 2 weeks. The cyclic AMP level of the latter group was also lower ($p < 0.1$) than the concentration 24.0 ± 1.1 of the control group consisting of 13 headache patients with normal findings on neurological examination.

TABLE 1. *The effect of anticonvulsants and convulsions on the CSF cyclic AMP concentration (nmoles/liter) in rabbits (means ± SE)*

Group	Basal	1 hr	3 hr	6 hr
Control (saline)	24.0 ± 2.2	37.7 ± 5.9	46.8 ± 7.0^a	31.0 ± 4.9^a
Phenobarbital	16.9 ± 1.9	25.2 ± 3.8^b	20.6 ± 3.4	21.4 ± 2.3
Diphenylhydantoin	18.5 ± 1.4	25.0 ± 3.0^b	22.1 ± 2.0	23.6 ± 2.8^b
Carbamazepine	17.9 ± 1.4	26.2 ± 1.9	27.9 ± 1.3^a	26.9 ± 2.2^a

$^a p < 0.005$ when compared with the respective basal value.
$^b p < 0.05$ when compared with the respective basal value. (paired t-test).

DISCUSSION

Biochemical abnormalities of brain have been increasingly implicated as possible mechanisms underlying the epileptic process. On the other hand, there are many observations regarding brain cyclic AMP in association with epilepsy:

1. In epileptic synaptic discharge, many transmitter substances are involved, including catecholamines and 5-hydroxytryptamine (Curtis, 1969), which are able to stimulate adenyl cyclase at least *in vitro* (Fumagalli et al., 1971).
2. In epileptic patients reduced CSF concentrations of 5-hydroxytryptamine and some other transmitters have been reported (Shaywitz et al., 1975).
3. Electroconvulsive treatment and anoxia increase the brain cyclic AMP content of experimental animals (Goldberg et al., 1970).
4. In experimentally induced epileptogenic focus, there is an increase in adenyl cyclase activity and a decrease in phosphodiesterase activity resulting in elevated cyclic AMP levels (Walker et al., 1973).

It is also possible that ischemic changes in neurons or glial cells associated with reduced energy state during convulsions lead to increased leakage of cyclic AMP into CSF. Enzymes of large molecular weight have been shown to be elevated in CSF after epileptic attacks (Miyazaki, 1958), so it is probable that cyclic AMP as an intracellular substance of rather low molecular weight is liberated more easily by cellular disturbances. Antiepileptic drugs caused a marked decrease in the basal CSF cyclic AMP levels of rabbits and partially inhibited the rise after convulsions. The low cyclic AMP concentration of patients free from attacks may also be due to the medical treatment. The possible mechanism may be a direct effect on the enzymes controlling cyclic AMP levels or a secondary effect caused by diminished synaptic transmission. The latter alternative is favored by the fact that cyclic AMP with enzymes adenyl cyclase and phosphodiesterase occurs in large amounts in synaptic membranes (e.g., Siggins et al., 1973).

It can be concluded that:

1. Electrically induced convulsions cause an increase in CSF cyclic AMP concentration in rabbits.
2. Treatment with phenobarbital, diphenylhydantoin, and carbamazepine decrease the basal CSF cyclic AMP levels and partially inhibit the rise after convulsions.
3. Epileptic attacks in man cause an increase in CSF cyclic AMP level lasting for about 3 days.
4. The results suggest the involvement of cyclic AMP in epileptic discharge and in the mechanism of action of anticonvulsants.

REFERENCES

Breckenridge, B. McL. (1970): Cyclic AMP and drug action. *Annu. Rev. Pharmacol.,* 10:19–34.
Broadus, A. E., Hardman, J. G., Kaminsky, N. I., Ball, J. H., Sutherland, E. W., and Liddle, G. W. (1971): Extracellular cyclic nucleotides. *Ann. N.Y. Acad. Sci.,* 185:50–66.

Curtis, D. R. (1969): Central synaptic transmitters. In: *Basic Mechanisms of the Epilepsies,* edited by Jasper, H. H., Ward, A. A., and—Pope, A. pp. 105–135. Churchill, London.

Fumagalli, R., Bernareggi, V., Berti, F., and Trabucchi, M. (1971): Cyclic AMP formation in human brain: An in vitro stimulation by neurotransmitters. *Life Sci.,* Part I, 10:1111–1115.

Gilman, A. G. (1970): A protein binding assay for adenosine 3′,5′-cyclic monophosphate. *Proc. Natl. Acad. Sci. U.S.A.,* 67:305–312.

Goldberg, N. D., Lust, W. D., O'Dea, R. F., Wei, S., and O'Toole, A. G. (1970): A role of cyclic nucleotides in brain metabolism. Role of cyclic AMP in cell function. *Adv. Biochem. Psychopharmacol.,* 3:67–87.

Krishna, G., Forn, J., Voigt, K., Paul, M., and Gessa, G. L. (1970): Dynamic aspects of neurohumoral control of cyclic 3′,5′-AMP synthesis in brain. Role of cyclic AMP in cell function. *Adv. Biochem. Psychopharmacol.,* 3:155–172.

Major, P. W., and Kilpatrick, R. (1972): Cyclic AMP and hormone action. *J. Endocrinol.,* 52: 593–630.

Miyazaki, M. (1958): Glutamic oxalacetic transaminase in cerebrospinal fluid. *J. Nerv. Ment. Dis.,* 126:169–175.

Rall, T. W., Sutherland, E. W., and Berthet, J. (1957): The relationship of epinephrine and glucagon to liver phosphorylase. IV: Effect of epinephrine and glucagon on the reactivation of phosphorylase in liver homogenates. *J. Biol. Chem.,* 244:463–475.

Shaywitz, B. A., Cohen, D. J., and Bowers, M. B. (1975): Reduced cerebrospinal fluid 5-hydroxyindole acetic acid and homovanillic acid in children with epilepsy. *Neurology (Minneap.),* 25:72–79.

Shimizu, H., and Daly, J. W. (1972): Effect of depolarizing agents on accumulation of cyclic adenosine 3′,5′-monophosphate in cerebral cortical slices. *Eur. J. Pharmacol.,* 17:240–252.

Siggins, G. R., Battenberg, E. F., Hoffer, B. J., and Bloom, F. E. (1973): Noradrenergic stimulation of cyclic adenosine monophosphate in rat Purkinje neurons: An immunocytochemical study. *Science,* 179:585–588.

Sutherland, E. W. (1970): On the biological role of cyclic AMP. *J.A.M.A.,* 214:1281–1288.

Sutherland, E. W., and Rall, T. W. (1957): The properties of an adenine ribonucleotide produced with cellular particles, ATP, Mg^{++}, and epinephrine or glucagon. *J. Am. Chem. Soc.,* 79:3608–3618.

Sutherland, E. W., Robison, G. A., and Butcher, R. W. (1968): Some aspects of the biological role of adenosine 3′,5′-monophosphate (cyclic AMP). *Circulation,* 37:279–306.

Walker, J. E., Lewin, E., Sheppard, J. R., and Cromwell, R. (1973): Enzymatic regulation of adenosine 3′,5′-monophosphate (cyclic AMP) in the freezing epileptogenic lesion of rat brain and in homologous contralateral cortex. *Neurochemistry,* 21:79–85.

Epilepsy, The Eighth International Symposium,
edited by J. K. Penry. Raven Press, New York
© 1977.

HL-A Antigens in Primary Generalized Epilepsy

Raffaella Scorza Smeraldi, Carlo L. Cazzullo, Giovanna Fabio,
Claudio Rugarli, Enrico Smeraldi, and Raffaele Canger

Policlinico di Milano, Milan, Italy

The major histocompatibility system of man, the HL-A system, is under the control of many closely linked genes controlling not only those cell surface determinants that behave as histocompatibility antigens, but also immune response differences, some components of complement, and perhaps other related functions. HL-A loci are highly polyallelic. The products of some of them (for example, of loci A and B) are easily identified by serological methods, whereas others (the locus D products) are, at the present time, mainly identified by the mixed lymphocyte reaction *in vitro,* for they are able to elicit the proliferation of allogenic lymphocytes (LD or lymphocyte-defined antigens).

The great polymorphism displayed by HL-A products confers to the system the character of a powerful genetic marker for those diseases in which inheritance plays a role. Moreover, some recent experimental and clinical data support the hypothesis that HL-A products are also important for the interactions between cells and external factors, as well as in cell-to-cell interactions (Svejgaard et al., 1975; Smeraldi et al., 1976*a;* Smeraldi and Scorza Smeraldi, 1976; Bellodi et al., 1977). This hypothesis is also indirectly supported by the associations found between HL-A alleles and several diseases in which alterations of cell surface determinants or of cell-to-cell interactions have been suggested to play a role (Cazzullo et al., 1974; Smeraldi et al., 1975; Smeraldi et al., 1976*b,* 1976*c;* Bennahum et al., 1976).

In the present work, we investigated whether some association exists between HL-A familial segregation and primary generalized epilepsy, a disease for which a strong genetic contribution is indicated by twins and family studies and for which an autosomal dominant inheritance has been suggested (Metrakos and Metrakos, 1961).

PATIENTS AND METHODS

The subjects of our investigation were the members of seven families, in which one or more members were affected by primary generalized epilepsy (grand mal, petit mal absences, Janz syndrome) and some displayed clinical and/or EEG patterns compatible with a higher susceptibility to convulsiveness (subclinical EEG epileptiform discharges and/or febrile convulsions). Whenever possible, the EEG of each family member included in our investigation was recorded.

All subjects were HL-A typed for the following HL-A specificities: A1, A2, A3, A9, A10, A11, A28, A29, AW19, AW25, AW26, AW30 of the first SD locus; B5, B7, B8, B12, B13, B14, B17, B18, B27, BW15, BW16, BW21, BW22, BW35, BW40 of the second SD locus. The technique was the microlymphocytotoxicity test by Mittal et al. (1968). The sera employed are listed elsewhere (Smeraldi et al., 1975). To detect the determinants controlled by the D locus (LD determinants), we tested each member of a family unit as stimulator and as responder in the one-way mixed lymphocyte cultures *in vitro* against the cells of the other members and against unrelated control cells, employing a technique described previously (Smeraldi et al., 1976*a*).

On the basis of HL-A typing and of the results of the mixed lymphocyte stimulation, HL-A haplotypes of each member of a single family were obtained (haplotype is the genetic information carried by a single chromosome).

In the present work, the individual LD determinants of the subjects investigated were not identified by "typing" the cells against a panel of known homozygous LD cells, but were identified arbitrarily by letters Da, Db, and so on in the the family segregation analysis.

RESULTS

The results are summarized in Table 1, in which relevant clinical data of the families investigated are reported, together with the HL-A haplotypes of each member.

Family IEL

The father, homozygous at loci B and D, had a Janz syndrome with spikes, polyspikes, and waves on the EEG. Both children had a history of febrile convulsions and presented grand mal seizures. They were discordant for both maternal and paternal haplotypes HL-A but shared both paternal antigens B13 and Dx.

Family LA BR

Both children showed epileptic symptoms and typical EEGs. They differed for the inheritance of paternal haplotype but shared the HL-A haplotype inherited from the mother. Both parents were clinically healthy and showed a normal EEG.

Family PAMP

The parents had no history of epileptic symptoms. The maternal EEG was normal; the paternal EEG was not recorded. The two children, who showed,

TABLE 1. *HLA haplotypes and clinical and EEG findings of 7 families*

Family	Age (yr)	HLA haplotypes	Clinical	EEG	Age at onset
IEL					
Father	32	A1, B13, Dx, A9, B13, Dx	Janz syndrome	Spikes, polyspikes, and waves	13 yr
Mother	32	A10, B-, Dz, A10, B17, Dd	—	Normal	—
Child #1	11	A1, B13, Dx, A10, B-, Dz	Febrile convulsions, grand mal	Spikes and waves	10 mo
Child #2	10	A9, B13, Dx, A10, B17, Dd	Febrile convulsions, grand mal	Spikes, polyspikes, and waves	2 yr
LA BR					
Father	40	A9, B7, Dx, A2, B13, Dy	—	Normal	—
Mother	43	A3, B-, Dz, B13, Dy	—	Normal	—
Child #1	17	A11, B-, Dd A2, B13, Dy, B-, Dd	Febrile convulsions, grand mal, petit mal	Spikes and waves	18 mo
Child #2	11	A9, B7, Dx, A11, B-, Dd	Petit mal	Spikes, polyspikes, and waves	10 yr
PAMP					
Father	38	AW25, B14, Dx, A-, B-, Dy	—	—	—
Mother	37	AW32, B13, Dz, A2, B13, Dd	—	Normal	—
Child #1	7	A-, B-, Dy, AW32, B13, Dz	Febrile convulsions, petit mal	Spikes, polyspikes, and waves	10 mo
Child #2	4	AW25, B14, Dx, A2, B13, Dd	Febrile convulsions	Spikes and waves	1 yr
ROV					
Father	38	A11, B5, Dx, A-, B-, Dy	—	—	—
Mother	37	A3, B7, Dz, A9, B12, Dd	Grand mal	Spikes and waves	13 yr
Child #1	8	A11, B5, Dx, A9, B12, Dd	—	Spikes and waves	—
Child #2	3	A11, B5, Dx, A9, B12, Dd	—	—	—

Family	Age (yr)	HLA haplotypes	Clinical	EEG	Age at onset
SANT					
Father	45	A2, B-, Dx, A9, B-, Dy	—	—	⊢
Mother	40	A3, B-, Dz, A10, B12, Dd	Grand mal	Spikes and waves	13 yr
Child #1	14	A2, B-, Dx, A10, B12, Dd	Petit mal, grand mal	Spikes and waves	7 yr
Child #2	8	A2, B-, Dx, A10, B12, Dd	—	Spikes and waves (?)	—
SPIN					
Father	37	A9, B12, Dx, A11, BW22, Dy	—	Normal	—
Mother	36	AW25, B17, Dz, A-, B17, Dd	—	Normal	—
Child #1	7	A11, BW22, Dy, AW25, B17, Dz	Petit mal	Spikes and waves	7 yr
Child #2	5	A9, B12, Dx, AW25, B17, Dz	Petit mal	Spikes and waves	3 yr
Child #3	3	A9, B12, Dx, A-, B17, Dd	—	Normal	—
TAZZ					
Father	55	A2, BW15, Dx, A3, B8, Dy	—	—	—
Mother	52	A1, B-, Dz, A11, B17, Dd	—	—	—
Child #1	29	A3, B8, Dy, A11, B17, Dd	Petit mal, grand mal	Spikes and waves	10 yr
Sibling #1	8	A3, B8, Dy, A3, B8, Db	—	Spikes and waves	—
Sibling #2	3	A3, B8, Dy, A3, B8, Db	—	Spikes and waves (?)	—
Child #2	27	A3, B8, Dy, A11, B17, Dd	—	Spikes and waves (?)	—
Sibling #1	8	A9, B8, Da, A11, B17, Dd	Febrile convulsions	Spikes and waves	9 mo
Sibling #2	4	A9, B8, Da, A11, B17, Dd	Febrile convulsions	—	—
Child #3	18	A3, BW15, Dx, A11, B17, Dd	Febrile convulsions	Spikes and waves	9 mo

respectively, febrile convulsions and petit mal absences or febrile convulsions only were completely different for HL-A constitution.

Family ROV

In this family, the father was clinically healthy but the EEG was not recorded. The mother displayed grand mal seizures and EEG spikes and waves. Child No. 1 was clinically healthy but displayed EEg spikes and waves. The EEG of the other child was not obtained. Both children were HL-A identical.

Family SANT

The father was clinically healthy; his EEG was not recorded. The mother displayed grand mal seizures and an altered EEG pattern. Child No. 1 showed petit mal absences and grand mal seizures. The second child had doubtful signs of spikes and waves on the EEG. The children were also HL-A identical.

Family SPIN

Both parents were clinically healthy and showed normal EEG patterns. Child No. 3 was healthy with a normal EEG, whereas child No. 1 and child No. 2 had a history of petit mal absences and showed EEG spikes and waves. Both shared the maternal haplotype HL-A AW25, B17, Dz but carried different paternal haplotypes. The healthy child differed from both for the maternal haplotype, whereas he shared with child No. 2 the paternal haplotype.

Family TAZZ

Both parents were clinically healthy, but their EEGs were not recorded. One of the mother's relatives had a history of "epileptic seizures" not better identified. Child No. 1 displayed petit mal absences and grand mal seizures with EEG spikes and waves. One of her children had no clinical symptoms but displayed spikes and waves on the EEG. The other one had only doubtful signs of EEG anomalies. Child No. 2 was clinically healthy but displayed doubtful spikes and waves on the EEG. Of her children, one had a history of febrile convulsions with EEG anomalies. The other one was normal but his EEG had not been recorded. Child No. 3 had febrile convulsions together with EEG anomalies. Child No. 1 and child No. 2 were HL-A identical; child No. 3 shared with them only the maternal haplotype. This same haplotype (HL-A A11, B17, Dd) was also present in both siblings of child No. 2 and was absent in those of child No. 1. These last were HL-A identical and homozygous at the two loci A and B.

DISCUSSION

These results are very preliminary, so we cannot draw definite conclusions about the existence of an association between HL-A segregation and disease predisposition.

With the small number of families studied, it is obvious that we could not calculate any abnormal frequency of any one HL-A allele or haplotype. Nevertheless, the affected subjects in an individual family tended to have the same HL-A segregation pattern. This would suggest that the HL-A region contains an epileptic connected locus strictly associated with loci A, B, and D, but not coinciding with them. Even though the parents in some of these families had no clinical signs of epilepsy and no specific EEG patterns or at least febrile convulsions, it must be kept in mind that these manifestations often disappear as the subject grows older.

Four of seven families demonstrated an agreement between segregation of the disease and that of the HL-A haplotypes. In family TAZZ, the disease seemed to segregate together with maternal HL-A A11, B17, Dd. The only discordant finding was the presence of EEG spikes and waves in the offspring of child No. 1. The anamnestic history of epileptic seizures in one maternal relative seemed to agree, on the other hand, with a maternal transmission. In family IEL, an apparent disagreement was found between HL-A and disease inheritance. However, in this family the father was homozygous for two of the three HL-A loci investigated. It could be possible that a similar homozygousness might exist at the epileptic connected locus and that both children inherited the same allele at this locus as they inherited the same alleles at the loci B and D. In the remaining family, a complete disagreement was found between HL-A and the disease inheritance pattern.

An autosomal dominant inheritance has been suggested for primary generalized epilepsy with age-dependent manifestations (Metrakos and Metrakos, 1961), and we stress that the same autosomal dominant inheritance is displayed by the HL-A products. Thus, we think that the connection suggested by our preliminary findings should be investigated in a larger number of families, making possible the calculation of concordance so that the common transmission hypothesis might be accepted or discarded.

SUMMARY

Seven families, in which one or more members were affected by primary generalized epilepsy (grand mal seizures, petit mal absences, or Janz syndrome) or showed febrile convulsions and/or asymptomatic EEG epileptiform discharges, were investigated for the possible association of the HL-A products segregation and the inheritance pattern of the disease. Five of these families showed a good agreement between HL-A and disease inheritance. In one case we observed a result which was possibly compatible with the association hypothesis, whereas in only one family a clear disagreement of HL-A and primary generalized epilepsy was observed. The meaning of these results is discussed.

REFERENCES

Bellodi, L., Scorza Smeraldi, R., Negri, F., Resele L., Sacchetti, E., and Smeraldi, E. (1977): Histocompatibility antigens and effects of neuroactive drugs on PHA stimulation of lymphocytes in vitro. *Arzneim. Forsch.,* 27:144.

Bennahum, D. A., Troup, G. M., Rada, R. T., Kellner, R., and Kyner, T. (1976): HL-A antigens in schizophrenic and manic depressive mental disorders. Paper presented to the First International Symposium on HL-A and Disease, Paris, June 23–25.

Cazzullo, C. L., Smeraldi, E., and Penati, G. (1974): The leucocyte antigenic system HL-A as a possible genetic marker of schizophrenia. *Br. J. Psychiatry,* 125:25.

Metrakos, K., and Metrakos, J. D. (1961): Genetics of convulsive disorders. II. Genetic and electroen-cephalographic studies in centrencephalic epilepsy. *Neurology (Minneap.),* 11:474.

Mittal, K. K., Mickey, M. R., Singal, D. P., and Terasaki, P. I. (1968): Serotyping for homotransplan-tation. XVIII. Refinement of the microdroplet cytotoxicity test. *Transplantation,* 6:91.

Smeraldi, E., Bellodi, L., Sacchetti, E., and Cazzullo, C. L. (1976*a*): The HLA system and the clinical response to treatment with chlorpromazine. *Br. J. Psychiatry,* 129:486.

Smeraldi, E., Bellodi, L., Scorza Smeraldi, R., Fabio, G., and Sacchetti, E. (1976*b*): HL-A SD antigens and schizophrenia: Statistical and genetical considerations. *Tissue Antigens,* 8:191.

Smeraldi, E., and Scorza Smeraldi, R. (1976): Interference between anti-HL-A antibodies and chlor-promazine. *Nature,* 260:532.

Smeraldi, E., Scorza Smeraldi, R., Cazzullo, C. L., Guareschi Cazzullo, A., Fabio, G., and Canger, R. (1975): Immunogenetics of the Lennox-Gastaut syndrome: Frequency of HL-A antigens and haplotypes in patients and first degree relatives. *Epilepsia,* 16:699.

Smeraldi, E., Scorza Smeraldi, R., Guareschi Cazzullo A., Cazzullo, C. L., Rugarli, C., and Canger, R. (1976*c*): Immunogenetics of Lennox-Gastaut syndrome: Search for LD determinants as genetic markers of the syndrome. Paper presented to the First International Symposium on HL-A and Disease, Paris, June 23–25.

Svejgaard, A., Platz, P., Ryder, L. P., Staub-Nielsen, L., and Thomsen, M. (1975): HL-A and disease associations: A survey. *Transplant. Rev.,* 22:3.

Epilepsy, The Eighth International Symposium,
edited by J. K. Penry. Raven Press, New York
© 1977.

Temporal Lobe Epilepsy: On Whom to Operate and When

Inge Jensen

University Clinic of Neurosurgery, Rigshospitalet, Copenhagen, Denmark

Temporal lobe epilepsy is an extremely severe type of epilepsy, which not seldom is socially invalidating. This is not only due to the seizures but predominantly is caused by the frequently accompanying psychiatric disorders. Fortunately, progress in pharmacotherapy, especially the introduction of carbamazepine, has relieved many patients from their epilepsy, but still the number of patients suffering from drug-resistant temporal lobe epilepsy is exorbitantly large.

Unilateral temporal lobe resection has, since first applied in 1948, proved to be an excellent treatment of drug-resistant temporal lobe epilepsy of unilateral or predominantly unilateral temporal origin. By the end of 1975 surveys from neurosurgical clinics all over the world covering more than 2,000 operations were available (Inge Jensen, 1975a; Van Buren et al., 1975). In summary, the outcome was that almost two-thirds of the patients at follow-up 1 to 10 years postoperatively had no or few seizures, and in more than three-quarters the operation could be designated as "worthwhile." Furthermore, over half of the patients who preoperatively displayed some psychiatric disorders were normalized or had markedly improved. The surveys also indicated that the outcome was better in operations performed in the more recent years than in those dating from the earliest period, and, further, that inclusion of the mesial structures in the resections favorably influenced the surgical prognosis.

The surgical treatment of drug-resistant temporal lobe epilepsy was instituted in Denmark in 1960, and by the end of March, 1975, a total of 106 patients had been submitted to an anterior temporal lobectomy at Rigshospitalet, Copenhagen. All operations but one were performed by the same neurosurgeon, K. Vaernet, who followed the principles laid down by Falconer (Falconer et al., 1955; Falconer, 1965), resecting the tip of the temporal lobe *en bloc,* including the mesial structures, so that the whole specimen was available for histological examination (Inge Jensen and Vaernet, *in press*).

The present chapter covers the first 74 consecutively operated patients (1960 through 1969). Neither before nor during the operation was any tumor or gross vascular malformation recognized in any of the patients. All patients suffered from psychomotor and/or focal seizures originating from the temporal lobe, and 55 of them also had grand mal. Their epilepsy was extremely severe, and preoperatively all of them were socially handicapped due to their frequent and severe seizures and/or psychiatric disturbances. In all patients a unilateral or predominantly unilateral spike-discharging temporal focus was revealed through routine EEG scalp recordings or through recordings with sphenoidal electrodes. The case material consists of 43 males and 31 females. At the time of the operation the ages of the patients ranged from 4 to 54 years, including 14 patients of 15 years or younger. In 60 of the patients the preoperative duration of epilepsy was more than 4 years.

A retrospective follow-up investigation was undertaken in 1970 and 1971. The median postoperative follow-up period was 5.1 years. The overall result of the operation on seizures was found to be that 61% of the patients became free from any seizures, 20% obtained a reduction in their seizure frequency by at least 75%, and the remaining 19% obtained only some reduction in seizure frequency or no change. In this last group, denoted "no change," there were also four postoperative deaths, which occurred 8 days, 2 months, and 3 and 5 years postoperatively.

The final outcome in 81% of the patients in the two best therapeutic groups compares favorably with the results published from other centers.

A unilateral temporal lobe resection in patients with temporal lobe epilepsy also favorably influences the postoperative psychiatric status. In the Danish case material roughly one-third of the patients were found to be without any psychiatric abnormalities at follow-up, as compared to one-eighth at the time of operation; a further one-third had improved, whereas only one-tenth had deteriorated. The normalization or improvement in psychiatric condition is apparently closely related to therapeutic success regarding relief from seizures or a marked reduction in the seizure frequency; but the conclusion is not statistically significant.

Information on operative complications is available from approximately half of the neurosurgical clinics performing unilateral temporal lobe resections. Based on these surveys it is possible to conclude that complications resulting in persistent inconvenience to the patient now are few and have become less severe (Inge Jensen, 1975a; Van Buren et al., 1975; Inge Jensen and Vaernet, *in press.*) Further, it must be observed that all operative deaths occurred early in the series, and that the last operative fatality was recorded in the early 1960s.

It is to be anticipated that in many cases an anterior temporal lobectomy will be followed by a partial homonymous hemianopia involving the upper quadrants (Falconer and Wilson, 1958). Accordingly, this sequel is not considered a complication, especially as the patient is not inconvenienced by the defect, and in most cases it remains unnoticed by him or her. Contrary to this a complete hemianopia presents considerable inconvenience to the patient, it even prevents him from obtaining a driver's license. Unfortunately, it is not possible to predict in which cases this comparatively infrequent complication will occur (Inge Jensen and Seedorff, 1976).

The mortality rate in an epileptic population is considerably greater than that in the general population with the augmentation depending on the severity of the epilepsy. The total mortality rate in an unselected Danish epileptic population

(Brink Henriksen et al., 1970) was found to be 59.4 deaths per 1,000, as compared to 2.9 per 1,000 in the general population in the age group 10 to 59 years. Surveys from 14 neurosurgical clinics supply information on late mortality, giving a mortality rate of 47.6 per 1,000 patients surviving á temporal lobe resection. Thus it can be concluded that a temporal lobectomy not only benefits approximately three-quarters of the patients by abolishing or reducing their seizure frequency, but it also markedly decreases the excess mortality postoperatively (Inge Jensen, 1975*b*). The late mortality is for one-third related to epilepsy, for another third due to suicide, and for the last third due to other causes. This high suicidal rate is in accordance with the most recent observations from the Guy's-Maudsley Hospital (D. Taylor, *personal communication*).

The neuropathological findings in the Danish study (Inge Jensen and Klinken, 1976) were 4 small tumors; 9 focal, well-defined, nonneoplastic changes (vascular malformation, porencephaly, atherosclerosis in the uncus, sequelae of toxoplasmosis, cortical dysplasia, heterotopia of nerve cells, meningocerebral scar, sequelae of ablation of a meningioma, and cystic gliosis); 7 nodular glioses; 14 cases of diffuse gliosis, satellitosis, and depletion of ganglion cells ("mesial temporal sclerosis"); 10 cases of perivascular lymphocytic and histiocytic infiltration; 17 equivocal changes (questionable gliosis or perivascular infiltration or no definite structural abnormality); and 13 sequelae of a previous iatrogenic insult. The eventual neuropathological conclusion was that the surgical outcome apparently is better the more focal and circumscribed the histological lesion; regarding relief from seizures this is but a trend, while the observation is statistically significant at the 5% level with regard to the psychiatric normalization and/or improvement. This observation is in full accordance with those of Morris (1956), Haberland (1958), Paillas (1958), Goldensohn (1962), Green and Scheetz (1964), Dill and Gulotta (1970) and Engel et al. (1975).

The criteria in selecting the patients for surgery have in the Danish case material been in accordance with the principles applied at the Montreal Neurological Institute (Rasmussen, 1969) and at the Guy's-Maudsley Hospital (Falconer, 1965). In summary, the requirements were that the patients suffered from epilepsy of long standing, which had proved resistant to medical therapy, and that a unilateral or predominantly unilateral temporal focus was found on the EEG. The Danish neurosurgeon, however, accepted patients with bilateral EEG abnormalities if there was a predominance over one temporal lobe, without any definite limitations as to the ratio in the distribution of the abnormalities in the two hemispheres. It is evident from our series that patients with an anterior temporal and/or sphenoidal electrode focus definitely have a more favorable result of the operation than patients with a mid- or posttemporal focus, with 80% and 48%, respectively, in the successful group. Diffuse slow-wave activity or diffuse paroxysmal activity, on the other hand, unfavorably influences the postoperative prognosis regarding relief from seizures.

In a few of the Danish patients it was not possible to maintain adequate medication because the patients developed drug intolerance, and in several patients progressive psychiatric disturbances provided an additional indication for operation. The indications for operation are in themselves of prognostic value: in all patients the main indication was resistance to medication; this alone or associated with a suspicion of tumor favorably influenced the postoperative prognosis, whereas an additional psychiatric indication had a less satisfactory prognosis (Inge Jensen and Vaernet, *in press*). The prognosis regarding relief from seizures is unfavorably influenced by a family history of several relatives suffering from neurological diseases localized to the central nervous system, and that of psychiatric normalization by major psychiatric disorders affecting first degree relatives. Apart from these observations, genetic and other etiological factors are found to be without significant prognostic importance (Inge Jensen, 1975*c*, 1976*a*).

All but one of the patients in the Danish case material suffered from psychomotor epilepsy, and the incidence of grand mal was 74%, which is quite comparable with other surveys. The occurrence of a single type of seizure is prognostically favorable, regarding both abolition of seizures and attainment of a psychiatrically normal status at follow-up. Preoperative presence of grand mal is highly unfavorable as only 51% of the patients with grand mal were free from any seizures and only 22% of them were psychiatrically normal at follow-up as compared to 89% and 53%, respectively, of the patients without grand mal. The type of psychomotor attack *per se* did not influence the postoperative prognosis regarding relief from seizures, whereas the presence of either ictal-affective attacks or automatisms of a complex nature unfavorably influenced the psychiatric status at follow-up. The previously published recordings on the prognostic value of the presence of the various types of seizures are not directly comparable, but on the basis of them and the present study it is possible to conclude that the preoperative presence of generalized seizures *per se* unfavorably influences the surgical prognosis (Inge Jensen, 1976*b*).

The age at onset of psychomotor or focal seizures does not influence the surgical or psychiatric prognosis, whereas onset of grand mal between the ages 5 and 19 years is prognostically highly unfavorable.

In the present study the preoperative duration of epilepsy in one-fifth of the patients was less than 5 years, and in another fifth, 20 years or longer. In accordance with Falconer and Serafetinides (1963) and Stepién et al. (1969) but in disagreement with Bengzon et al. (1968), the prognosis is observed to be favored by a preoperative duration of epilepsy of 4 years or less. If grand mal is present the preoperative duration of this specific type of epilepsy should preferably not exceed 1 year. With a preoperative duration of psychomotor epilepsy of 10 years or longer the number of satisfactory operative results decreases.

When comparing the few records of age at temporal lobectomy and the eventual outcome of this treatment, it seems obvious that this operation preferably should be performed in childhood, adolescence, or early adulthood, and at any rate as soon as this specific type of epilepsy has proved to be resistant to medication (Falconer and Serafetinides, 1963; Bengzon et al., 1968; Shefer et al., 1970; Inge Jensen, 1976*b*).

The most important aspect in the treatment of these patients is to relieve them of their seizures and improve their psychiatric status, and quite naturally complete or partial social rehabilitation is the secondary aim after the achievement of a good surgical result. A Danish social investigation (Inge Jensen, 1976c) has confirmed the observations by Taylor (Taylor and Falconer, 1968; Taylor, 1972) that patients with temporal lobe epilepsy are born into lower social classes than expected from the social stratification in the general population. Further, it revealed that these patients are subjected to downward social mobility and that this must be caused by their epilepsy and accompanying psychiatric disorders, as their siblings who represent the same age groups and who are raised under the same social conditions have experienced an upward social mobility. The patients' social decline is partly caused by their impaired schooling and further education. The age at which the temporal lobe resection is performed is of considerable importance, as 61% of the patients operated on at age 17 years or younger were working full-time at follow-up, as compared with 30% of the patients who were older.

Unilateral temporal lobe resection in patients fulfilling the operative criteria might effectively prevent this social decline, especially if the resection is performed in childhood or adolescence, or at any rate as soon as the epilepsy has proved resistant to medication.

SUMMARY

During the last 25 years unilateral anterior temporal lobectomy has proved to be an excellent treatment of drug-resistant temporal lobe epilepsy. On a global basis (2,484 operations), approximately half of the patients become free from any seizures and in two-thirds the operation can be characterized as "worthwhile" regarding relief from seizures. The Danish figures were 61% and 88%, respectively. The operation favorably influences the psychiatric status, which in the Danish case material is found closely related to relief from seizures. The operative complications are few and have become less severe. The operative mortality, which always has been very low, can now be regarded as negligible, as no fatality has been recorded since the early 1960's. The mortality rate in an epileptic population is considerably greater than that in the general population, dependent on the severity of the epilepsy. Apparently, a temporal lobectomy decreases the mortality rate. The criteria in selecting the patients for operation have been drug-resistant epilepsy of long standing and a unilateral or predominantly unilateral temporal spiking focus on the EEG. The present Danish investigation has proved that the presence of a single type of seizure and a short duration of epilepsy, especially of grand mal, favorably influence the postoperative prognosis. Further, it has shown that the social rehabilitation is found to be significantly improved by operation at an early age. Genetic and etiological factors are observed to be without significant prognostic importance. The eventual neuropathological outcome was that the more specific and circumscribed the histological abnormality, the better the final outcome. It must therefore be concluded that unilateral temporal lobectomy ought to be taken into consideration at a much earlier moment and should not be considered a treatment applied as an ultimum refugium.

ACKNOWLEDGMENTS

This study was supported by grants from the Danish Epilepsy Association and the Danish Foundation for the Advancement of Medicine.

REFERENCES

Bengzon, A. R. A., Rasmussen, T., Gloor, P., Dussault, J., and Stephens, M. (1968): Prognostic factors in the surgical treatment of temporal lobe epileptics. *Neurology (Minneap.),* 18:717–731.

Brink Henriksen, P., Juul-Jensen, P., and Lund, M. (1970): The mortality of epileptics. In: *Life Assurance Medicine. Proceedings of the 10th International Congress,* edited by R. D. C. Brackenridge, pp. 139–148. Pitman Co., Ltd., London.

Dill, R., and Gullota, F. (1970): Pathomorphologische Befunde bei Temporallappenepilepsien. *Schweiz. Arch. Neurol. Neurochir. Psychiatr.* 106:241–255.

Engel, J., Jr., Driver, M. V., and Falconer, M. A. (1975): Electrophysiological correlates of pathology and surgical results in temporal lobe epilepsy. *Brain,* 98:129–156.

Falconer, M. A. (1965): The surgical treatment of temporal lobe epilepsy. *Neurochirurgia (Stuttg.),* 8:161–172.

Falconer, M. A., Hill, D., Meyer, A., Mitchell, W., and Pond, D. A. (1955): Treatment of temporal-lobe epilepsy by temporal lobectomy. *Lancet,* 1:827–835.

Falconer, M. A., and Serafetinides, E. A. (1963): A follow-up study of surgery in temporal lobe epilepsy. *J. Neurol. Neurosurg. Psychiatry,* 26:154–165.

Falconer, M. A., and Wilson, J. L. (1958): Visual field changes following anterior temporal lobectomy. *Brain,* 81:1–14.

Goldensohn, E. S. (1962): Temporal lobe epilepsy: Neurological and electrical aspects. *Bull. N. Y. Acad. Med.,* 38:653–661.

Green, J. R., and Scheetz, D. G. (1964): Surgery of epileptogenic lesions of temporal lobe. *Arch. Neurol.,* 10:135–148.

Haberland, C. (1958): Histological studies in temporal lobe epilepsy based on biopsy materials. *Psychiatr. Neurol. (Basel),* 132:12–29.

Jensen, Inge (1975*a*): Temporal lobe surgery around the world. Results, complications, and mortality. *Acta Neurol. Scand.,* 52:354–373.

Jensen, Inge (1975*b*): Temporal lobe epilepsy. Late mortality in patients treated with unilateral temporal lobe resections. *Acta Neurol. Scand.,* 52:374–380.

Jensen, Inge (1975*c*): Genetic factors in temporal lobe epilepsy. *Acta Neurol. Scand.,* 52:381–394.

Jensen, Inge (1976*a*): Temporal lobe epilepsy. Aetiological factors and surgical results. *Acta Neurol. Scand.,* 53:103–118.

Jensen, Inge (1976*b*): Temporal lobe epilepsy. Types of seizures, age, and surgical results. *Acta Neurol. Scand.,* 53:335–357.

Jensen, Inge (1976*c*): Temporal lobe epilepsy. Social conditions and rehabilitation after surgery. *Acta Neurol. Scand.,* 54:22–44.

Jensen, Inge, and Klinken, L. (1976): Temporal lobe epilepsy and neuropathology. *Acta Neurol. Scand.,* 54:391–414.

Jensen, Inge, and Seedorff, H. H. (1977): Temporal lobe epilepsy and Neuro-ophthalmology. Ophthalmological findings in 74 temporal lobe resected patients. *Acta Ophthalmol. Scand.,* 54: 827–841.

Jensen, Inge, and Vaernet, K. (1977): Temporal lobe epilepsy. Follow-up investigation of 74 temporal lobe resected patients. *Acta Neurochir. (Wien) (in press).*

Morris, A. A. (1956): Temporal lobectomy with removal of uncus, hippocampus and amygdala. *Arch. Neurol. Psychiatry,* 76:479–496.

Paillas, J. E. (1958): Aspects cliniques de l'épilepsie temporale. In: *Temporal Lobe Epilepsy,* edited by M. Baldwin and P. Bailey, pp. 411–439. Charles C. Thomas, Springfield, Ill.

Rasmussen, T. (1969): The role of surgery in the treatment of focal epilepsy. *Clin. Neurosurg.,* 16:288–314.

Shefer, D. G., Belyaev, Y. I., Bein, V. N., and Boreiko, V. B. (1970): Remote results subsequent to surgical treatment of temporal epilepsy through partial resection of the temporal lobe. *Vopr. Neirokhir.,* 34:17–24.

Stepién, L., Bidziński, J., and Mazurowsky, W. (1969): The results of surgical treatment of temporal lobe epilepsy. *Pol. Med. J.,* 8:1184–1190.

Taylor, D. C. (1972): Mental state and temporal lobe epilepsy. *Epilepsia,* 13:727–765.

Taylor, D. C., and Falconer, M. A. (1968): Clinical, socio-economic, and psychological changes after temporal lobectomy for epilepsy. *Br. J. Psychiatry,* 114:1247–1261.

Van Buren, J. M., Ajmone-Marsan, C., Mutsuga, N., and Sadowsky, D. (1975): Surgery of temporal lobe epilepsy. In: *Neurosurgical Management of the Epilepsies. Advances in Neurology, Vol. 8,* edited by D. P. Purpura, J. K. Penry, and R. D. Walter, pp 155–196. Raven Press, New York.

Epilepsy, The Eighth International Symposium,
edited by J. K. Penry. Raven Press, New York
© 1977.

Chronic Cerebellar Stimulation in the Treatment of Epilepsy: A Preliminary Report

G. W. Fenton, P. B. C. Fenwick, G. S. Brindley, M. A. Falconer, C. H. Polkey, and D. N. Rushton

Maudsley Hospital and Institute of Psychiatry, University of London, England

Irving Cooper (1973, 1974) was the first person to use the technique of chronic cerebellar stimulation in the treatment of epilepsy. The rationale for this approach was based on the observations that cerebellar stimulation can often inhibit clinical and electrographic seizure activity caused by epileptogenic lesions of the cerebral cortex in rats and cats, whereas ablation of the cerebellum can make the experimental epilepsy worse (Grabow et al., 1974). The finding that diphenylhydantoin and phenobarbital, both effective anticonvulsant drugs, increase the Purkinje cell firing rates was taken as further supporting evidence (Halpern and Julien, 1972). It should be noted, however, that Puro and Woodward (1973) were able to confirm this finding using only toxic doses of diphenylhydantoin. Cooper's initial reports in a small series of patients with differing types of seizure patterns were impressive, some subjects showing a marked reduction or even total abolition of seizures.

Since Cooper's technique seemed a promising new approach to the treatment of epilepsy, we decided to apply it to a number of patients with seizures intractable to other forms of therapy. One patient has now been treated for 20 months. A second has had cerebellar electrodes implanted and has recently commenced a stimulation program. This chapter describes the clinical features and outcome of the first patient and presents some observations on the electrical activity of the cerebellum.

CASE REPORT

The first patient is a 29-year-old girl of dull intelligence (WAIS full-scale IQ 75, verbal 88, performance 64) and immature, dependent personality. There is no behavior disorder but she has suffered from intractable epilepsy since the age of 12 years with generalized convulsions, transient drop attacks, and brief petit mal absences. There is a history of status epilepticus at the age of 6 years with a transient left hemiparesis of 1 week's duration.

She lives with her parents, both school teachers in their early fifties. Her brother died at the age of 15 years of congenital heart disease. There is no family history of epilepsy.

EEG recordings, performed during both wakefulness and quinalbarbitone-induced sleep carried out over a number of years showed frequent generalized spike-and-wave complexes with independent right and left posterior, mid, and anterior temporal focal spike discharges, most marked in the left posterior temporal region. The EEG background was diffusely abnormal with a generalized excess of theta and delta frequencies and little alpha rhythm. A marked asymmetry was present in the temporal areas with more beta and alpha rhythm on the right side and more theta and delta activity on the left. Plain x-rays of the skull showed a small middle fossa on the left. However, a left carotid arteriogram and pneumoencephalogram were normal.

The seizures had remained intractable to therapy with all the usual anticonvulsant drugs in varying combinations, with the exception of clonazepam and sodium valproate, given in sufficient dosage to ensure serum concentrations within the therapeutic range. Close outpatient observation over 5 years revealed an average seizure frequency of 60 drop attacks and 88 petit mal attacks each month and one grand mal seizure every 2 months. No periods of spontaneous or drug-induced remission had occurred.

Cerebellar Electrode Implant Procedure

She was considered a suitable candidate for chronic cerebellar stimulation because of the severe and intractable nature of the epilepsy. Four electrode arrays, each consisting of eight platinum electrodes mounted on a silicone rubber base, were constructed by one of the authors (G.S.B.) and his team in the M.R.C. Neurological Prostheses Unit at the Institute of Psychiatry. These were essentially similar to those used by Cooper. It was arranged that two arrays should be placed over the medial and lateral aspects of the superior surface of each cerebellar hemisphere. Each was to be connected by a lead passing through a suboccipital burr hole via the subcutaneous tissues of the neck to a radio receiver placed subcutaneously in the left pectoral region.

The operative procedures involved in inserting the electrodes were carried out in several stages. During the first operation bilateral suboccipital craniectomies were carried out and the anterior surface of the cerebellum was exposed. The electrodes were placed without difficulty and the posterior fossa incision closed. The connecting leads were brought to a point in front of the anterior border of the left sternomastoid. The patient was then retowelled in the supine position and the leads brought down through the subcutaneous tissue of the neck to the left pectoral region. The suboccipital, neck, and left pectoral wounds were then sutured. The patient made an uneventful recovery from this operation. Eleven days later the distal ends of the leads were externalized for 48 hr through the left pectoral skin incision in order to permit recording from the cerebellar electrodes, testing of the electrodes, and calibration of the stimulus parameters using an external stimulator.

Electrophysiological Recording

The spontaneous activity from the cerebellar and scalp electrodes was recorded during the waking state by an SLE 16-channel electroencephalograph using a bipolar recording technique. Six channels from the cerebellar and scalp leads were tape recorded using an F.M. recorder for off-line computer analysis. The spontaneous background activity from the cerebellar electrodes had an amplitude of between 50 and 100 μv and was of only slightly higher amplitude than the scalp EEG activity. It is thus of much lower voltage than the usual human electrocorticogram. The frequency spectra of both the cerebellar and scalp channels, computed by power spectral analysis using the Fast Fourier Transform of 30-sec epochs of recorded activity, were essentially similar. Eye opening and closure had no effect on the activity from the cerebellar electrodes; neither did auditory or visual stimulation. Neither voluntary nor passive limb movement, including fist clenching, altered the cerebellar activity.

Diphasic transients with a lambdoid waveform appeared synchronously from the right and left centroparietal scalp channels and the right and left medial and lateral cerebellar leads from time to time. The scalp distribution of these potentials was over the frontocentral areas of both cerebral hemispheres with little spread posteriorly. They were apparently spontaneous in occurrence and were presumably transmitted from the cerebellum via the ascending efferent connections between the deep cerebellar nuclei and areas 4 and 6 of the cerebral cortex (Truex and Carpenter, 1969).

Intermittent high-voltage atypical spike-and-wave complexes appeared synchronously from both the scalp and cerebellar channels. During epochs when frequent spike and spike-and-wave discharges were recorded from the scalp, delta waves were prominent in the cerebellar leads.

Because of the similarity in amplitude and frequency profile of the activity recorded from the cerebellar leads to that of the scalp EEG, it is tempting to regard the potential changes recorded from the cerebellar leads as merely occipital cortex activity transmitted by volume conduction through the tentorium cerebri. However, the evidence against this hypothesis is as follows: (1) crosscorrelograms between the cerebellar channels and the centroparietal scalp leads in our patient indicate a high correlation with no phase shift between the ipsilateral cerebellar and centroparietal scalp EEG activity and a low correlation between the cerebellar and the contralateral centroparietal scalp EEG activity; (2) Papakostopoulos et al. (1976), using a similar technique, have found a low correlation between the cerebellar rhythms and the ipsilateral scalp occipital EEG activity; (3) cerebellar activity shows a lack of response to eye opening; and (4) transients with a lambdoid waveform occur synchronously in the cerebellar and centroparietal scalp EEG leads in the absence of spread to the occipital region of the scalp. Thus, it seems more probable that the potential changes recorded from the cerebellar electrodes represent the intrinsic activity of the cerebellar cortex. The high correlation between the cerebellar activity and the ipsilateral central area of the cerebral cortex may be due to spread of potential changes along the efferent pathways from the deep nuclei of the cerebellum to areas 4 and 6 of the cerebral cortex.

Insertion of the Receivers

After the 48-hr recording period, the left pectoral incision was reopened. Eight miniature radio receivers (two for each electrode array) were connected to the cerebellar leads via a silicone rubber block and placed beneath the skin in the pectoral region above the left breast. The skin incision was then resutured and healed quickly. The patient was able to leave the neurosurgical ward within 15 days of the final operation.

Therapeutic Stimulation Procedure

Stimulation with 10-Hz unidirectional square wave pulses was commenced shortly afterwards using a radio transmitter, the transmitting coils being strapped to the skin covering the receivers. The current used was adjusted to that just below the threshold which caused stimulation of the fifth and seventh cranial nerves. This electrical stimulation alternated continuously between the right and left medial cerebellar electrodes (7 min right and 7 min left). For the first 2 months the stimulation was carried out continuously throughout nocturnal sleep only (12 to 15 hr daily). Subsequently, for the last 18 months, the stimulation was performed continuously throughout the 24 hr period using a portable transmitter, first carried in a satchel by the patient but later modified so that it could be worn in a belt around the waist.

Apart from intermittent, throbbing frontal headaches for the first few weeks after the onset of the continuous cerebellar stimulation program, no side effects have been reported. No nystagmus, ataxia, or other clinical evidence of cerebellar dysfunction has been observed throughout the 20 months of stimulation. The patient is freely mobile during the day and wears the stimulator in a belt around her waist. The transmitting coils are kept in position over the implanted receivers by the use of a specially tailored brassière. At night the transmitter batteries are recharged by mains voltage while the stimulation continues. The patient sleeps with the transmitting coils strapped to the left pectoral region with microphone adhesive. At times during the night the coils slip from this position when she rolls over in sleep.

Effect of Treatment after 20 Months

Seizure Frequency

The changes in seizure frequency are displayed in Fig. 1 in histogram form, each column representing the number of attacks (major, drop, and petit mal seizures) during successive 4-month periods. The base-line period consisted of

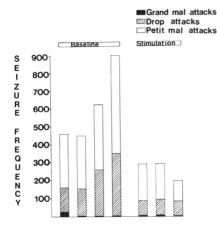

FIG. 1. Continuous cerebellar stimulation in an epileptic patient. Each column represents the number of seizures in a 4-month period.

16 months' observation prior to hospital admission. The stimulation period covers the 12-month period since discharge from hospital. There has been no appreciable change in major seizure frequency. However, a significant reduction in both the drop attacks (mean before treatment of 270 per month and after treatment of 80 per month) and petit mal seizures (mean per month before treatment of 380 and after treatment of 125). A change in character of the drop attacks has also been noticed, with these attacks being less abrupt in onset.

EEG Recordings

Regular routine waking recordings were performed at two to four weekly interviews for 5 months before the implant operation. Since the operation nine recordings have been performed at intervals of 1 to 2 months. The number of bursts of generalized spike-and-wave activity of an amplitude greater than 80 μv and lasting more than 5 sec were counted during a standard period of 17 min recording on each occasion. The mean value before operation was 22 and after operation was 3. This difference is significant at the 0.01 level using a t-test (two-tailed). This change was gradual and became apparent only 3 months after the operation. Since then the change has been sustained.

Cognitive Function

Psychometric testing 6 months after the operation revealed no change in the full-scale WAIS IQ (75), but the performance scale IQ had increased from 64 to 80. However, the most dramatic change was a striking improvement of performance in tests of verbal and visual learning. In the Wechsler Logical Memory subtest, the correct delayed recall of the test material expressed as a percentage of the correct immediate recall was 59% before the operation as compared to 90% afterwards. Performance on the Rey-Osterreith test, a measure of visual retention, was also improved, the percentage of correct recall increasing from 47 to 65%.

Behavior

Since the operation she has been observed to be more alert and socially more competent, showing a greater degree of maturity in her dealing with other people. She is now able to be more independent of her parents. A reflection of this improvement is the fact that she is now actively involved in the management of the local handicapped persons club, of which she is secretary.

DISCUSSION

Quite clear and sustained reductions in seizure frequency and rate of occurrence of EEG spike-and-wave complexes have been demonstrated in our patient following chronic cerebellar stimulation over a 20-month period. These have been accompanied by an improvement in cognitive function with better performance of tasks involving the learning of new material, both verbal and nonverbal. The patient has also become more alert and socially competent. These changes have been achieved without alteration in anticonvulsant medication. Although this definite clinical improvement coincides with the cerebellar stimulation procedure, it is premature to assume a direct causal relationship. A number of alternative explanations must be considered.

The clinical changes may be totally unrelated to the electrical stimulation. During the past 2 years the patient, who previously lived a lonely life with few social contacts outside the family circle, has been the focus of interest of the therapeutic team involved in the project. She has had much social and personal interaction with the various members of the team and has identified closely with them and their therapeutic aims. The consequent intense and continuous social stimulation may have influenced the outcome. However, such social factors can hardly explain the sustained and cumulative nature of the improvement. In any case she had previously taken part in an anticonvulsant drug trial over a 2-year period and hence was the subject of much clinical interest and investigation. This project involved frequent visits to the epilepsy clinic and much personal contact with several therapists concerned with the trial assessments. No change in seizure frequency or behavior occurred during this time.

Having rejected the social stimulation hypothesis, we must consider the effect of the electrical stimulation on the brain. This may have acted directly on the cerebellum, influencing Purkinje cell discharge patterns, as suggested by Cooper (1973). However, it has not been possible to demonstrate any clinical evidence of change in cerebellar function by electrical stimulation. Unilateral electrical stimulation of the cerebellar cortex with ten 1-msec pulses per second of a strength (usually 5 to 10 mA) near the threshold for causing headache had no effect, ipsilaterally or contralaterally, on limb muscle tone, tendon reflexes, gait, speed or accuracy of rapid repetitive movement, latency of hand movement in response to a visual signal, or long latency stretch reflex in the thumb. Handwriting (right hand) was also unaffected. No nystagmus was caused other than that clearly attributable to cranial nerve stimulation. The normal nystagmus on extreme deviation of the eyes was unaffected. When stimulation caused no headache or cranial nerve effects, the patient was unaware of it. Effects apparently due to spread of current to the ipsilateral fifth, sixth, or seventh nerves or nuclei could be elicited from seven of the eight electrode sets; thresholds were from 3 to 15 mA (Brindley et al., 1976*a*). Averaged scalp evoked responses to electrical stimulation of the cerebellum were recorded over the contralateral sensorimotor area, through electrodes arranged to minimize stimulus artifact. These were of 40 to 45 msec latency. The strength of cerebellar stimulation required was only a little below the range in which facial paresthesiae occurred, and the size of the evoked potential increased rapidly in this range of stimulus strength, although remaining of the same latency and general form. These responses may well have been evoked by weak stimulation of the trigeminal nerve root. (Brindley et al., 1976*b*.). Stimulation during prolonged episodes of spike-and-wave discharge has no effect on the spike-wave complexes. Thus, as well as there being no evidence of alteration of cerebellar function following stimulation, no unequivocal evidence of a functional cerebellar output could be demonstrated. Hence, the hypothesis that the cerebellar electrode stimulation acts by a direct effect on the cerebellum receives scant support.

There is no doubt, however, that the current generated by the stimulation spreads widely throughout the brainstem, affecting the fifth and seventh cranial nerves. Therefore, the therapeutic action of the stimulation may be mediated through stimulant effects on the reticular formation caused by the current spread. Chronic reticular activation may lead to a higher level of cortical arousal with increased alertness and improved learning ability, features shown by our patient. Increased alertness tends to inhibit the development of seizures and could account for the improvement in seizure frequency. Such a mechanism could also explain the gradual development of the therapeutic effect. Against this arousal system hypothesis is the observation that the stimulation procedure had no obvious effect on her nocturnal sleep pattern.

On the available evidence, the nonspecific reticular formation stimulation hypothesis seems the most plausible. Clearly, more work is required using both primate models and patients along the lines proposed by Grabow et al. (1974).

ACKNOWLEDGMENTS

The authors wish to thank Mr. John Cooper and Mr. Peter Donaldson of the M.R.C. Neurological Prostheses Unit for their work in construction of the electrode arrays and maintenance of the stimulation equipment, and the medical and technical staff of the Department of Clinical Neurophysiology, Maudsley Hospital for their invaluable assistance with the recordings.

REFERENCES

Brindley, G. S., Falconer, M. A., Fenton, G. W., Fenwick, P. B. C., Polkey, C. H., and Rushton, D. N. (1976a): Immediate effects of cerebellar stimulation in an epileptic patient. *Electroencephalogr. Clin. Neurophysiol.*, 41:539.

Brindley, G. S., Falconer, M. A., Fenton, G. W., Fenwick, P. B. C., Polkey, C. H., and Rushton, D. N. (1976b): Scalp evoked responses to cerebellar stimulation in man. *Electroencephalogr. Clin. Neurophysiol.*, 41:539–540.

Cooper, I. S. (1973): *Effect of chronic stimulation of anterior cerebellum on neurological disease. Lancet,* 1:206.

Cooper, I. S. (1974): *The Cerebellum, Epilepsy and Behaviour.* Plenum Press, New York.

Grabow, J. D., Ebersold, M. J., Albers, J. W., and Schima, E. M. (1974): Cerebellar stimulation in the control of seizures. *Mayo Clin. Proc.,* 49:759–774.

Halpern, L., and Julien, R. (1972): Augmentation of cerebellar Purkinje cell discharge rate after diphenylhydantoin. *Epilepsia,* 13:377–385.

Papakostopoulos, D., Cooper, R., Cummins, B., and Winter, A. (1976): Evoked and intrinsic activities in the cerebellum of conscious man. *Electroencephalogr. Clin. Neurophysiol.,* 41:538.

Puro, D. G., and Woodward, D. J. (1973): Effects of diphenylhydantoin on activity of the rat cerebellar Purkinje cells. *Neuropharmacology,* 12:433–440.

Truex, R. C., and Carpenter, M. B. (1969): *Human Neuroanatomy.* Williams & Wilkins Co., Baltimore.

Epilepsy, The Eighth International Symposium,
edited by J. K. Penry. Raven Press, New York
© 1977.

Multiple Sclerosis and Seizures

* Marta Elian and Geoffrey Dean

Midland Centre for Neurology and Neurosurgery, Smethwick, Worcestershire, England; and Medico-Social Research Board, Dublin 2, Ireland

A possible causal relationship between multiple sclerosis (MS) and epilepsy was first suggested 106 years ago by Leube (1871). The various publications during the century that followed were able to neither prove nor disprove the suspected causal relationship.

The opportunity to study this problem further arose for us when investigating the incidence of MS in immigrants from low prevalence areas. We reviewed 2,400 case notes from patients suffering from multiple sclerosis in the West Midland region of England. The notes in which fits, faints, seizures, or their synonyms were mentioned were studied in detail; the family physician was asked to fill in a questionnaire and was contacted by telephone for additional information and discussion. When possible, the patient was seen. After elimination of the doubtful cases, we found 27 patients who suffered from both MS and seizures: 20 females and 7 males. The following summarizes our findings.

FINDINGS

Regarding the *multiple sclerosis*, about half of the patients suffered from a severe form of MS leading to partial or total incapacitation, three patients died from the consequences of MS. None of the patients had the purely spinal form of MS, and all patients had a variety of clinical signs as evidence of multiple cerebral demyelinating foci. No definite correlation could be found between the appearance of fits and the exacerbation of the symptoms of MS, although in some of the patients the two dates coincided.

From the point of view of the *seizures*, the majority of the patients (sixteen) had generalized convulsions only, seven patients had both generalized convulsions and focal seizures, and only four patients had purely focal seizures. None were found to have petit mal. In six patients the onset of the seizures preceded that of the other symptoms of MS—in two of these there was no history of trauma or other central nervous system disease to explain the epilepsy. In four patients the onset of seizures was concomitant with the appearance of other symptoms

---

* Present address: Department of Neuro-Sciences, St Bartholomew's Hospital, West Smithfield, London E.C.1, England.

TABLE 1. *Severity of epilepsy according to frequency of seizures*

Frequency	No. of patients
One isolated fit	3
One isolated series of fits	3
Several isolated fits every few years	10
Several series of fits every few years	5
Three or more fits per year	6

of MS. In the remaining 17 patients, 1 to 22 years elapsed between the first symptoms of MS and the seizures which followed them. Table 1 shows the severity of the seizure disorder, as revealed by the frequency of the seizures.

The *EEG* examinations were not timed to correlate with a certain stage of the MS nor with that of the seizures—this being a restrospective study with variable hospital facilities. We obtained 27 records from 16 patients; nine of these tracings were considered to be within normal limits, 4 showed lateralizing focal features in the form of slow waves and spikes, and 14 records revealed bilateral abnormalities with diffuse nonspecific slowing.

Of the 27 patients, 21 had *psychiatric symptoms* severe enough to warrant consulting a psychiatrist. Only two were euphoric; the remaining nineteen patients showed depressive symptomatology. Six people attempted suicide one or more times; in one patient this was successful. All suicide attempts were made by barbiturate overdose, alone or in combination with other anticonvulsant drugs. The question arises whether or not a causal relationship between multiple sclerosis and epilepsy exists.

DISCUSSION

In order to answer this question we must first examine the availability of statistical evidence for it. The incidence of epilepsy among MS patients varies in the published reports from 0.5% to over 10%. Epilepsy among the general population varies between 0.3 and 0.5% (Lennox, 1960). Even if we take the higher number as a base line, from the 2,400 patients with MS the maximum number of patients who would be expected to suffer from epilepsy as well would be 12. We have found 27 or 1.1%, i.e., more than double the expected number. It seems the greater the number of MS patients in a given series, the lower the relative number of patients with seizures among them. In our opinion the statistical evidence, although suggestive, is not enough to support the assumption that there is a causal relationship between the two diseases.

Alternatively, three points serve as circumstantial evidence that the MS determines the epileptic symptomatology, to some extent at least.

1. Other paroxysmal phenomena in addition to the seizures, such as paroxysmal dysarthria, paroxysmal pain in the limbs, and paroxysmal dysesthesia along with trigeminal neuralgia, are not infrequent symptoms of MS.

TABLE 2. *Seizures among patients with MS—review of literature*

No. of patients with seizures	No. of patients with MS	%	
8	74	10.8	Fuglsang-Frederiksen and Thygesen, 1952
10	132	8	Trouillas and Courjon, 1972
13	216	6	Storring, 1941
13	268	4.85	Bau-Prussak and Prussak, 1929
13	289	4.5	Drake and Macrae, 1961
3	80	3.7	Feldman, 1957
28	793	3.5	Muller, 1949
17	500	3	Cendrowski and Majkowski, 1972
27	2,400	1.1	This study
19	4,000	0.5	Hopf et al., 1970

2. The male : female ratio in epilepsy is 1:1 with perhaps a slight male preponderance. In our series, as in several other series in the literature (Hopf et al., 1970), the female : male ratio in patients who suffered from the two diseases was found to be 3:1, thus indicating that the sex ratio is determined by MS.

3. When epilepsy occurs in patients with MS, the type and course of the seizures differ from that usually seen in the general population: more generalized convulsions and no petit mal are seen; the course of epilepsy is more benign with fewer seizures—in clusters—that often do not require treatment. All patients agreed that epilepsy is the lesser evil of the two diseases—and this is in agreement with the findings in the literature (Müller, 1949; Table 2).

The psychiatric symptomatology seems to be determined by the epilepsy because not the euphoria commonly seen in patients with MS but the depression prevails. The number of patients suffering from psychiatric symptoms and especially the suicide rate are higher than in the sufferers of either disease alone.

SUMMARY

We found that 27 patients or 1.1%, as opposed to the "expected" 0.5%, of the 2,400 patients suffering from MS in the West Midland region had seizures.

The epilepsy when combined with MS tended to be milder and had a better prognosis, often not requiring treatment. Of these 27 patients, 23 had generalized convulsions, 4 had focal seizures only, and none had petit mal. Instead of euphoria often seen in patients with MS, the patients affected with both epilepsy and MS tended to suffer from depression. This and the easy availability of drugs, especially barbiturates, increased the risk of suicide.

REFERENCES

Bau-Prussak, S., and Prussak, L. (1929): Ueber Epileptische Anfalle bei multipler Sklerose. *Z. Neurol.,* 122:410–524.
Cendrowski, W., and Majkowski, J. (1972): Epilepsy in multiple sclerosis. *J. Neurol. Sci.,* 17:389–398.

Drake, W. E., and Macrae, D. (1961): Epilepsy in multiple sclerosis. *Neurology (Minneap.)*, 11:-810–816.

Feldman, S. (1957): Convulsions in multiple sclerosis. *J. Nerv. Ment. Dis.*, 125:213–220.

Fuglsang-Frederiksen, V., and Thygesen, P. (1952): Seizures and psychopathology in multiple sclerosis. An electroencephalographic study. Discussion of pathogenesis. *Acta Psychiatr. Neurol. Scand.*, 27:17–41.

Hopf, H. C., Stamatovic, A. M., and Wahren, W. (1970): Die cerebralen Anfalle bei der Multiplen Sklerose. *Z. Neurol.*, 198:256–279.

Lennox, W. G. (1960): *Epilepsy and Related Disorders,* pp. 497, 1015. J. & A. Churchill, Ltd., London.

Leube, W. (1871): Ueber multiple inselformige Sklerose des Gehirns und Ruckenmarks. *Dtsch. Arch. Klin. Med.*, 8:1–5.

Müller, R. (1949): Studies in disseminated sclerosis. *Acta Med. Scand. [Suppl.]*, 222:3–214.

Storring, G. E. (1941): Epilepsie und Multiple Sklerose: Zugleich ein Beitrag zur Differential diagnose der Epilepsie. *Arch. Psychiatr. Nevenkr.*, 112:45–75.

Trouillas, P., and Courjon, J. (1972): Epilepsy with multiple sclerosis. *Epilepsia,* 13:325–333.

Epilepsy, The Eighth International Symposium,
edited by J. K. Penry. Raven Press, New York
© 1977.

Epileptic Seizures During Sleep in Children

*C. A. Tassinari, **G. Terzano, †G. Capocchi, ‡B. Dalla Bernardina, §F. Vigevano, ‖O. Daniele, C. Valladier, C. Dravet, and
J. Roger

*Centre St. Paul and INSERM (U_6); Marseille, France; *Neurologic Clinic, Bologna, It-
aly; **Neurology Clinic, University of Parma, Parma, Italy; †Neurology Clinic, University of Ancona, Ancona, Italy; ‡Pediatric Clinic, University of Verona, Verona, Italy;
§Neurologic Clinic, Roma, Italy; and ‖Neurologic Clinic, Palermo, Italy*

The aim of this chapter is to give the clinician some clues for the diagnosis
of sleep-related epileptic seizures, occurring mainly in children. The data are
drawn from our experience with 300 epileptic patients who had seizures during
nocturnal polygraphic recordings. The patients were mostly children from the
Centre Saint-Paul of Marseilles, a special center for epilepsy, where children with
severe epilepsy, often associated with mental retardation, are observed. Exhaustive reviews on epileptic seizures and sleep may be found in the works of Daly
(1973), Janz (1974), and Hara and Wada (1974).

MYOCLONUS AND SLEEP

Epileptic Myoclonus on "Falling Asleep"

The main clinical symptoms in five patients were isolated, repeated myoclonic
jerks usually occurring in the evening on falling asleep. Careful questioning,
however, revealed that myoclonic jerks were also present during the day. In all
cases, primary generalized epilepsy was characterized on the waking EEG as
normal background activity with bursts of *generalized multiple spikes, occurring
only when the patients' eyes were closed.* Such discharges were usually accompanied by generalized myoclonic jerks. Intermittent photic stimulation evoked
in four patients both the paroxysmal discharges on the EEG and the generalized
myoclonias.

It was evident that myoclonus was related to closure of the eyes and not to
the sleeping-waking cycle. When the eyes were closed, the myoclonus was equally
present during the day and the evening. Obviously, the eyes were more likely to
be closed on falling asleep than during the daytime.

Three conditions can be evoked for a differential diagnosis: "nocturnal myoclonus," "restless legs syndrome with myoclonus," and "physiological myoclonus" on falling asleep.

The nocturnal myoclonus described by Symonds (1953) is unlikely to correspond to the epileptic myoclonus observed in our cases. In Symonds' cases, the absence of any EEG paroxysmal discharge (frequent and easily observed in our cases) and the clinical findings make unlikely the hypothesis of myoclonus of epileptic nature. Such cases suggest to us the diagnosis of restless legs syndrome of the myoclonic variety (Ambrosetto et al., 1965) or of physiological myoclonus of sleep (Oswald, 1959), both manifestations of a nonepileptic nature.

From our experience, as well as from the investigations of Lugaresi and colleagues (1970), we conclude that there is no evidence for a type of epilepsy having as a *sole symptom* the occurrence of epileptic myoclonias on falling asleep or during sleep.

Epileptic Myoclonus During Sleep

Epileptic myoclonias were recorded during sleep in patients having myoclonias accompanied by other epileptic manifestations that were usually more evident and frequent during wakefulness.

Isolated epileptic myoclonic jerks were observed in light sleep stages (stages I or II) or during arousal periods of deep sleep in patients with primary generalized epilepsy (and also with myoclonic jerks, isolated or associated with grand mal seizures, during wakefulness or awakening). Such myoclonias were usually accompanied by bursts of multiple spikes on the EEG, and only rarely did they awaken the subjects and produce an evident myoclonic movement. Myoclonic jerks related to bursts of multiple spikes were also observed in the Lennox-Gastaut syndrome, even if less frequently than in primary generalized epilepsy.

In absences with important clonic and tonic components (myoclotonic absences) during wakefulness (Tassinari et al., 1969), brief bursts of rhythmic, 3 cps myoclonic jerks can occur during stages I through III of sleep.

In degenerative diseases, such as the Unverricht-Lundborg and Ramsay Hunt syndromes, in which epileptic myoclonic jerks are also evident during wakefulness, the myoclonias with concomitant discharges on the EEG were particularly frequent during slow sleep stages. The myoclonias, however, were less frequent than in wakefulness and more frequent than in primary generalized epilepsy. In Ramsay Hunt disease, as well as in syndromes with postanoxic intention myoclonus, myoclonias can be present during REM sleep concomitantly with multiple spike discharges involving the somatomotor central and midline regions (Tassinari et al., 1973a, 1973b, 1974a).

GENERALIZED SEIZURES ON MORNING AWAKENING OR ON AROUSAL FROM SLEEP

The seizures most frequently observed on early morning awakening were related to very different types of epilepsy.

Spasms or brief tonic contractions occurred in children with *hypsarrhythmia* or West syndrome presenting with the usual clinical and EEG aspects. The spasms very often repeated in long series, at times with pseudoperiodic repetition, lasting for periods of 10 to 20 min.

Similar spasms were also observed in a small series of children (aged 3 to 6 years) who had severe encephalopathy with psychic impairment and various ictal and interictal EEG features, with different etiologic factors (birth trauma, anoxia, metabolic encephalopathies, Batten disease).

In patients with *primary generalized epilepsy,* seizures were recorded immediately after awakening in the morning. It was a matter of either repeated generalized myoclonus (see Janz, 1962), sometimes followed by a tonic-clonic seizure, or prolonged (10 to 20 min) twilight status accompanied on the EEG by continuous diffuse spike-and-wave discharges ("petit mal status" or "absence status"). Almost all of the patients with myoclonic jerks on awakening had a photosensitive epilepsy.

Generalized clonic seizures with or without impairment of consciousness were observed (Tassinari et al., 1973*b*) in a patient with *dyssynergia cerebellaris myoclonica* (Ramsay Hunt syndrome) and in three patients with primary generalized epilepsy and tonic-clonic seizures.

During the night, particularly on *arousal from slow sleep* (stages II to III), generalized myoclonus, "absence status," and generalized clonic seizures, as described above, were observed. The usual sequence was a progressive increase of generalized interictal spikes and waves with a concomitant arousal pattern in the EEG, leading to a clinical awakening of the patient and subsequently to the clinical seizures.

GENERALIZED SEIZURES DURING SLEEP

Only five patients had *generalized tonic-clonic seizures* (one seizure each) without focal onset during slow sleep. The electroclinical features were the same as in a typical grand mal seizure during wakefulness, with the tonic-clonic phase and the postictal EEG depression with the late facial tonic contraction. The patients did not awake and normal sleep patterns reappeared on the EEG 10 to 20 min after the end of the seizures.

Secondarily generalized tonic-clonic seizures were observed in patients with partial epilepsy. Clinically, the seizures during sleep could not be distinguished from generalized tonic-clonic seizures without focal onset. The sleep concealed the first clinical motor symptoms, such as versive movements and unilateral clonias, which were present in the seizures during wakefulness.

Tonic seizures were the most frequently observed ictal discharges during sleep. Recording of such seizures in children constitutes an element of positive diagnosis of the Lennox-Gastaut syndrome (Gastaut et al., 1966), since tonic seizures are extremely rare in other types of epilepsy in children.

Clinically, it is useful to know that tonic seizures, contrary to tonic-clonic seizures, are frequently repeated during the night (exceptionally, there is only one seizure). Their motor expression becomes attenuated with the deepening of sleep, often being limited to a slight arm elevation or to opening of the eyes, whereas during wakefulness the tonic contraction is usually quite diffuse and severe. Tonic seizures, if particularly frequent, can disrupt the sleep organization with a decrease or disappearance of REM sleep and stages III and IV. This can provoke daytime sleepiness, which in turn will facilitate tonic seizures.

PARTIAL SEIZURES DURING SLEEP

Among a large variety of partial seizures with various etiologic factors, topography, and clinical expression that were recorded, we will discuss only two types of seizures of which knowledge can be most useful in clinical practice.

Partial Sleep Seizures in the Syndrome of Benign Epilepsy with Rolandic or Midtemporal Spikes

This is a frequent type of epilepsy (at least as frequent or probably more so than petit mal with typical absences) which occurs in otherwise normal children, with seizures appearing in 80% of the cases during sleep. Seizures are usually manifested in orofacial clonias of one side (often with salivation and gasping noises), which can also occasionally involve the arm and the leg of one side and eventually become a generalized motor seizure.

The interictal EEG shows frequent high-voltage spikes and spikes and waves around the rolandic or midtemporal regions. Ictal features of such seizures are illustrated in Fig. 1 (also see Dalla Bernardina and Tassinari, 1975).

Knowledge of such nocturnal seizures (Lombroso, 1967; Loiseau and Beaussart, 1973) greatly facilitates the diagnosis of this benign form of epilepsy, allowing a confident prediction of only rare and likely nocturnal seizures that will disappear in a few years without leaving any psychic impairment.

Seizures with Complex Symptomatology During Sleep

In rare instances (a dozen cases) seizures were recorded during sleep with particularly complex behavioral and psychic manifestations (screaming and agitation, a fearful expression, prolonged confusion). Such seizures were due to prolonged ictal discharges, maximal over the frontotemporal regions. The ictal symptomatology alone could be misleading with nonepileptic sleep behavioral manifestations, such as pavor nocturnus or sleepwalking (see Jovanovic, 1970; Tassinari et al., 1975).

It should be noted that seizures with similar symptomatology also occurred in our patients during the daytime. In our experience, we have never exclusively observed nocturnal seizures with such complex symptomatology. From a practical point of view, we suggest a very cautious attitude before making the diagnosis of epileptic seizures *(even if the interictal records show abnormalities)* in patients with *only* nocturnal complex behavioral manifestations. We strongly suggest

(Tassinari et al., 1972, 1974*b*) that the clinician require direct proof (recordings) of such seizures before accepting them as epileptic, unless similar epileptic seizures also occur during the day.

NONEPILEPTIC PAROXYSMAL NOCTURNAL BEHAVIORAL MANIFESTATIONS

Episodes of pavor nocturnus, night sleepwalking (and eventually somniloquia, jactatio capitis somniloquia) should never be considered as epileptic seizures or "equivalent." In a previous paper (Tassinari et al., 1972) we demonstrated, and we confirm this with four additional cases, that such episodes are not of epileptic origin even if they occur in epileptic patients with nocturnal seizures. The same holds true for other manifestations, such as enuresis nocturna. It is significant that of more than 90 patients with enuresis nocturna in whom we recorded nocturnal epileptic seizures, only 1 patient had an episode of enuresis as a sole symptom related to an epileptic seizure during sleep. In all of the other cases in which epileptic nocturnal seizures were recorded, either enuresis did not occur on the particular night of the recording or, if it did occur, it was unrelated to the seizures.

These data enable us to consider that there is no relationship between epileptic seizures and the above-mentioned nocturnal manifestations. Obviously, the real or supposed "EEG abnormalities" which could eventually be distinguished in the EEGs of patients with enuresis, pavor nocturnus, and somnambulism, for example, do not imply a relationship of these manifestations to epilepsy.

EPILEPTIC ENCEPHALOPATHY DURING SLOW SLEEP WITH SUBCLINICAL EPILEPTIC STATUS (E.S.E.S.)

This particular and probably rare condition is characterized by status epilepticus with continuous spikes and waves which occur as soon as the patient falls asleep. To date, we have observed 15 cases in 800 epileptic patients studied during sleep, including the first 5 cases described by one of the authors in collaboration with Patry and Lyagoubi (Patry et al., 1971). Laurette and Arfel (1976) have also recently observed the condition in one patient.

EEG sleep recording is necessary for the diagnosis of E.S.E.S. (Fig. 2). During wakefulness, the EEG abnormalities are of various types, usually atypical spikes and waves, focal or diffuse. As soon as the patient falls asleep, continuous high-voltage, diffuse, slow (2 to 2½ cps) spike-and-wave discharges appear and persist throughout the non-REM sleep. The continuous discharges make it impossible to distinguish slow sleep as stages I, II, III, and IV. REM sleep phases are present in normal percentage and can be easily detected because the status epilepticus disappears during this stage. Status epilepticus during sleep is a constant feature which persists for years and occurs every time the patient falls asleep. Electroclinical seizures or paroxysmal discharges other than the diffuse spikes and waves

A

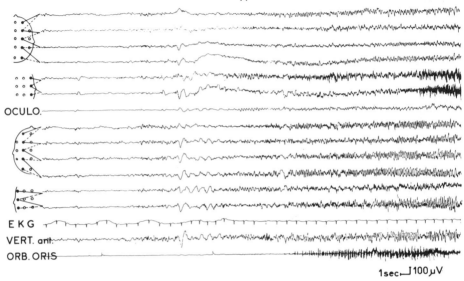

OCULO.

EKG
VERT. ant.
ORB. ORIS

1sec 100μV

B

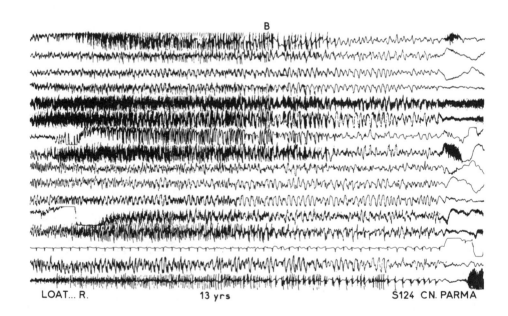

LOAT... R.   13 yrs   S124 CN. PARMA

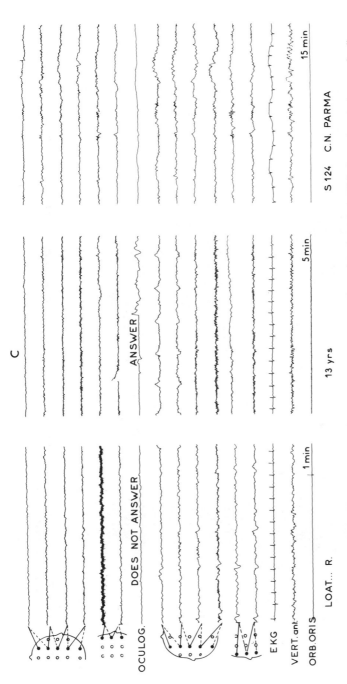

FIG. 1. Benign epilepsy of childhood with centrotemporal spikes with rare nocturnal seizures. Interictal EEG showed centrotemporal spikes. **A:** Seizure onset with fast rhythmic activity beginning and predominant over the left hemisphere and **B:** Ending with slow wave with left predominance. **C:** One minute after the end of the seizure there was slowing on the left hemisphere, maximal over the temporal region. The patient could not answer questions. A few minutes later the EEG became normal *(mid-strip)*, the patient was able to answer, and subsequently resumed sleep *(right)*. Clinically, the patient had right facial myoclonias (on the orbicullaris oris recording), hypersalivation, and gasping noises. The patient was awakened by the seizure; consciousness was not impaired.

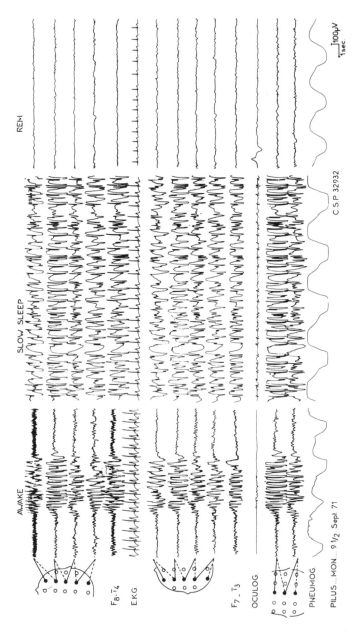

FIG. 2. E.S.E.S.: Bursts of diffuse spikes and waves during wakefulness. During sleep the spikes and waves become continuous and disappear only during REM periods.

were not recorded during sleep. Clinical features and the evolution of the E.S.E.S. syndrome can be divided into three periods:

1. Onset of 4 to 10 years, with various types of rare nocturnal seizures (frequently orofacial) and/or diurnal absences (usually atypical absences). One of our patients, however, never had an evident seizure.

2. Status characterized by severe *psychic impairment* with complex features consisting mainly of lack of interest in the surroundings, prepsychotic-like behavior, inability to carry on normal duties or scholastic activity, with an important decrease in IQ scores. Slow sleep constantly shows the presence of status epilepticus during this period. The status phase usually lasts from 2 to 5 years.

3. Period of remission when spontaneous seizures, if still present, disappear. There is a progressive but never complete remission, with improvement in behavior, social performance, and IQ scores. At this time, EEGs during sleep no longer show continuous spikes and waves.

The data, although still incomplete, suggest a close relationship between the presence of the status epilepticus during sleep and the psychic syndrome. The "substitution" of the continuous spike-and-wave discharges for the normal physiological sleep pattern of slow sleep could be the cause of the appearance of severe psychic disturbances.

E.S.E.S. is probably the unique syndrome of a truly sleep-related epilepsy and is probably the only form in which a sleep recording is absolutely essential for its diagnosis.

REFERENCES

Ambrosetto, C., Lugaresi, E., Coccagna, G., and Tassinari, C. A. (1965): Clinical and polygraphic remarks in the syndrome of restless legs. *Riv. Patol. Nerv. Ment.,* 86:244–252.

Dalla Bernardina, B., and Tassinari, C. A. (1975): EEG of a nocturnal seizure in a patient with "benign epilepsy of childhood with rolandic spikes." *Epilepsia,* 16:497–501.

Daly, D. D. (1973): Circadian cycles and seizures. In: *Epilepsy: Its Phenomena in Man,* UCLA Forum in Medical Sciences, No. 17, edited by M. A. B. Brazier, pp. 215–233. Academic Press, New York.

Gastaut, H., Roger, J., Soulayrol, R., Tassinari, C. A., Régis, H., Dravet, C., Bernard, R., Pinsard, N., and Saint-Jean, M. (1966): Childhood epileptic encephalopathy with diffuse slow spike-waves (otherwise known as "petit mal variant") or Lennox syndrome. *Epilepsia,* 7:139–179.

Hara, T., and Wada, T. Eds. (1974): *Circadian Rhythm and Epilepsy.* Japanese Branch of the ILAE, Tokyo.

Janz, D. (1962): The grand mal epilepsies and the sleeping-waking cycle. *Epilepsia,* 3:69–109.

Janz, D. (1974): Epilepsy and the sleeping-waking cycle. In: *Handbook of Clinical Neurology, Vol. 15,* edited by P. J. Vinken and G. M. Bruyn, pp. 457–490. Elsevier, Amsterdam.

Jovanovic, U. J. (1970): Somnambuli psychomotorische Epilepsie. *Dtsch. Z. Nervenheilkd,* 197: 181–191.

Laurette, G., and Arfel, G. (1976): "État de mal" electrographique dous le sommeil d'apres-midi. *Rev. Electroencephalogr. Neurophysiol. Clin.,* 6:137–139.

Loiseau, P., and Beaussart, M. (1973): The seizures of benign epilepsy with rolandic paroxysmal discharges. *Epilepsia,* 14:381–389.

Lombroso, C. T. (1967): Sylvian seizures and mid-temporal spike foci in children. *Arch. Neurol.,* 17:52–59.

Lugaresi, E., Coccagna, G., Mantovani, M., Berti-Ceroni, G., Pazzaglia, P., and Tassinari, C. A. (1970): The evolution of different types of myoclonus during sleep: A polygraphic study. *Eur. Neurol.,* 4:321–331.

Oswald, I. (1959): Sudden bodily jerks on falling asleep. *Brain,* 82:92–99.

Patry, G., Lyagoubi, S., and Tassinari, C. A. (1971): Subclinical "electrical status epilepticus" induced by sleep in children. *Arch. Neurol.,* 24:242–252.

Symonds, C. P. (1953): Nocturnal myoclonus. *J. Neurol. Neurosurg. Psychiatry,* 16:166–171.

Tassinari, C. A., Bureau-Paillas, M., Dalla Bernardina, B., Grasso, E., and Roger, J. (1974*a*): Etude électroencéphalographique de la dyssynergie cérébelleuse myoclonique avec épilepsie (syndrome de Ramsay-Hunt). *Rev. Electroencephalogr. Neurophysiol. Clin.,* 4:407–428.

Tassinari, C. A., Bureau-Paillas, M., Dalla Bernardina, B., Mancia, D., Capizzi, G., Dravet, C., Valladier, C., and Roger, J. (1974*b*): Generalized epilepsies and seizures during sleep: A polygraphic study. In: *Brain and Sleep,* edited by H. M. Van Praag and H. Meinardi, pp. 154–166. De Erven Bohn BV, Amsterdam.

Tassinari, C. A., Coccagna, G., Mantovani, M., Dalla Bernardina, B., and Roger, J. (1973*a*): Polygraphic study of dyssynergia cerebellaris myoclonica (Ramsay-Hunt syndrome) and of the intention myoclonus (Lance-Adams syndrome) during sleep. *Eur. Neurol.,* 9:105–120.

Tassinari, C. A., Dalla Bernardina, B., Bureau-Paillas, M., Dravet, C., Ambrosetto, G., and Roger, J. (1975): Nocturnal epileptic seizures with exceptional clinical symptomatology (resembling pavor nocturnus, terrific dreams, enuresis and sleep walking). *Electroencephalogr. Clin. Neurophysiol.,* 39:217.

Tassinari, C. A., Dalla Bernardina, B., Coccagna, G., Mantovani, M., and Roger, J. (1973*b*): A specific EEG pattern in the intention myoclonus syndrome during sleep: A polygraphic study in 14 subjects. *Electroencephalogr. Clin. Neurophysiol.,* 34:760.

Tassinari, C. A., Lyagoubi, S., Santos, V., Gambarelli, F., Roger, J., Dravet, C., and Gastaut, H. (1969): Etude des décharges de pointes ondes chez l'homme. Les aspects clinique et électroencéphalographiques des absences myocloniques. *Rev. Neurol. (Paris),* 121:379–383.

Tassinari, C. A., Mancia, D., Dalla Bernardina, B., and Gastaut, H. (1972): Pavor nocturnus of non-epileptic nature in epileptic children. *Electroencephalogr. Clin. Neurophysiol.,* 33:603–607.

THE NEEDS OF DEVELOPING COUNTRIES

Epilepsy, The Eighth International Symposium,
edited by J. K. Penry. Raven Press, New York
© 1977.

Epilepsy in Developing Countries

C. L. Bolis

*Neurosciences Program, Division of Mental Health, World Health Organization,
Geneva, Switzerland*

The history of epilepsy is as old as man, and the disorder was for a long time, and unfortunately sometimes still is, framed in a superstitious atmosphere, where magic signs and magic remedies and rituals were seen as the only form of treatment. Hippocrates, 25 centuries ago, was the first to oppose the divine and sacred theory of the epilepsies, but only a century ago, Jackson in 1874 was able to give a more scientific approach to the description of epilepsy. He defined epilepsy as "a *sudden, excessive,* and *rapid* discharge of grey matter of some *part* of the brain; it is a *local* discharge" (Taylor, 1931). Locock in 1857 introduced potassium bromide for the treatment of the epilepsies, and only in the nineteenth century was it possible to remove epileptic patients from insane asylums, with the intervention of Esquirol (1938). Finally, the twentieth century is the era of classification, differentiation, and treatment of the different forms of the epilepsies, but only in these last decades has an appropriate treatment been possible.

Nevertheless, the differentiation of the different forms of the epilepsies and their prevention and treatment are not yet possible in all continents. Lack of information to the general public, lack of preparation of physicians and paramedical workers, and deficiencies in the possibility and availability of preventive treatment are the major causes for this situation.

The World Health Organization since 1957 has been concerned with the problem of the epilepsies, convening meetings and trying to develop a common and accepted language in the field of the epilepsies. The *Dictionary of Epilepsy* (Gastaut, 1973) is an example of efforts in the latter area. Recognizing that the needs of developing countries in this field are immense and growing, the WHO has recently established a special program in the neurosciences, which has among its priorities the problem of the epilepsies.

One of the main constraints is the lack of epidemiological knowledge about the epilepsies in developing countries. Health services are not available in a majority of the populations of many countries, and the size of the problem is therefore often judged on contact with the relatively few hospitals and specialized institutions.

Epidemiological studies certainly will contribute to our knowledge about the major causes of the epilepsies in developing countries. All of the studies conducted in Africa, for example, report that generalized tonic-clonic seizures (grand mal) predominate in comparison to absence (petit mal) seizures and that the prevalence is higher in males than in females. It is difficult to interpret these findings because the lower incidence of petit mal epilepsy can be related to the fact that these patients are not usually seen and treated. Epidemiological research is important in regard to not only the number of patients but to the types of epilepsy and their pathogenesis, and this can certainly be of great help for the possible prevention of the disease.

In developing countries, the incidence of epilepsy after infectious disease is higher than in countries such as the United States and France (e.g., 10% in Africa versus 1 or 2% in the latter countries). Parasitic infections of the brain may be an underlying cause of epilepsy in more than 10% of cases in many developing countries. The WHO Expanded Immunization Program will be instrumental in the prevention of several infectious diseases such as measles, tuberculosis, tetanus, and possibly cerebrospinal meningitis.

Malnutrition also seems to play an important role in the pathogenesis of the epilepsies. This should be investigated even if it may offer some technical difficulties. The effect of malnutrition in brain development is clear, and nutritional encephalopathies may be at the origin of certain types of epilepsies.

Cerebrovascular disease is also an important aspect in the incidence of the epilepsies, and its study should be extended to children in a systematic way. Indeed, no data related to this pathology are available. An additional area for study relates to the genetic traits of the epilepsies in developing countries.

Another objective of the WHO Neurosciences Program is to develop training programs for physicians and other health personnel. Because very few specialists in neurology and practically no child neurologists are available in developing countries, such training programs could be instrumental in prevention of the epilepsies, especially those epilepsies that are sequelae of febrile convulsions, which are increasing in number. Training activities have already been implemented by the WHO, and short courses and fellowships for training on theoretical or practical aspects of control programs for the epilepsies are being organized for medical doctors. Similar training courses will be organized for paramedical staff who, if well trained, will be very important in the control of epilepsy, especially in those areas of the world which are underserved by health services.

A third priority area in this field, in addition to research and training, is treatment. It seems clear that epileptic seizures can be controlled by a very few drugs, the first among these being phenobarbital. Thus, a limited number of drugs should be available in rural areas so that patients can be treated by local health services before being referred, if necessary, to the hospital for assessment, therapy, or even control of drug level in the blood. Since in many developing countries the availability of drugs is very limited, promotion of the production of useful drugs locally and stimulation of the production of long-acting drugs are important measures that must be undertaken simultaneously with efforts to improve health services. The WHO is contributing in this field by publication of a paper prepared by the WHO Collaborating Centres for Research and Training in the Neurosciences in Marseilles and Ibadan (Gastaut and Osuntokun, 1976).

Education of the family and the community plays a major role in rehabilitation of the epileptic patient. In many developing countries, the beliefs about the divine and sacred nature of epilepsy make treatment difficult and diminish possibilities of success. In school or at work the epileptic is left alone and feels guilty and discouraged. Health education should therefore be vigorously undertaken. The general knowledge must be put, with great enthusiasm and efficiency, at the disposal of all countries in the world, and in this field the impact of the WHO is crucial.

REFERENCES

Esquirol, E. (1938): *Des Maladies Mentales-medicales; Higieniques et Medico-Legal, Vol. 1.* J. B. Baillière, Paris.

Gastaut, H. (1973): *Dictionary of Epilepsy, Part I: Definitions.* World Health Organization, Geneva.

Gastaut, H., and Osuntokun, B. O. (1976): Proposals on antiepileptic pharmacotherapy for use in developing countries. *Epilepsia,* 17:355–360.

Locock, C. (1857): Contribution to discussion on paper by E. H. Sieveking. *Lancet,* 1:528.

Taylor, J. (Ed.) (1931): *Selected Writings of John Hughlings Jackson, Vol. 1, On Epilepsy and Epileptiform Convulsions.* Hodder and Stoughton, London.

Epilepsy, The Eighth International Symposium,
edited by J. K. Penry. Raven Press, New York
© 1977.

Epilepsy in India

G. Arjundas

Institute of Neurology, Madras Medical College, Madras, India

The developing countries can be classified into two distinct categories: (1) those which during their long tenure of existence once enjoyed an acme of glory and grandeur and then in sequence touched the rock bottom of privation and poverty and are doing their best to rise again; and (2) those with largely an aboriginal population whose development has been a continuous process and who have yet to benefit from the fruits of modern civilization.

Both of these groups are in the grip of hardship emanating from their tradition and taboos, which leave them stunted in creative thinking. Economic and political colonialism has further aggravated the situation in some of these regions. For its survival, such a population becomes a victim of two evils: adaptation to a lower standard of living, and an increase in fertility and procreation for a feeling of security in numbers against disease and death. Thus, a vicious cycle of excess population and further poverty and starvation is set up. The growth of science is completely in shambles; homeostasis of idleness and sloth due to underemployment and unemployment reigns supreme; drive and motivation are at their lowest ebb.

INDIA'S POPULATION

India has a population of 550 million living in 3.3 million square kilometers (1971 census). Of this population, 20% (110 million) is congregated in urban areas, which consists of only 1.4% of the total land area. Adequate medical facilities are available to this urban population. About 55 million living in the larger rural areas also have available some kind of organized and centralized medical facility. This leaves 385 million spread over vast areas who do not have access to any reasonable medical facilities unless they travel long distances.

HOW MANY EPILEPTICS ARE THERE IN INDIA?

Although epidemiological studies may be applied to 165 million by random sampling of the population, it is almost impossible at present to apply this to the 385 million in rural areas. However, a random sampling of some of these villages, which are spread all over India, when added to the figures available from areas with organized medical services, gives some idea of the number of epileptics. At present, collection of data has been going on:

1. *In major hospitals of India and in epilepsy centers on a hospital-based population.* These hospitals are used mainly by the poorer classes of people, primarily the working population, and hence results cannot be generalized. However, the hospital-based study has been useful in analyzing (1) types of epileptic seizures; (2) types of treatment and their results; (3) attitudes of relatives, teachers, employees, and patients to their epilepsy; (4) types of follow-up necessary for different types of epilepsy; and (5) results in children in regard to education capacities, intelligence, and so forth, before and after treatment.

2. *Among organized labor.* Most of organized labor, especially in large urban areas, is looked after by medical officers. These in turn are supplemented by the state insurance coverage. These medical officers belong to the Federation of Association of Occupational Health.

The members of the association have been requested to collect similar data among the staff and their relatives working in their organization.

3. *In mini health centers in villages adjoining the cities.* About 16 mini health centers have been started in areas surrounding Madras City, covering a rural population of about 100,000 family units. The staff managing these health centers are paramedical persons who have been trained to give first-aid therapy to anyone who presents with a medical problem, and to arrange for further examination in a nearby (within 5 to 6 miles) well-equipped hospital.

Similar mini health centers are operating at present on a trial basis in other parts of the state. These mini health centers are being supported as follows: one-third recurring expenses come from voluntary contributions from the people living in the areas, one-third recurring expenses are subsidized by the state government, and one-third recurring expenses are subsidized by the federal government.

What do we propose to do about dissemination of knowledge regarding treatment, education of the afflicted regarding the nature of their disorder, rehabilitation of those affected in near normal or sheltered jobs, and collection of information from the vast rural areas now beyond medical reach?

Dissemination of knowledge is relatively simple and is carried out by specialists at medical and nonmedical meetings of the Indian Medical Association which involves people in general practice who are the closest individuals to distant villages.

Education is being accomplished at meetings of nongovernmental agencies such as the Rotary Club and Lions Club, where employers and professionals meet; specialists or doctor members of these organizations are induced to speak on this disorder. These agencies are present in smaller towns, but the members control large rural populations in some form or another.

Rehabilitation of the epileptic is being encouraged by members of the Indian Association and Occupational Health. This is an association of doctors who are in charge of large industrial populations and plantations with good medical facilities, supplemented by the State Health Insurance Hospitals. The main difficulty regarding jobs in the urban centers is caused by keen competition and fear of accidents, compensation claims, and so forth. Members of this association have frequent meetings with experts in the epilepsies and members of the Indian Epilepsy Association and are educated in rehabilitation of the affected. In some cases the Indian Epilepsy Association has coerced industries to rehabilitate epileptics. In rural areas, there is no problem because whole families work in the fields and the epileptics do as much work as others except when they have an attack and are allowed to rest and are looked after by the family.

Some progress has been made in collecting and disseminating information to the vast rural areas beyond the medical reach at present. After several years of assessment and thinking, the Government of India has come forward with schemes to organize day-to-day first-aid treatment by training an educated resident of the village. Although at present this lot is supposed to fall on the postman or teacher, it is postulated to enlarge this scheme by taking nongovernmental educated persons for this work. With the rapid spread of education there are always one or more school final residents in all villages.

OCCUPATION AND EPILEPSY

About 33% of the population of 550 million are in the working force. The rest are classified as dependents. The sex ratio of the working force is 4.5 to 1 in favor of males, with only 123 million men and 27 million women employed. Occupation and rehabilitation of epileptics present no serious problems in the rural population. Many of these epileptics are productive and well cared for by their families. Their main needs are education about epilepsy and the availability of regular treatment, mostly free of charge, if possible.

In contrast, the main problems with occupation and rehabilitation are in the urban population. Here, medical facilities and drugs are available but jobs are difficult to get and retain. In the hospital-based population, a detailed study was made of the occupation of 2,222 patients. Of these, 40% were students and 10% were housewives, comprising half the patients without income.

ADJUSTMENT WITH OCCUPATION AND EPILEPSY

About 70% of epileptics made a good adjustment in their occupation despite their seizure disorder. About 25 to 30%, however, did deteriorate in their occupation. This may be related to lack of understanding on the part of the employers or to a deficit in the patients' work capacity produced either by an attack or by drugs. This group needs multidisciplinary assistance for better rehabilitation in their work.

EDUCATION

The literacy in India has almost quadrupled since 1891, having risen from 6 to 29% in 1971, with a male to female ratio of 2:1. Education makes possible communication and acquisition of knowledge, especially through mass media such as newspapers, wireless, and television. In the hospital-based studies of 2,216 epileptics, about 66% were students at school or university and 16% were semiliterate, reflecting the higher incidence of literacy in towns and cities. A follow-up of students after the onset of epilepsy at four centers in India showed no gross change in over 50% of these. With better education of teachers and better control of epilepsy, this should increase considerably, as has been seen in the excellent work of Virmani and colleagues at New Delhi.

SOCIAL SYSTEMS

Joint Family Concepts

One of the saving graces in the rural population is the continuing joint family concept. This also exists in the cities, but it is changing fast as the result of migration and separation of families for job opportunities. A joint family system enables better and more sympathetic care for children and adults who suffer from epilepsy, and rehabilitation is no problem in the rural areas. In the hospital-based study of 2,216 epileptics, it was found that 84% of the patients were urban, and 37% of all cases had a joint family base.

Parental Consanguinity

The gross differences in social customs in various parts of India are illustrated by the fact that certain communities sanction intermarriage among maternal cousins, for example, uncle and niece in South India. The Muslims and Parsees carry this further to first-degree consanguinity of paternal cousins. On the other hand, in greater parts of Northern India it is a sacrilege to marry even a very distant relative. Although the geneticists have pronounced an increased incidence of hereditary disorders in offspring of consanguinous union, our experience in South India does not bear this out. The concepts are correct in a broad sense that idiopathic epilepsy is a hereditary disorder and that the gene can be diluted by marrying into nonepileptic families. However, the details of heredity are not firm and clear.

In the hospital-based study, the incidence of consanguinity, a family history of seizures, and a past history of febrile seizures were identical in the so-called genetic epilepsies and the acquired focal epilepsies. The significance of this is not clear.

TYPES OF EPILEPSIES

Education, employment, and social life are the spheres most affected by epilepsy, and these depend on the types of seizures as much as on their control. Patients with absence seizures (petit mal) showed the lowest incidence, with problems occurring mainly during school age. The idiopathic grand mal group showed an incidence of 45%. These are the patients, who if therapy is regular and adequate, can in a majority of cases progress to normal physical and mental development. Temporal lobe seizures occurred in 26%. These invariably have behavior disorders and their seizures are poorly controlled with available drugs. They form the most difficult group. In several cases, however, neurosurgery has been of benefit. Other types of focal seizures were evident in 23%, and these are the ones who need intensive and thorough study with costly equipment in well-equipped neurology centers to detect a curable focal cause for their fits. Hence, only about half of the epileptics need specialized assessment and one-fourth need greater detailed study. Proper advice and treatment produce rewarding benefit, as seen in the hospital-based studies.

PRECIPITATING FACTORS

Epilepsy is only a disorder, and in a majority of cases a carefully obtained history may bring to light a nonspecific or specific precipitating factor. The elucidation of this precipitating factor can lead to the correct dispensation and minimization of medication. Dr. Jeavons, for example, has shown in his studies of attacks precipitated by television viewing that all the patient has to do to reduce attacks is to view with one eye only. In our study, no precipitating factors were found in 58% of the patients. Emotional factors were present in 11%, sleep in 7%, lack of sleep in 5%, fatigue in 5%, menstruation in 2%, fever in 2%, lunar cycle in 2%, bath in 3%, and omission of drugs in 6%. The relationship of fits to the various phases of the moon and to the taking of a bath are under further study.

PERSONALITY AND EPILEPSY

In an intrinsic brain disorder such as epilepsy and in the interaction between an epileptic and society, one expects many personality problems. In a study of 2,457 hospital-based patients suffering from various types of seizure disorders, premorbid personality (i.e., before treatment) was assessed. More than 80% of all patients were normal. As expected, behavior disorders were highest in those with temporal lobe seizures. Total personality adjustment was good in about two-thirds of the cases.

MENTAL STATUS

In a study of 2,457 hospital-based cases of seizures, evaluation of mental status revealed a similar incidence of mental retardation in all groups, being maximum in the petit mal group. Mental deterioration after onset of seizures was also noted maximally in this group (23%).

GENERAL IQ AND EPILEPSY

The broad statement that epileptics tend to be geniuses or degenerates is not borne out by our study. There was an equal percentage of patients with superior intelligence in genetic and nongenetic types of seizure disorders. Just over 50% in each group were of average intelligence.

STUDIES AND EPILEPSY

Many school teachers remain uninitiated in the various aspects of epilepsy. The moment a child has a fit he is sent home and declared unfit to study further. Our study of students with epilepsy shows that epilepsy *per se* delayed education in a very small percentage of cases (less than 10%). There was, however, deterioration in the studies of about one-third of the cases (maximum in petit mal group, 42%). With adequate therapy and understanding from the teacher, this can be reduced to a much lower percentage. Hence, the education of teachers in handling students with correctable diseases should form a part of their training in teaching. Only about 17% of the students had to leave their studies because of epilepsy.

SUMMARY

The problems of epilepsy in India are highlighted. It is important to realize that epilepsy in most of the cases is a chronic, nonurgent disorder that needs prolonged therapy with a minimum of guidance and follow-up. Thus, epilepsy can be grouped under other chronic health problems, such as parasitic infestations and malnutrition, in India, and steps undertaken for the latter will be quite adequate for epilepsy as well. More difficult are the social problems of stigma and superstitions, and hence the tendency to hide the disorder. With an increase in literacy and mass media communication to the distant parts of the country, progressive educative programs are being established. It will take a long time but with the dedicated efforts of the Indian Epilepsy Association and with guidance from international bodies against epilepsy, we expect a rapid change and improvement in knowledge and care of epileptics in our country.

Epilepsy, The Eighth International Symposium,
edited by J. K. Penry. Raven Press, New York
© 1977.

Epilepsy in the African Continent

B. O. Osuntokun

Neurology Unit, Department of Medicine, University College Hospital, Ibadan, Nigeria

In Africa neurology is still in its early developing phase, and trained personnel in most African countries are extremely few. For example, in Nigeria, a country with an estimated population of 80 million—a quarter of the population of Africa—and occupying a land area of 356,000 square miles, there are only seven neurologists and five neurosurgeons and they are concentrated mainly in two university teaching hospitals at Ibadan and Lagos. Yet in this respect of health manpower, Nigeria is relatively better off than most other black African nations. In Ghana, with an estimated population of eight million, there are one neurosurgeon and one neurologist. The situation in the francophone West African countries and in East Africa is similar, although facilities for dealing with neurological diseases have existed for some two decades in teaching hospitals in the capital cities of most of the countries. Authentic reports on neurological disorders including convulsive disorders in the Africans in most countries are understandably of recent origin.

MEDICAL SERVICES IN DEVELOPING COUNTRIES IN AFRICA

In developing countries in Africa, medical services are provided mainly by a chain of district, general, and specialist hospitals, which are maintained and run either by the government or by voluntary agencies such as the various missionary societies. In some countries there are a number of private hospitals. Dispensaries, maternity centers, and rural health centers, manned by non-doctor personnel and visited occasionally by itinerant doctors, often constitute the only health care delivery system for populations in the rural areas. The apex of the health care delivery system is constituted by the university teaching hospitals of the medical schools, which two decades ago included those at Dakar (Senegal), Ibadan (Nigeria), and Makerere, Kampala (Uganda); by 1976, there were 21 university teaching hospitals (6 in Nigeria alone) in black Africa (excluding those of Hamitic African countries).

In developing countries in Africa, there is a shortage of health personnel of all types. The doctor:population ratio in most countries is less than 1 to 20,000; most of the doctors available are found in cities. For example, in Nigeria the doctor:population ratio is 1:22,000, but four-fifths of the doctors available live in the cities of Ibadan, Lagos, Kaduna, Zaria, Kano, Benin, and Enugu (with a total estimated population of about five million).

Apart from inadequacy of health personnel, the annual per capita income in developing countries is low, ranging from about 100 to 1,000 U.S. dollars. The percentage of the gross national product spent on health services is of the order 5.0%. The health care delivery system is therefore hampered, apart from nonavailability of health personnel, by lack of equipment and drugs. For example, in the Western State of Nigeria with a population of eleven million and which has one of the best health services in black Africa, the annual budget for drugs for 1972 and 1973 was 1.2 million U.S. dollars. Although the socioeconomic status of Nigerians has improved considerably in the last 4 years due to the oil boom in most developing countries in Africa, money for financing health care delivery is still a major constraint.

It is against the background described above that we should consider the needs of developing countries in Africa in the management of convulsive disorders.

EPIDEMIOLOGY OF EPILEPSY IN DEVELOPING COUNTRIES IN AFRICA

Lack or inadequacy of accurate epidemiological data has grossly impaired the planning and execution of effective health care delivery in many parts of Africa. Most of the information available is derived from hospital-based data, which usually constitute the "tip of the iceberg": this applies particularly to available data on convulsive disorders in the African. In the last two decades, several authors who have reported on Africans who suffered from convulsive disorders include Carothers (1953) from Kenya; Gelfand (1957), Levy, Forbes, and Parirenyatwa (1964) from Southern Rhodesia; Smartt (1959) and Aall-Jilek (1965) from Tanzania; Hurst, Reef, and Sachs (1961), Bird, Heinz, and Klintworth (1962), and Cosnett (1964) from South Africa; Piraux (1962) from Congo; Collomb, Zwingelstein, and Seck (1963) and Collomb et al. (1970) from Senegal; Dada and Odeku (1966), Dada (1970a), and Osuntokun and Odeku (1970) from Nigeria; Giel (1968) from Ethiopia; Billington (1968), Billinghurst (1970), and Orley (1970) from Uganda; Compere and Compere (1970) from Zaire; and Edoo and Haddock (1970) from Ghana.

INCIDENCE AND PREVALENCE RATES

There is no study reported, so far, on the incidence of epilepsy in the African. Prevalence rates in the Africans based on surveys of defined communities (distinct from hospital population) have been reported—4 per 1,000 in Congolese (Piraux, 1960), Bantus in South Africa (Bird et al., 1962), Ghanians (Haddock, 1973), and Ugandans (Orley, 1970). Levy et al. (1964) found a prevalence rate of 7.4 per 1,000 in the Semokwe area of Southern Rhodesia. Giel (1968) reported prevalence rates of 5 per 1,000 in an urban area and 8 per 1,000 in a rural community of Ethiopia. Collomb et al. (1970) gave a prevalence rate of 3 to 8 per 1,000 for Senegalese. Dada (1970*a*) obtained a computed rate of 13 to 15 per 1,000 in Nigerians living in Lagos, although the actual rate found in a survey was 3 per 1,000. In great contrast to the finding of Smartt (1959) who reported a prevalence rate of 1 per 1,000 among Tanzanians, Jilek and Jilek-Aall (1970) found a prevalence rate of 20 per 1,000 (and probably higher, since this was based on voluntary attendance at the clinic) among a Wapogoro tribe in Tanzania. Epilepsy appears to be more common in some African populations than in Caucasians: in the latter the prevalence rate is usually 4 to 6 per 1,000 (Kurland, 1959; Lancet, 1961).

The frequencies in hospital population indicate the size of the problem constituted by epilepsy and vary from country to country depending on availability of health facilities, extent and degree of health education of the populace, and willingness of the patients to use available facilities. In most African countries, epilepsy still is regarded as a terrible disease, and the epileptic is socially stigmatized and abhorred. Many Africans believe that only the witch doctor or the native medicine man is capable of unravelling its cause and treating it. In the rural areas parents and patients alike may accept it as a misfortune and never seek modern medical treatment. Frequency rates reported in hospital populations include 0.09% in Bantus in Johannesburg, South Africa (Hurst et al., 1961), 10% among the Zulus in South Africa (Cosnett, 1964), 0.33% in Ghanians Haddock, 1967), 0.4% in Nigerians (Osuntokun, 1971, 1972), and 19.65% in Zaireans (Dechef, 1970). Apart from infections affecting the nervous system, epilepsy is the commonest disease of the nervous system in the Africans.

Age and Sex Distribution

The age and sex distribution of 1,923 Nigerians suffering from epilepsy [23 patients whose epilepsy followed wounds sustained during the Nigerian civil war, 1967 to 1970, and described elsewhere by Adeloye and Odeku (1971) were excluded] and evaluated in the University College Hospital (UCH), Ibadan, is shown in Table 1, which epitomizes the patterns reported in the Africans by several authors previously referred to. The age distribution in Africans who suffer from epilepsy is similar to that described in Caucasians. In this largest series of epileptics in the Africans reported, in 85% of the patients the onset age was below

TABLE 1. *Age and sex distribution of 1,923 Nigerians with epilepsy*

Age groups (years)	0–9	10–19	20–29	30–39	40–49	50–59	60–69	70+	Total
Males	362	424	222	83	50	27	10	3	1,181
Females	274	239	125	53	26	12	11	2	742
Total	636	663	347	136	76	39	21	5	1,923

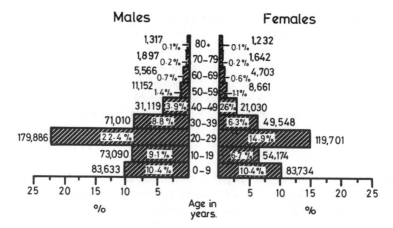

FIG. 1. Population of Ibadan, 1973. Distribution by age and sex. Total population 803,098 (From Statistics Division, Ministry of Economic Planning, Ibadan).

30 years—the same as in Dada's (1970*a*) smaller series of 117 Nigerian patients. In 67%, the onset age was in the first and second decades of life. However, it should be noted that in developing countries in Africa, life expectancy is still low—of the order of 40 years only—and this explains the usual age distribution of the population, of which Fig. 1 showing age and sex distribution for the population of Ibadan, Nigeria, is typical. It should be noted that for Ibadan, the age groups under 30 represent 41.9 and 32% of the male and female population, respectively.

Males predominate among African epileptics as reported by several authors (Gelfand, 1957; Piraux, 1960; Levy et al., 1964; Dada, 1970*a*; Osuntokun and Odeku, 1970; Billinghurst, 1970; Edoo and Haddock, 1970). This is also true of many (nongynecological) diseases [in neurology, the notable exceptions are migraine and polymyositis according to Osuntokun (1971)]. Perhaps partly for socioeconomic reasons, in most parts of Africa, males more readily come to the hospital and hence predominate in the hospital populations in Africa. Besides, illiterate African patients value more the male than the female child. However, Orley (1970) from Uganda and Hurst et al. (1961) from South Africa reported female preponderance in small series of 83 (38 males and 45 females) and 50 (21 males and 29 females).

Etiology

Idiopathic epilepsy is the commonest cause of epilepsy in all age groups below 40 years, beyond which the frequency of symptomatic epilepsy rises sharply to reach 100% in the eighth decade (Osuntokun and Odeku, 1970). Excluding the report of Piraux (1960) in which symptomatic epilepsy accounted for 75% in 209 patients, idiopathic epilepsy constitutes 55 to 80% of epilepsy reported in the Africans.

Major etiological factors in symptomatic epilepsy include sequelae of infections (10 to 20%), vascular lesions (6 to 20%), trauma (4 to 12%), cerebral tumors (3 to 10%), metabolic derangements (1 to 2%), and birth injuries (1 to 2%).

The commonest cause of symptomatic epilepsy is infective and infectious disease of the central nervous system. Epilepsy followed recovery from meningitis, encephalitis, or cerebral abscess or was associated with tuberculoma of the brain and neurosyphilis. Parasitic infections, such as cysticercosis in association with epilepsy, and believed to be etiologically related to epilepsy in 6 to 16% of Bantus and Southern Rhodesians who suffer from epilepsy (Gelfand, 1957; Bird et al., 1962; Levy et al., 1964; Powell et al., 1966), are not important in the etiology of epilepsy in West Africans. Schistosoma granuloma was a cause of epilepsy in 2 Nigerian patients in a series of 1,923 patients seen in UCH, Ibadan, from 1957 to 1976. In an autopsy survey in Nigerians, the brain was rarely (0.02%) involved in schistosomal infections (Edington et al., 1975). There is no evidence that other parasitic infections such as toxocariasis, ascariasis, and filariasis cause epilepsy in the Africans (Dada, 1970*b*).

In Nigerians who suffer from epilepsy, a history of febrile convulsions is obtained in a relatively high proportion—20% (Osuntokun and Odeku, 1970), 26% (Dada, 1970*a*), and 23% (J. B. Familusi, 1976 *personal communication*). Followed up for 5 years, 21.4% of Nigerian children who presented with febrile convulsions developed epilepsy or recurrent seizures in the absence of febrile episodes (J. B. Familusi, 1976, *personal communication*). Febrile convulsions are common in the African child: 5% of all children under the age of 10 seen in UCH, Ibadan, suffer from febrile convulsions (Osuntokun et al., 1968). Febrile convulsions constitute 20% of the 4,000 pediatric emergencies seen annually in UCH, Ibadan (J. B. Familusi, 1976, *personal communication*).

The commonest causes of fever in children suffering from febrile convulsions are malaria, bronchopneumonia, and gastrointestinal infections (Osuntokun et al., 1968; Familusi and Sinnette, 1971). Livingston (1960) and Lennox (1953) state that in 50 to 90% of children with febrile convulsions a recurrence will occur, and that recurrent seizures will become established in between 10 and 20%. Various other authors (Thom. 1942; Shanks, 1949; Peterman, 1952; Keith, 1963; Hamill and Carter, 1966) estimate that between 3 and 76% of childhood febrile seizures presage adult epilepsy. The prevalence rate of epilepsy among the Wapogoro tribe of Tanzania is one of the highest in the world: febrile convulsions are said to be very common in childhood (Jilek and Jilek-Aall, 1970). In the African child who is also likely to be malnourished, febrile convulsion does not carry a good prognosis and may possibly result in some damage to the brain, predisposing to recurrent seizures in childhood or later in life. Febrile infantile convulsions occurred significantly more commonly in Nigerian epileptics, especially those who suffered from temporal lobe epilepsy, than in matched controls

(Dada et al., 1969; Osuntokun, 1972). This probably explains why in 98% of Nigerians who suffer from temporal lobe epilepsy no demonstrable structural lesion is found—a finding similar to the experience of Williams (1975) among Caucasians. Febrile episodes constitute the commonest precipitating factor of seizure in adult Nigerian epileptics (Osuntokun and Odeku, 1970).

In some parts of Nigeria, crude "resuscitative" measures —such as thrusting limbs into fire, rubbing pepper on the eyes and face, or forcing down the throat of the unconscious child and concoction containing as the main ingredient cow's urine—produce a high mortality and morbidity due to induced hypoglycemia and aspiration bronchopneumonia (Osuntokun and Odeku, 1970).

In developing countries in Africa, poor antenatal and obstetric care is responsible for a high frequency of birth injury to infants from prolonged labor. Prolonged labor is believed to predispose to epilepsy especially of the temporal lobe type— common in Africans—by producing sclerosis of Ammon's horn in the temporal lobe (Aird et al., 1967).

Posttraumatic epilepsy is becoming increasingly common in the developing countries in Africa. Nigeria and the East African countries have the highest rate in the world of automobile accidents per million vehicle miles (Schram, 1969): in UCH, Ibadan, head injury is very common, and about 150 patients with severe head injury are seen annually.

There is no convincing evidence of any racially determined predisposition to epilepsy among Africans, and neither are racial traits such as hemoglobinopathy and glucose-6-phosphate deficiency of any etiological significance. Positive family history of epilepsy was obtained in 6 to 18% of African patients who suffered from centrencephalic epilepsy (Piraux, 1960; Haddock, 1967; Dada, 1970a; Osuntokun and Odeku, 1970) compared with 1% or less in symptomatic epilepsy. Some authors have reported a high familial tendency in some African populations: Levy et al. (1964) reported a positive family history of 20% in urban and 85% in rural black Rhodesians, and Hurst et al. (1961) and Bird et al. (1962) found 28.3 and 20% of Bantu patients in South Africa with positive family history of epilepsy.

Types of Epilepsy

Accuracy of type diagnosis of epilepsy in many and earlier reported series of epilepsy in the Africans has been doubted because until recently in many centers type diagnosis has been based on clinical features alone. From the published reports, in many based mainly on clinical evidence (Hurst et al., 1961; Osuntokun and Odeku, 1970; Dada, 1970a; Billinghurst, 1970; Levy, 1970), grand mal attacks constitute 60 to 92%. Petit mal attacks appear to be relatively uncommon—reported as 2% (Piraux, 1960), 3% (Dada et al., 1969), 4% (Hurst et al., 1961; Levy et al., 1964; Osuntokun and Odeku, 1970; Osuntokun et al., 1974), and 5% (Collomb et al., 1963; Dada and Odeku, 1966). It is possible that the rarity of petit mal epilepsy in the Africans may be more apparent than real in that the brief attacks of petit mal epilepsy are not readily recognized as significant or serious enough to make the parents or patients seek help in a hospital. Temporal lobe epilepsy (clinical) is common—10 to 20% (Dada, 1970a; Osuntokun and Odeku, 1970). However, electroencephalographic findings present a different type pattern of epilepsy in the Africans (Mundy-Castle, 1970; Osuntokun et al., 1974), with focal and diffuse abnormalities predominating. Of the 1,180 patients seen at UCH, Ibadan, since 1970, who suffered from epilepsy and who had an electroencephalographic examination, 40% showed focal abnormalities in the temporal lobes; 26% had focal abnormalities in sites other than the temporal lobes with or without secondary centrencephalic discharges; 8% had primary centrencephalic discharges (half of these showed petit mal features); 16% showed diffuse and nonspecific abnormalities; and 10% had normal EEGs.

PROBLEMS IN MANAGEMENT OF EPILEPSY IN THE DEVELOPING COUNTRIES IN AFRICA

Accuracy of Diagnosis

For obvious reasons stated earlier, only a small proportion of the epileptics in developing countries can be seen and treated by trained personnel. It is well known that, clinically, brief attacks of impaired consciousness in temporal lobe epilepsy may mimic petit mal attacks, and misdiagnosis may occur in the absence of facilities for adequate and appropriate investigation. The drug treatment of petit mal epilepsy is different from that of temporal lobe epilepsy, and mistaken treatment of one for the other may make a patient worse. In 5 to 15% of African patients suffering from epilepsy, a treatable cause such as a meningioma or tuberculoma is present, but facilities for diagnosis and treatment are confined to only a few centers in Africa.

Drug Treatment

Drug treatment of epilepsy in the Africans has been reported by several authors to be very effective if the patient can be convinced to take the drug(s) regularly according to instructions and return to the clinic for follow-up. Although the defaulting rate of patients in terms of returning to the clinic may be as low as 5% (Osuntokun, 1972), many patients stop taking their drugs of their own accord when they have been free of seizures for a few weeks despite repeated injunctions that treatment with drugs should be stopped only at the discretion of the doctor. Drug treatment should be made as simple as possible, and preferably drugs should be prescribed to be taken once or at the most twice daily except in the case of educated patients. Phenobarbital is much cheaper than phenytoin sodium, more suitable for prescription as a single daily dose, and preferred as the "front-line" drug in the treatment of grand mal attacks and temporal lobe epilepsy. Monitoring of serum levels of anticonvulsants known to be of great value in the management of epilepsy in developed countries (because chronic overdosage with antiepileptic drugs can cause an increase in frequency of seizure as well as a whole range of psychiatric disorders) is not available as of now in any center in developing countries in Africa.

For economic reasons and effectiveness, it is desirable to limit the drug armamentarium to six or seven named drugs for treatment of epilepsy, viz: phenobarbital, phenytoin sodium with primidone, sulthiame, and carbamazepine as "reserves" for major and focal epilepsies; ethosuximide with clonazepam and sodium valproate as adjuncts or substitutes when necessary for petit mal; and diazepam for status epilepticus. In Africa, except in teaching hospitals and in the big cities, these drugs are not always available.

Side effects of anticonvulsants are relatively uncommon in the Africans. Megaloblastic anemia is extremely rare, and the black skin and abundant sunshine seem to protect against anticonvulsant-induced osteomalacia (Apantaku et al., 1975). Osteomalacia, for similar reason, is rare even in pregnant African women (Olatunbosun et al., 1975).

Surgical Treatment

Surgical treatment of epilepsy is available in only four countries in developing countries in Africa—Nigeria, Ghana, Kenya, and Senegal. Temporal lobectomy is not practiced because of lack of adequate facilities for appropriate investigations: the same is true of cerebellar stimulation.

SOCIAL PROBLEMS OF THE EPILEPTIC IN DEVELOPING COUNTRIES IN AFRICA

Epilepsy is a dreaded "disease." The epileptic is ostracized. The family is shunned. Epilepsy in many communities in developing countries in Africa is regarded as a sign or a manifestation of visitation of the devil (Dada and Odeku, 1966; Billington, 1968; Osuntokun, 1975), the effect of witchcraft, the revenge of an aggrieved ancestral spirit, or consumption of something harmful while *in utero* (Gelfand, 1973). In Madagascar an epileptic is refused burial in the family grave. The saliva of the epileptic is believed by many Nigerians and other Africans to transmit the disease. In many countries in Africa, the epileptic is an outcast as vividly described by Giel (1968), writing about Ethiopians. Suicide or attempted suicide is not uncommon among Nigerians who suffer from epilepsy (Osuntokun, 1972). The epileptic is likely to drop out of school, lose his or her job, find it impossible to marry, lose his wife or her husband, and be tormented to the extent of becoming "psychiatric" and a vagabond. Levy (1970) and Jilek and Jilek-Aall (1970) described severe burns as frequent complications of epilepsy in Southern Rhodesian Africans and the Wapogoro tribe of Tanzania. This was as a result of patients falling into domestic fires around which the family gathers every evening. Staring into flames appears to precipitate seizures possibly by photic stimulation, and relations would not pull patients from the fire for fear of contracting the disease through the foaming saliva.

WHAT CAN BE DONE TO HELP THE EPILEPTIC IN DEVELOPING COUNTRIES IN AFRICA

Prevention

Ideally, the best way to eradicate or limit the morbidity or mortality imposed by a disease is to attempt to prevent the disease. In the developing countries and in the context of epilepsy, this approach cannot prove very effective, for many types of epilepsy have no known cause, although the frequency of head injury in automobile accidents can be reduced by certain measures (such as compulsory wearing of seat belts, and imposition of speed limits). It is also possible to reduce the prevalence of infections such as meningitis (especially acute meningococcal meningitis which occurs in epidemics nearly every year in a belt running across Africa, just south of the Sahara).

Specifically, however, reduction in the frequency of febrile convulsions in childhood by control of malaria and measles (which predisposes to bronchopneumonia) and prevention of malnutrition in the child would be beneficial. A child in tropical Africa who has had more than one febrile convulsion should receive continuous prophylactic antimalarial chemotherapy until the age of 6 and treatment with an anticonvulsant (preferably phenobarbital) for a minimum of 3 years after the last attack of convulsion. In addition, the parents should be instructed to give an antipyretic such as aspirin (in a single adequate dose) as soon as febrile illness occurs, and be instructed how to "cool" the child. Parents should be educated that febrile convulsion may be a sign of infections of the nervous system—such as meningitis or encephalitis—and should seek advice in hospital. Vaccination of children against measles and whooping cough (in addition to poliomyelitis, smallpox, and tetanus) should be mandatory.

Improved obstetric, maternal, and infant child care would reduce the frequency of prolonged labor, birth injury, malnutrition, and neonatal infections.

Genetic counseling is not feasible in many developing countries in Africa but may be relevant in the few cases of "centrencephalic" epilepsy and epilepsy due to malformations inherited as autosomal dominants, such as tuberous sclerosis, which have been reported in the Africans (Osuntokun, 1971). Phenylketonuria, fortunately, is very rare in the Africans.

Integration of Management (in Simple Terms) of Neurological Disorders into the Basic Health System

For some decades to come, there is bound to be inadequate personnel in clinical neurosciences in developing countries in Africa. In Nigeria today there are probably 640,000 epileptics. Most of these will never have access to modern methods of treatment applied by a "western-trained" doctor. It is important therefore to incorporate management in simple terms of neurological disorders into the training program of those who man the basic health units (the medical auxiliaries, dispensary attendants in Nigeria, medicine Africain in Senegal, rural medical practitioner in Tanzania, community health officer in Ethiopia, medical assistant in Sudan, Kenya, Malawi, and Uganda, and health center superintendent in Ghana). The basic approach to the diagnosis and management of epilepsy should be taught to these non-doctor personnel, who after appropriate evaluation can be allowed to prescribe, for example, only phenobarbital for major epilepsies and diazepam (administered preferably intravenously, but it can be given rectally as well) for status epilepticus before seeking a doctor's opinion at the earliest opportunity. They will not be allowed to prescribe ethosuximide, since they may find it difficult to distinguish petit mal from some form of temporal lobe epilepsy. Such non-doctor personnel could also be used to achieve a limited community diagnosis of convulsive disorders (by acting as front-line agents or scouts) and, more importantly, to carry out intensive health education of the community on convulsive disorders.

Developing countries in Africa should be encouraged to embark on training programs to produce high level and skilled manpower in neurosciences. Each country should have at least one center at the apex of the health care delivery system fully equipped to deal with neurological problems and to promote and coordinate basic clinical and epidemiological research as well as train personnel in neurosciences. In this respect the effort of the World Health Organization is laudable, for its neurosciences program places great emphasis on the training of health personnel in developing countries and on stimulating research in neurological disorders in the tropics, especially in centers of excellence, which are designated WHO Collaborating Centers in Neurosciences (Ibadan is the only center so far designated as such in Africa).

Workshops and seminars on epilepsy in developing countries should be encouraged. They have "multiplying" effects, especially in developing countries such as those in Africa, where trained personnel in neurosciences are very scarce. Such workshops when and where they have been held in the recent past (as in African countries and India by a traveling team sponsored by the International Bureau for Epilepsy and the International Epileptic Association) have proved very successful and have been widely attended by doctors, nurses, social welfare officers, and schoolteachers.

Epileptic Clinics

Where the personnel are available as in teaching hospitals in developing countries, serious consideration should be given to establishment of special clinics to deal with convulsive disorders. Such clinics, despite possible unequivocal and incontrovertible disadvantages such as a tendency to "treat the disease rather than the patient," offer enormous opportunity for expert care, for periodic clinical and ancillary reexaminations to lay the ghost of structural diseases, and for research, especially in therapeutic trial. Ideally, the work in such clinics should be performed by a team including neurologist, psychiatrist, social worker, and welfare officers.

Health Education and Voluntary Organizations

Health education of the community is vital to eliminate the social stigmatization of epilepsy. Voluntary organizations interested in this aspect can help tremendously to augment the efforts of hospitals and government agencies—especially in the area of education of the public, obtaining suitable employment for epileptics, and in general minimizing the social, psychological, and economic consequences which represent a significant or major part of the disability of the epileptic. Unfortunately, in the developing countries in Africa, efforts to form voluntary organizations to augment governmental efforts in the care of epilepsy have not yielded encouraging results. The Epilepsy Bureau for Africa formed in 1968 has not made any impact. An attempt was made in 1969 to launch a Nigerian Epilepsy Association without much success. However, these attempts are worth repeating, for experience in the developed countries has shown that voluntary organizations can contribute a lot to improvement of opportunities for the proper treatment and management of epilepsy, promotion of better understanding of epilepsy by the populace, and stimulation of research in epilepsy.

In developing countries in Africa [with the exception of South Africa (Minde, 1975)], there are no special centers for epileptics (in contradistinction to leprosaria for leprosy, which is a less feared or dreaded disease). This is not a deliberate act. It appears that the authorities are not aware that establishment of special epilepsy centers as found in the developed countries (e.g., York in the United Kingdom) or special schools for the severely handicapped epileptic child (Stores, 1976) is one of the most appropriate ways of helping some intractable epileptics.

Long-Acting Anticonvulsants

The high defaulting rate of epileptics from medical clinics is a cause of concern, and deaths of patients with idiopathic epilepsy are more often due to status epilepticus than to any other: in our experience the mortality rate of status epilepticus is 50% (Osuntokun, 1972). There are now available for the treatment of schizophrenia long-acting neuroleptics—which can be administered parenterally (such as perphenazine enanthate, fluphenazine decanoate) or orally (e.g., pimozide). It will be a happy day for epileptics in the developing countries when such preparations are available for the effective treatment of epilepsy. Unfortunately, as Levy (1970) points out, the pharmaceutical companies in developed countries are not interested in research in this direction.

SUMMARY

Epilepsy is by far the commonest chronic neurological disorder in the developing countries in Africa, in nearly all of which delivery of health care especially in the rural areas is grossly inadequate where the doctor:population ratio may be as low as 1 to 100,000, although it is as high as 1 to 5,000 in some cities. In addition, there is a great dearth of trained personnel in clinical neurosciences: for example, in Nigeria, with an estimated population of eighty million, there are five neurosurgeons and seven neurologists, mostly domiciled in two cities whose combined population is three million.

The prevalence of epilepsy in developing countries in Africa is probably higher than in the Caucasians, although accurate epidemiological data for most of these countries are lacking; yet the practice of modern clinical neurosciences in Africa is less than two decades old. A brief review of the available and relevant epidemiological data on epilepsy in the Africans is presented and discussed against the background of our experience involving 1,923 patients seen in the University College Hospital, Ibadan, 1,180 of whom had electroencephalographic examination.

Males predominate (male:female ratio, 3:2). Eighty-five percent are under the age of 30 at onset with peak incidence of age of onset in the second decade. In 60% of the patients, no cause is found. Sequelae of infections, vascular lesions and trauma, cerebral tumors, metabolic derangements, and birth injuries in descending order of frequency are the major causes of symptomatic epilepsy. Febrile convulsions in African children are probably potent precursors to epilepsy in later life, and malaria and bronchopneumonia are the commonest causes of febrile convulsions. On clinical and electroencephalographic evidence, petit mal epilepsy is relatively uncommon (4%).

The problems in the management of epilepsy in the Africans are discussed and include lack of facilities and personnel for accurate diagnosis and treatment, inadequate supply or nonavailability of drugs, high defaulting rate of patients, and the adverse and often pernicious social stigmatization of epileptics. Possible solutions to some of these problems discussed include integration of management (in simple terms) of convulsive disorders into the basic health system, aggressive pursuit of health education of the public by governmental and nongovernmental agencies, active and intense promotion of training of health personnel in neurosciences, and research aimed at producing long-acting anticonvulsants.

ACKNOWLEDGMENTS

The assistance of my colleagues Professor A. Adeloye, Drs. O. Bademosi, J. B. Familusi, and A. Olumide in the preparation of this chapter and under whose care many of the patients were seen in UCH, Ibadan, is hereby gratefully acknowledged. Mr. Felix Oke and Mrs. C. O. Aderanti performed the electroencephalographic examinations. I thank Mrs. Beatrice Oso for secretarial assistance.

REFERENCES

Aall-Jilek, L. M. (1965): Epilepsy in the Wagoporo tribe in Tanganyika. *Acta Psychiatr. Scand.,* 41:57–86.

Adeloye, A., and Odeku, E. L. (1971): Epilepsy after missile wounds of the head. *J. Neurol. Neurosurg. Psychiatry,* 34:98–103.

Aird, R. B., Venturini, A. M., and Spielman, P. M. (1967): Antecedents of temporal lobe epilepsy. *Arch. Neurol.,* 16:67–73.

Apantaku, J. B., Afonja, O. A., and Boyo, A. E. (1975): The effect of long term anticonvulsant therapy on serum calcium, phosphate and alkaline phosphatase in Nigerian epileptic patients. *Trop. Geogr. Med.,* 27:418–421.

Billinghurst, J. R. (1970): Epilepsy in Uganda (urban). *Afr. J. Med. Sci.,* 1:149–154.

Billington, W. R. (1968): The problem of the epileptic patient in Uganda. *East Afr. Med. J.,* 45: 563–569.

Bird, A. V., Heinz, H. J., and Klintworth, G. (1962): Convulsive disorders in Bantu mine-workers. *Epilepsia,* 3:173–187.

Carothers, J. C. (1953): The African mind in health and disease (a study in ethnography). WHO Bulletin, No. 17.

Collomb, H., Zwingelstein, J., and Seck, I. (1963): Assistance aux malades mentaux et aux epileptiques au Senegal. III emes Journees Medicales de Dakar. Colloque de Sante Publique, pp. 51–56.

Collomb, H., Dumas, M. Ayats, Viriev, R., Simon, M., and Roger, J. (1970): Epidemiologie de l'epilepsie au Senegal. *Afr. J. Med. Sci.,* 1:125–148.

Compere, A., and Compere, J. (1970): Premiere estimation des problems poses par l'epilepsie dans l'est de la Republic Democratique du Congo. *Afr. J. Med. Sci.,* 1:201–205.

Cosnett, J. E. (1964): Neurological disorders in the Zulu. *Neurology (Minneap.),* 14:443–454.

Dada, T. O. (1970*a*): Epilepsy in Lagos, Nigeria. *Afr. J. Med. Sci.,* 1:161–184.

Dada, T. O. (1970*b*): Parasites and epilepsy in Nigeria. *Trop. Geogr. Med.,* 22:312–322.

Dada, T. O., and Odeku, E. L. (1966): Epilepsy in the Nigerian patient: A review of 234 cases. *W. Afr. Med. J.,* 15:153–163.

Dada, T. O., Osuntokun, B. O., and Odeku, E. L. (1969): Epidemiological aspects of epilepsy in Nigeria: A study of 639 patients. *Dis Nerv. Syst.,* 30:807–813.

Dechef, G. (1970): Notions sur l'epidemiologie de l'epilepsie au Congo (Kinshasha). *Afr. J. Med. Sci.,* 1:309–314.

Edington, G. M., Nwabuebo, I., and Junaid, T. A. (1975): The pathology of schistosomiasis in Ibadan, Nigeria with special reference to the appendix, brain, pancreas, and genital organs. *Trans. R. Soc. Trop. Med. Hyg.,* 69:153–162.

Edoo, B. B., and Haddock, D. R. (1970): Epilepsy in Accra, Ghana: A report on classification and aetiology. *Afr. J. Med. Sci.,* 1:207–212.

Familusi, J. B., and Sinnette, C. H. (1971): Febrile convulsions in Ibadan children. *Afr. J. Med. Sci.,* 2:135–149.

Gelfand, M. (1957): Epilepsy in the African. *Cent. Afr. J. Med.,* 3:11–12.

Gelfand, M. (1973): The traditional concept of the Shona to epilepsy. *Cent. Afr. J. Med.,* 19:184–187.

Giel, R. (1968): The epileptic outcast. *East Afr. Med. J.,* 45:27–31.

Haddock, D. R. W. (1967): An attempt to assess the prevalence of epilepsy in Accra. *Ghana Med. J.,* 6:140–141.

Haddock, D. R. W. (1973): Neurological disorders in Ghana. In: *Tropical Neurology,* edited by J. D. Spillane, pp. 143–160. London, Oxford University Press.

Hamill, J. F., and Carter, S. (1966): Febrile convulsions. *N. Engl. J. Med.,* 274:563–564.

Hurst, L. A., Reef, H. E., and Sachs, S. B. (1961): Neuropsychiatric disorders in the Bantu. *S. Afr. Med. J.,* 35:750–754.

Jilek, W. G., and Jilek-Aall, L. M. (1970): The problem of epilepsy in a rural Tanzanian tribe. *Afr. J. Med. Sci.,* 1:305–307.

Keith, H. M. (1963): *Convulsive Disorders in Children with Reference to Treatment with Ketogenic Diet,* p. 37. Little, Brown and Co., Boston.

Kurland, L. T. (1959): The incidence and prevalence of convulsive disorders in a small urban community. *Epilepsia,* 1:143–161.

Lancet (1961): Annotation: A survey of epilepsy. *Lancet,* 1:438.

Lennox, W. G. (1953): Significance of febrile convulsions. *Pediatrics,* 35:341–357.

Levy, F. (1970): Epilepsy in Rhodesia, Zambia and Malawi. *Afr. J. Med. Sci.,* 1:291–303.

Levy, L. F., Forbes, J. I., and Parirenyatwa (1964): Epilepsy in Africans. *Cent. Afr. J. Med.,* 10: 241–249.
Livingston, S. (1960): Management of the child with one epileptic seizure. *J.A.M.A.,* 175:135.
Minde, M. (1975): History of mental health services in South Africa: Part VIII: Services for epileptics. *S. Afr. Med. J.,* 49:1968–1972.
Mundy-Castle, A. C. (1970): Epilepsy and the electroencephalogram in Ghana. *Afr. J. Med. Sci.,* 1:221–236.
Olatunbosun, D. A., Adeniyi, F. A., and Adadevoh, B. K. (1975): Serum calcium, phosphorus and magnesium levels in pregnant and non-pregnant Nigerians. *Br. J. Obstet. Gynaecol.,* 82:568.
Orley, J. (1970): Epilepsy in Uganda (rural): A study of eighty-three cases. *Afr. J. Med. Sci.,* 1: 155–160.
Osuntokun, B. O. (1971): The pattern of neurological illness in tropical Africa: Experience at Ibadan. *J. Neurol. Sci.,* 12:417–422.
Osuntokun, B. O. (1972): Epilepsy in the developing countries: The Nigerian profile. *Epilepsia,* 13:107–111.
Osuntokun, B. O. (1975): The traditional basis of neuropsychiatric practice among the Yorubas of Nigeria. *Trop. Geogr. Med.,* 27:422–430.
Osuntokun, B. O., Bademosi, O., Familusi, J. B., and Oke, F. (1974): Electroencephalographic correlates of epilepsy in Nigerian children. *Dev. Med. Child Neurol.,* 16:659–663.
Osuntokun, B. O., and Odeku, E. L. (1970): Epilepsy in Ibadan, Nigeria. *Afr. J. Med. Sci.,* 1:185–200.
Osuntokun, B. O., Odeku, E. L., and Sinnette, C. H. (1968): Convulsive disorders in Nigerians: The febrile convulsions (an evaluation of 195 patients). *East Afr. Med. J.,* 46:385–394.
Peterman, M. G. (1952): Febrile convulsions. *J. Pediatr.,* 41:536–540.
Piraux, A. (1960): Les epilepsies en Africa Centrale. *World Neurol.* 1:510–522.
Piraux, A. (1962): Epilepsies in Central Africa. In: *First Pan African Psychiatric Conference,* edited by T. A. Lambo, pp. 95–99. Government Printer, Ibadan, Nigeria.
Powell, S. J., Proctor, E. M., Wilmot, A. J., and MacLeod, I. N. (1966): Cysticercosis and epilepsy in Africans: A clinical and serological study. *Ann. Trop. Med. Parasitol.,* 60:152–615.
Schram, R. (1969): Accident services and protection in Africa with special reference to Uganda road accidents. In: *Integrating Rehabilitation in Africa,* edited by B. O. Barry. National Fund for Research into Crippling Diseases, London.
Shanks, R. A. (1949): Nature of infantile convulsions. *Am. J. Dis. Child.,* 78:763–774.
Smartt, C. G. F. (1959): Epilepsy in Tanganyika and its treatment with primidone. *East Afr. Med. J.,* 36:91–98.
Stores, G. (1976): The investigation and management of school children with epilepsy. *Public Health,* 90:171–177.
Thom, D. I. (1942): Convulsions in early life and their relationship to chronic convulsive disorders and mental defect. *Am. J. Psychiatry,* 98:574–580.
Williams, D. (1975): The border-land of epilepsy revisited. The Seventh Gowers Memorial Lecture. *Brain,* 98:1–12.

Epilepsy, The Eighth International Symposium,
edited by J. K. Penry. Raven Press, New York
© 1977.

Epilepsy, Health, and Underdevelopment

R. Rada

Faculty of Medicine, University de Los Andes, Mérida, Venezuela

The underdeveloped territories in Africa, Asia, and Latin America that nurtured the wellsprings of civilization have emerged in contemporary history as the underdeveloped areas of the modern world, culturally dependent on and economically exploited by the countries of the northern hemisphere. This situation is the outcome of the industrial revolution, basically of the development of world capitalism.

At the present moment in history, a change in the relations between countries is being witnessed, as the underdeveloped nations begin the search for an autochthonous style, which, if apprehended consciously, could provide the basis for a real "national project," with a clear ideological basis, capable of shaping a coherent policy in industrial and agrarian spheres as well as in services for the community, including education and health. Institutional organization would take place in accordance with comprehensive development, and production and social relations would bypass the obsolete structures of neocolonialism or so-called "nationalist development" *(desarrollismo).*

The health sector cannot be isolated from other areas in a national framework of sectoral relations, but in our countries—in Latin America—such relations are fortuitous and the functioning of the health system is chaotic, in the throes of a crisis that could be characterized in regard to my own country, Venezuela, by the following features: 1) the high cost of health care; 2) the excessive cost of medicines; 3) emphasis on curative over preventive action; 4) inequality of access to health services; 5) unequal geographic distribution of services; 6) unequal geographic distribution of doctors; 7) unsatisfactory ratio of doctors to nurses; 8) unequal and inappropriate distribution of doctors by specialities; 9) shortage of hospital beds; 10) shortage of qualified workers; 11) lack of reliable information; 12) excessive bureaucracy; 13) lack of coordination; 14) lack of control (external and internal); 15) inefficiency and ineffectiveness; 16) widespread corruption; 17) lack of State policy in regard to health; 18) lack of integration of the sector in national development policy.

Within this context, a form of medical private enterprise is developing that battens on the state in direct proportion to the rate at which technical development of modern medicine and medical institutions is imposed. Just as in the old Greek model, there are different services for the poor and for the rich; charity subsists as an ethical value invested with a sense of Christian submission and abnegation.

The word epidemiology has imitated the word ecology in its semantic evolution. Both are charged with mythical overtones in the world today and thereby run the risk of lack of effectiveness and consequent loss of prestige. The prevailing epidemiological practice in Latin America is based on the traditional methods used for infectious-contagious diseases, supported by sanitary environmental health measures. Modern epidemiology directed toward the study of the ". . . distribution and determinants of states of health in human populations . . ." and stressing causality, mainly based on multifactor models, for the prevention, surveillance, and control of health disorders in human populations, is awaiting official discovery and meanwhile is thrust into the background. Epidemiological studies such as the one promoted by the Pan American Health Organization (PAHO) on the prevalence of the epilepsies among school children in three Latin American countries (Chile, Mexico, and Venezuela) will produce figures and assess the extent of the problem, and this is important as a first step. As a result of my own study in Mérida, Venezuela, however, I forecast the ultimate failure of this project because of the apathy in official support from sanitary authorities, the limitation created by not linking this research with a wider program of research in mental health, and worst of all, the failure to provide health services for detected cases, children demanding a solution to their problems, and the prospect of more cases when the study is made known in the community. The research team cannot cope with even a reasonable demand on the part of the population.

Referring to the "team," I am convinced—and this is not new—that any approach to epilepsy has to be a multidisciplinary effort, involving not a mere assembling of individuals from different disciplines but the agreement of institutions, through their personnel, on a clear goal, extended in time, and on far-reaching and comprehensive objectives.

HEALTH AS AN OPERATIONAL ENTITY

An international working group sponsored by the World Health Organization (November 1975) has tried to solve the nonoperational component of the universal definition of health—that synonymous with happiness. The group has designed a system broken down into subsystems in which the equilibrium would correspond to the actual state of health and an unbalance would generate the state of disease. The subsystems, shown in Fig. 1, are individual or psychobiologic, "natural," and social. Each subsystem has components (Fig. 2) that might be identified as "indicators" or parameters for particular situations in particular social groups in accordance with decisions produced by the state. The individual is considered within this comprehensive system, integrated with the natural and social systems, interacting and reacting toward the use of health services, and showing different degrees of social participation, depending on disease and health.

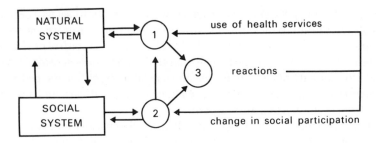

(1) PSYCHOBIOLOGICAL SYSTEM OF THE INDIVIDUAL	disease as a psychobiological state (medical nosography).
(2) INDIVIDUAL SOCIAL RELATIONS	disease as a social state.
(3) INDIVIDUAL CONSCIOUSNESS	disease as perceived state; perceived nosology.

FIG. 1. Simplified process where disorder corresponds to individual disease. [From Economic Planning Center, Finland (November 1975). *Health: A System Analysis Study.*]

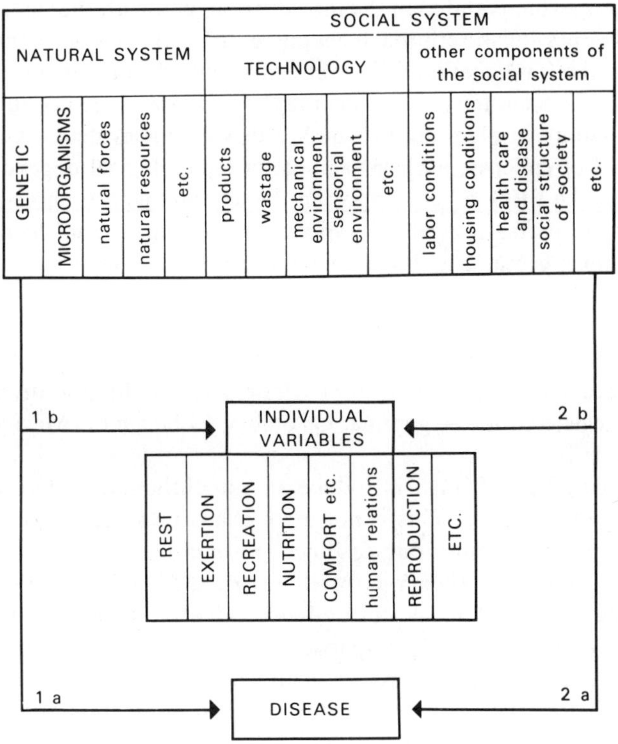

FIG. 2. Schematic description of disease etiology. [From Economic Planning Center, Finland (November 1975).]

It is possible for governments or government agencies to select specific ends and goals for a health policy directed toward prevention or toward the treatment of any particular state of health, including such items as: 1) control of risk factors; 2) prevention of traumas; 3) early detection of diseases: mass screening methods; 4) basic care for patients, using, for example, general practitioners, pediatricians, and internists; 5) specialized care: specialities in medical care and research; 6) study of the social participation of patients.

Within such a model system, with clearly defined items and indicators, international action could be conceived as assessment of the initial design of the program for the study of epilepsy, including periodic evaluation, and information to the government offices designated to supervise the project on the progress of the action undertaken. This work, to be done by health planners and epidemiologists, would be the basis for developing a data control system on epilepsy and related disorders, and for preparing studies in the field of descriptive epidemiology (magnitudes) or analytical epidemiology related particularly to causality.

OBSTACLES AND DEPENDENCE

Following up what is stated in the introduction, and with the same critical and perhaps rather pessimistic approach, let me return to the obstacles that are bound to aggravate the fundamental failure already pointed out: the absence of a national scheme for scientific development in the underdeveloped countries in question, where failure in planning for the health sector is evident.

In the field of epilepsy, a clear example of technological dependence is seen in the case of the EEG, a very important factor in diagnostic assessment. EEG machines, spare parts, or even the paper for recording, are not locally available and contact must be made with American, European or Japanese manufacturers. Again, most of the anticonvulsant drugs come from foreign firms, with consequent distortion of the pharmaceutical market, a game played with all the rules of free enterprise of the capitalist system, where our countries are the exploited. [In this regard see the *Anticonvulsant Glossary* (1971) for the diverse types of hydantoins registered for Argentina, Colombia, El Salvador, Mexico, Uruguay, and Venezuela.]

At this point, I feel I must introduce an autochthonous note on epilepsy in underdeveloped countries. This is not mere chauvinism. It is, on the contrary, a deliberate protest against our readiness to assimilate, at least in part, and superficially, all that in theory is produced in the "scientific centers" of the northern hemisphere. This is cultural dependence, without critical analysis through study, research, and comparison with our own situation for purposes of creativity and efficiency. There are many cultural, geographic, anthropologic and genetic factors that give credence to such an autochthonous outlook. The treatise written by Federico Sal y Rosas, a Peruvian physician descended from the Incas, who devoted more than 30 years of his life to a wide and meticulous study of epilepsy, contains an extensive bibliography and a clear-cut theoretical position on the physiological, clinical and socioepidemiological aspects of epilepsy, but it is practically unknown in most Latin American centers involved in any approach to epilepsy. It might be feasible to collect and distribute all this material and to promote seminars and discussions among health personnel.

Medical care undoubtedly occupies a prominent position in the health services. Specialization in medicine emerges as a consequence of technological progress and in response to an apparent division of labor in a complex modern process. But instead of such principles of organization, what we are faced with is a fierce struggle among physicians that promotes a false territoriality where the perplexed human being we call the "patient" finds himself at the vortex of a kafkaesque drama. The specialist, on the other hand, is a privileged physician with social and professional status, guided by the tenets of "free enterprise" and by the traditional saying that "no price is too high for the doctor's services"; but these tend to be increasingly costly, and greed for money is tending to bring corruption into medical practice. It has already been mentioned that specialists are poorly distributed geographically. Corruption, irresponsibility, and idleness are also in evidence. Let us give an example: 80 percent of the records in some Latin American EEG laboratories indicate "cortical irritability" or "dysrhythmia," followed by recommendations for treatment and periodic evaluation. Reluctance to be specific may well play a part in the situation; this is private practice, and there is no control of medical care.

There is no mechanism for protecting the patient's rights. The medical associations are zealous in defending the rights and wrongs of the medical profession, which only serves to perpetuate the crisis in the health sector and to maintain their members' earnings at a high level.

Perhaps an international advisory group could be useful in developing a realistic plan based on the WHO health criteria designed particularly for epilepsy, and in this, the International League Against Epilepsy could be of assistance. Periodic evaluation would result in a progressive program of education, achieving at least a partial if not an absolute change of attitude towards epilepsy. A definitive solution would have to come within the general context of a sociopolitical change that is beyond the scope of this introduction to a regional problem in regard to epilepsy.

REFERENCES

Economic Planning Center, Finland (November 1975): *Health: A System Analysis Study,* Draft for WHO. World Health Organization, Geneva.

International Bureau for Epilepsy (1971): *An International Glossary of Anticonvulsants,* IBE, London.

Epilepsy, The Eighth International Symposium,
edited by J. K. Penry. Raven Press, New York
© 1977.

Sociocultural and Economic Implications of Epilepsy in India

Vimla Virmani, V. Kaul, and S. Juneja

Department of Neurology, All-India Institute of Medical Sciences, New Delhi, India

With the effective medical control of epilepsy, there is increasing interest in the disturbances of affective cognitive functions in epileptic patients. Studies on the social aspects have indicated widespread social prejudices against epileptic patients (Bagley, 1972; Hartlage and Green, 1972; Rodin et al., 1972). The significance of modifying public attitudes toward the disease and the diseased and obtaining gainful employment for them has been stressed by Gregoriades (1972) and by Caveness and colleagues in their serial surveys from 1949 to 1974. The mysterious nature of the phenomenon and the social prejudices adversely affect the patients' sense of well-being. In the author's experience, about 18% of all epileptic patients have subjective complaints of impairment of memory, work efficiency, and intellectual functions. In a multicultured society such as India, educational and rehabilitation problems of these patients pose a special challenge.

PATIENTS AND OBSERVATIONS

The present observations were based on a study of 560 epileptic patients attending the epilepsy clinic in the hospital of the All-India Institute of Medical Sciences between 1965 and 1973. All types of epileptic patients fulfilling the following criteria were accepted: (1) age between 15 and 40 years, (2) minimum education of 8 years, and (3) average intelligence on clinical evaluation and confirmed by testing on the Wechsler Adult Intelligence Scale (WAIS). Grossly brain damaged patients and those whose fits were secondary to intracranial space-occupying lesions, infection of the central nervous system, or cerebrovascular diseases were excluded by relevant clinical and laboratory investigations.

Psychosocial data were obtained in a "funnel" type of interview, that is, the initial inquiries were general, pertaining to such factors as age, address, education, and occupation. Gradually, more personal information was sought, relating to academic achievement, hobbies, aspirations, and personality and/or mood changes. This was followed by a deeper probing into family, marital, social, and vocational aspects. Patients were followed at intervals of 6 months to a year for a period of 2 to 8 years. The effect of medical treatment and psychological advice given to them and the family was noted.

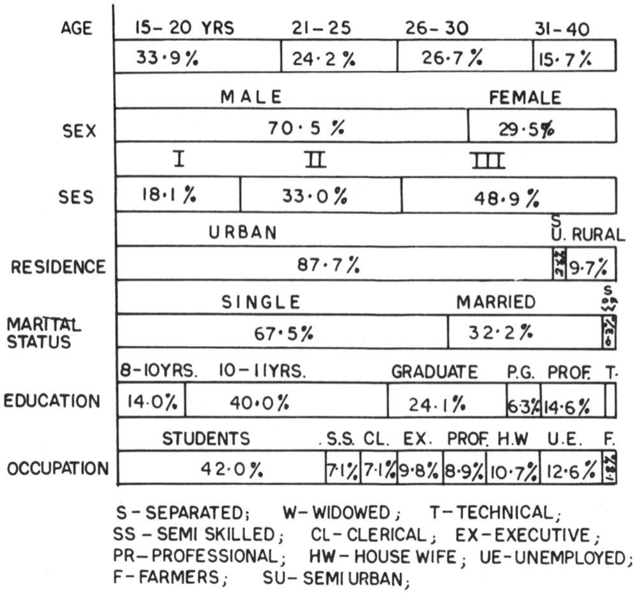

FIG. 1. Biodata of the patients.

The socioeconomic status of the patients, based on analysis of income, education, and occupation (Neki and Kapoor, 1963), was grouped from class I to V, I being the highest and V the lowest. The majority of the patients (58.1%) were between 15 and 25 years old, and 84% were below 30 years of age; 42% were students. The male:female ratio in this study was 2.4:1. In the epilepsy clinic at our hospital, the male:female ratio of all epileptics is 1.8:1. About half (48.9%) came from social classes III and IV and one-third from class II. Those in class I were in a relative minority (18.1%) (Fig. 1).

Only 25% of the patients felt that the illness had no adverse effect on their daily activities. Involvement of general health was complained of by about 45%, career by 35%, and studies by 30%. Restriction of social activities was felt by 27%, and 24% suffered from fear of ridicule (Table 1).

TABLE 1. *Effect of epilepsy on the patient's life*

	No. of patients	%
General health affected	250	44.6
Studies affected	168	30.0
Career affected	195	35.0
Social life restricted	150	27.0
Fear of ridicule	135	24.0
Lack of confidence	20	3.6
No effect	140	25.0

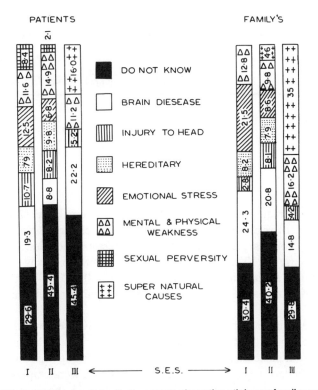

PATIENTS

FAMILY'S

DO NOT KNOW

BRAIN DIESEASE

INJURY TO HEAD

HEREDITARY

EMOTIONAL STRESS

MENTAL & PHYSICAL
WEAKNESS

SEXUAL PERVERSITY

SUPER NATURAL
CAUSES

I   II   III   ⟵ —————— S.E.S. —————— ⟶   I   II   III

FIG. 2. Patients' and familys' concept about the etiology of epilepsy.

One of the important factors which determines the effect of the disease on the patient is his own and his family members' concept about the nature of the illness. This information is given in Fig. 2. Comparison of this information showed that emotional stress as an etiological factor was mentioned more often by the family members, particularly of the upper social strata. Sexual perversity was conceived of by the patients themselves and not by the relatives, implying the disease, in the patient's opinion, to be a form of punishment for guilt.

Based on detailed probing, including leading questions, the information obtained from patients and relatives was categorized as showing normal concern, excessive anxiety, indifference, or negativism (Tables 2 and 3). We found that 48% of the patients had a normal attitude, 12% showed excessive anxiety, 18% were indifferent, and 22% were negativistic. There was no significant correlation between the patients' attitudes and their socioeconomic status. For the patients' relatives, the corresponding figures were 53%, 10%, 29%, and 8%. Normal attitudes among the relatives were significantly more frequent in classes I and II (76% and 81%, respectively) as against class III (24%) ($p < 0.01$). It is noteworthy that 53% of the relatives in class III were indifferent, compared to 9% and 5% in classes I and II, respectively. In the patient group, 74% averred that the disease had not interfered with their aspirations in life, 14% felt that

TABLE 2. *Patient's attitude toward epilepsy*

	Class I		Class II		Class III	
	No. of patients	%	No. of patients	%	No. of patients	%
Normal concern	42	39.6	93	50.0	134	50.0
Excessive anxiety	21	19.8	14	7.5	32	11.9
Indifference	22	20.8	24	12.9	56	20.8
Negativism	21	19.8	55	29.6	46	17.3
Total	106		186		268	

the disease had reduced their aspirations, and the remaining 12% had lost all interest in life. In relation to hobbies, 60% had no change, 20% had to change for less taxing hobbies, and 14% had lost all interest in hobbies. The group with onset of epilepsy at 10 to 20 years of age reported no change in aspirations significantly more often than did the others ($p < 0.05$) (Fig. 3). However, presence or absence of change in hobbies showed no significant relationship with the age at onset.

More patients in classes I and II sought medical advice early with a consequent relief of symptoms and better social adjustment, especially with regard to hobbies. But social strata made no appreciable difference regarding aspirations, especially with regard to career (Fig. 3). Only 35% of patients were employed, and these were not particularly handicapped by the attitudes of their employers or colleagues.

A notable observation in the present study was that although the disease had some detrimental effect on the patient's personal, social, and vocational life, the marital adjustment was not adversely affected if one of the partners developed fits. On the contrary, there was improvement in the harmonious marital relationship, epilepsy notwithstanding. This was significantly more marked in the higher social strata (Fig. 4). In the course of the follow-up, 68 subjects were married on our advice. All but five concealed their illness from their prospective spouses

TABLE 3. *Family members' attitude toward epilepsy*

	Class I		Class II		Class III	
	No. of patients	%	No. of patients	%	No. of patients	%
Normal concern	81	76.4	150	80.6	65	24.3
Excessive anxiety	11	10.3	22	11.8	22	8.2
Indifference	10	9.4	10	5.3	143	53.3
Negativism	4	3.9	4	2.3	38	14.2
Total	106		186		268	

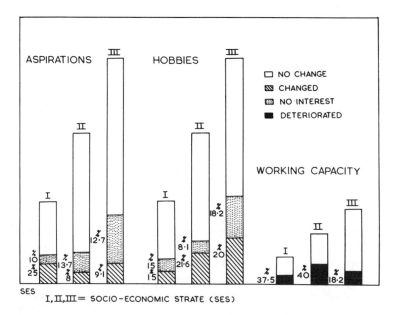

FIG. 3. Changes in aspirations, hobbies, and working capacity with respect to socioeconomic status.

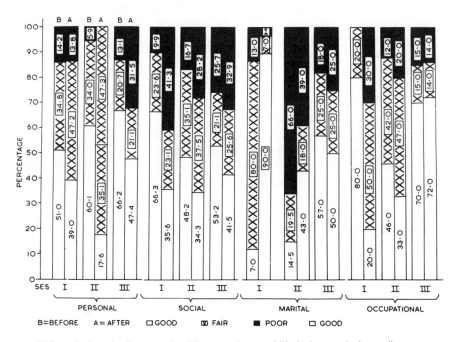

FIG. 4. Patients' adjustment in different spheres of life before and after epilepsy.

and their families, yet only two were subsequently deserted (in neither case for reasons related to the disease).

DISCUSSION

The present study was biased in favor of males, an urban population, and a middle social class. The highest and lowest classes were in the relative minority.

Differences in the concept of the etiology of the disease in different socioeconomic strata were compatible with the educational and social sophistication of the patients. Better acceptability with a consequent better attitude toward adaptation was found compatible with higher education and higher standards of living. This was in accordance with the observation made by Caveness and co-workers (1974) in their serial surveys of public attitudes toward epilepsy in the United States. Concepts about the nature of the disease, to a large extent, determine the attitude of the family and society toward the disease and the diseased. The patient's own concept about the disease and attitude toward it determine his/her reaction toward self, aspirations in life, and attitude toward the environment, both physical and social. Patients were more reluctant than the family members to accept the disease because of the deep-rooted fear of rejection and threat to their personal integrity. A large number (53.3%) of the family members of the lower socioeconomic strata showed an attitude of indifference. A relatively large number of patients in all three social strata showed indifference and negativistic attitudes toward the disease and themselves. Their new identity as afflicted individuals created conflicting emotional responses such as shame, inferiority, insecurity, fear of ridicule, and in some cases rebellion against the overprotective and subtly ambivalent attitudes of the parents and/or siblings and peers.

Normal concern about the diseased was shown by a majority of the family members in the upper strata (classes I and II), but less so in the lower stratum (class III). Excessive concern and anxiety were shown by 8.2 to 11.8% of family members in the different strata (Table 3).

The employed patients were not particularly handicapped by an adverse attitude of their employers or colleagues and felt no threat to their job stability. On the contrary, they received sympathy and consideration. It is characteristic of Indian culture that irrespective of the initial resistance or rejection, if an idea or a person happens to penetrate into a situation, the subsequent acceptance is devoid of controversy. Epileptic patients tend to stick to their job because of inherent feelings of insecurity and inability to find alternative employment. This attitude helps them to derive more job satisfaction than the nonepileptic population of comparable education and social standing. The dissatisfaction complained of by a small number of patients was not related to the disease. Deterioration in work efficiency and output was experienced by 35% of all the employed patients. It was much more obvious in the upper and middle social strata, in which the nature of occupation is usually more demanding. No change was observed in the lower stratum.

The relative stability of the institution of marriage in our culture, feelings of compassion and sympathy for the sick partner, and a better defined dominant-dependent axis due to one partner's being chronically ill accounted for the improved marital relationship and outweighed any feelings of repugnance or rejection in the spouse. Before a matrimonial alliance is made, the knowledge of the disease is a great hurdle to the relationship's materializing in India, where marriages are still mostly arranged by the parents. If the couple is married, however, the fact that the disease is partially or wholly concealed does not affect the subsequent harmonious marital relationship.

The diversity in educational standards, social customs, beliefs, and cultural background in the Indian society is unmatched. The problem of educating the public is, therefore, a challenging one and requires not only knowledge and skill but an implicit understanding of the special needs of the individual patient. Conceptualization of the basic nature of the disease is the single most important factor that determines the long-term prognosis of the epileptic patients. Social stigma, feelings of inferiority, and insecurity lower self-esteem and confidence and aggravate any cognitive disturbances that the epileptic patients may have, either because of incipient brain damage or as a result of prolonged administration of anticonvulsants. Educating the patients, the family members, and the community and giving proper perspective of the disease help in inculcating healthier attitudes and consequently better adaptation and socialization of the patient.

Premorbid personality, cultural background of the patients and their families, economic security, and family integration were some factors determining the quality of personal, educational, and vocational adaptations achieved by the patients. Rapport with the treating physician and the interest taken by the psychologist and the social workers were found to be very helpful in the total management.

SUMMARY

Study results confirmed that epilepsy has a detrimental effect on personal, social, academic, and occupational adjustments in varying proportions. Deterioration of memory, although a common complaint, was not borne out on serial psychometric evaluations. The level of anxiety, however, was high and accounted for the subjective memory deficit. Deterioration in personal, social, and occupational adjustment was more marked in the middle social strata, which are characterized by a high level of expectation and relatively limited resources. In the upper strata, where social demands are high, deterioration in the personal and social adjustment was more noticeable. Despite the prevailing social prejudices, it was notable that the marital adjustment of the couples showed improvement in all the social classes. This was attributable to the relative stability of the institution of marriage in India.

ACKNOWLEDGMENT

We are grateful to the Indian Council of Medical Research for their generous grant for carrying out this study.

REFERENCES

Bagley, C. (1972): Social prejudice and the adjustment of people with epilepsy. *Epilepsia,* 13:33–45.

Caveness, W. (1949): A survey of public attitudes toward epilepsy. *Epilepsia,* Series 2, 4:19–26.

Caveness, W. (1954): A survey of public attitudes toward epilepsy. *Epilepsia,* Series 3, 3:99–102.

Caveness, W. F. (1959): Trend in public attitudes toward epilepsy over the past decade. *Epilepsia,* 1:385–393.

Caveness, W. F., Merritt, H. H., and Gallup, G. H. (1969): A survey of public attitudes toward epilepsy in 1969 with an indication of trends over the past twenty years. *Epilepsia,* 10:429–440.

Caveness, W. F., Merritt, H. H., and Gallup, G. H., Jr. (1974): A survey of public attitudes toward epilepsy in 1974 with an indication of trends over the past twenty-five years. *Epilepsia,* 15:523–536.

Caveness, W. F., Merritt, H. H., Gallup, G. H., and Ruby, E. H. (1965): A survey of public attitudes toward epilepsy in 1964. *Epilepsia,* 6:75–86.

Gregoriades, A. D. (1972): A medical and social survey of 231 children with seizures. *Epilepsia,* 13:13–20.

Hartlage, L. C., and Green, J. B. (1972): The relation of parental attitudes to academic and social achievement in epileptic children. *Epilepsia,* 13:21–26.

Neki, J. S., and Kapoor, R. K. (1963): Social stratification of psychiatric patients. *Indian J. Psychiatry,* 5:76–86.

Rodin, E., Rennick, P., Dennerll, R., and Lin, Y. (1972): Vocational and educational problems of epileptic patients. *Epilepsia,* 13:149–160.

Epilepsy, The Eighth International Symposium,
edited by J. K. Penry. Raven Press, New York
© 1977.

The Epilepsies: Clinical and Epidemiological Aspects/Availability and Desirability of Services

Tarik I. Hamdi, Ala A. Al-Husaini, and Faiq Al-Hadithi

Department of Neuropsychiatry, College of Medicine, Baghdad, Iraq

The purpose of this study is to throw some light on the clinical and epidemiological aspects of epilepsy, to evaluate the efficiency of the services now available to manage epilepsy, and to outline the desired services according to the present status of the problem.

It is difficult to undertake an accurate epidemiological survey of epilepsy in Iraq, not only because of technical and personal limitations, but because of the cultural stigma that makes people reluctant to admit this problem. This means that the observed magnitude of the problem in a community like ours is much less than the actual truth (Rose et al., 1973).

The data outlined resulted from the study of 100 consecutive epileptics admitted to the Neuro-Psychiatric Unit, College Medical Centre, Baghdad. We hope that the result of the work will enlighten our way to a better understanding of epilepsy and hence better programs for its prevention, treatment, and rehabilitation.

GENERAL CONSIDERATIONS

Iraq has a population of ten million and about 30 neuropsychiatrists. Rapid improvement in the social, economic, and educational standards is putting a heavy burden on the medical services, as the concept of disease is changing.

The country is developing an industrialized and westernized way of life, which carries with it more road traffic accidents and hence more epileptics. Longer spans of life mean more cerebral atherosclerosis, cerebral vascular accidents, and more epilepsy.

The family and religious cohesions are very strong pillars that prevent deterioration of the epileptics. Families take good care of their patients, even the chronic and disturbed ones, which is a great help to the medical and social services in relieving much of their responsibilities.

The 5 epileptics per 1,000 population (50,000 epileptics) in this country are also looked after by various governmental hospitals and departments in which all services are free, but private services also exist. No facilities are available to rehabilitate the epileptics.

EPILEPSY IN IRAQ

This study was carried out in the Department of Neuropsychiatry, Baghdad Medical Centre, in a 53-bed unit within a 1,080-bed general hospital. The work includes the study of 100 epileptics admitted consecutively to the unit from January, 1974 until July, 1975.

The types of epileptics admitted were: (1) those with status epilepticus (25 patients), (2) those who were refractory to the conventional modes of treatment, with frequent daily attacks (44 patients), and (3) those who had had a fit for the first time and were in need of being investigated (31 patients).

Patients with febrile convulsions were excluded from the study. Investigations commenced with a full history and clinical examination. All patients underwent complete blood studies, urinalysis, stool examination, Wasserman reaction, and Kahn test for blood and CSF, general CSF study, and skull and chest X-rays. All patients also had EEG studies.

Other evaluations, such as glucose tolerance test, liver function, or neurosurgical procedures, e.g., air encephalography, ventriculography, and angiography, were proposed when indicated.

RESULTS

Most of the patients (68%) were in the first two decades of life (Table 1), and most had had epilepsy for many years (Table 2). The patients came to us because of uncontrolled fits, mostly due to ignorance. Either they failed to take their medication regularly or they regarded the cause of their illness as supernatural and due to powers, the ghost, or the devil eye. In the latter case, the mode of treatment would definitely be through native healers by means of exorcism, for example, and consequently fits would persist.

Sex Incidence

The patients included 63 males and 37 females. This does not reflect a higher incidence of epilepsy among males, because many families refuse to admit their

TABLE 1. *Age on admission*

Age (years)	No. of patients
< 1–10	15
11–20	41
21–30	18
31–40	11
41–50	7
51–60	5
60–> 60	3
Total	100

TABLE 2. *Age at onset of fits*

Age (years)	No. of patients
< 1–10	30
11–20	38
21–30	16
31–40	4
41–50	4
51–60	5
60–> 60	3
Total	100

young females to the hospital and may even hide their patients because of the stigma attached to epilepsy.

Family History

Eight percent of our patients did have a family history of epilepsy in spite of the high frequency of consanguinity among the general population.

Laboratory Findings

Many of our patients were anemic (20%), and some were infested with helminths, e.g., ancylostoma, bilharzia (10%).

Cerebrospinal fluid was abnormal in 18% of the cases, and none of our patients showed a positive Wasserman reaction or Kahn test for the blood or CSF.

The EEG was positive in 76% of the patients and negative in 24% despite the witnessed attacks.

The modes of clinical expression shown in Table 3 were the major presenting types of seizures. Ten percent of the patients showed mixed attacks, mostly major and minor fits.

TABLE 3. *Mode of expression of epilepsy*

Clinical seizure type	No. of patients
Major fit (with aura)	20
Centrencephalic	51
Myoclonic epilepsy	10
Absence attack	4
Jacksonian attack	4
Akinetic attack	5
Familial myoclonus	2
Salaam attack	1
Psychomotor attack	3
Total	100

TABLE 4. *Etiology of epilepsy*

Etiology	No. of patients
Epileia	2
Posttraumatic	5
Strokes	4
Brain tumors	4
Primary	2
Secondary	2
Encephalitis	7
S.S.P.E.	7
Postmeningetic	2
Cerebral palsy	1
Hypertensive encephalopathy	2
Mental retardation	10
Diabetes	2
Mercury poisoning	1
Contraceptive pills	1
Total	48

Causes of Epilepsy

Fifty-two patients were considered to have an idiopathic type of epilepsy. The remaining 48 were considered to suffer epilepsy secondary to a specific illness or an associated condition. Table 4 shows the different etiological causes.

Treatment and Prognosis

The conventional means of therapy were used: a single drug, a combination of drugs, the addition of a diuretic.

Phenobarbital, phenytoin, tridione, ethosuximide, sulthiame, carbamazepine, nitrazepam, and clonazepam were used in their appropriate indications.

Thirty-five of our patients, most of them suffering from generalized seizures, were on a combination of drugs. Four received no treatment because they had had a fit for the first time, all investigations were negative, and the fit did not occur again. The remaining 61 patients received a single medication. The usual procedure that we follow is to start treatment after the third documented attack, despite negative clinical and EEG findings.

TABLE 5. *Follow-up results*

Result	Percentage of patients
No more attacks	78%
Decreased frequency	7%
No improvement	5%
Referred to neurosurgical hospital	6%

The routine procedure in the department is to keep the patients 2 weeks after good stabilization. The results are summarized in Table 5.

DISCUSSION

Epilepsy among the Iraqi patients differs in no way from that seen among people in other parts of the world. Levy et al. (1964), reviewing epilepsy in Africans (great similarities to Iraqies), found no special etiological factors for the Africans.

The age incidence of idiopathic epilepsy in Iraq is in keeping with the finding that the peak is in the first two decades of life (Andreas and O'Doherty, 1961).

None of our cases showed atrophic lesions, which have a low incidence in Africa but a high incidence in Europe and America (Piraux, 1961).

Toxoplasmosis does not seem to be a factor in the causation of epilepsy in Iraq, as the incidence is the same in both the general population and epileptics (Saffar and Hamdi, 1968).

Two of our female patients developed schizophrenia-like psychosis on complete suppression of the fits. Two patients developed ataxia and other cerebellar symptoms while they were on hydantoin. The symptoms disappeared on changing to sulthiame.

Serum calcium level was estimated in 25% of patients who were on hydantoin for a long time. None of them developed disturbance in serum calcium level.

The 8% family history of epilepsy among our patients, despite the high incidence of consanguinity, indicates that the genetic background is not a major contributing factor for the development of epilepsy in Iraq (or that some patients do not divulge the presence of epilepsy in other members of the family).

Overprotection is very marked in this country, and most people are obsessed with the hereditary nature of the illness. The same belief is held by Nigerians (Dada and Odeku, 1966).

The possibility that amebiasis and other tropical diseases might induce epilepsy through the production of a generalized toxic state may contribute to some of our cases (Tsiminakis and Divolia, 1973). The same hypothesis may contribute with regard to bilharziasis (Taher et al., 1973), but our technical limitations did not allow us to clarify these hypotheses.

The facilities available for the management of epilepsy are hardly sufficient. Moreover, industrialization of the country will bring more patients to medical attention than are now recognized in the agricultural societies. Rehabilitation centers and employment services are important facilities that ought to be founded for better attention to people with epilepsy. Although the facilities at hand are deficient, the strong family cohesion helps to prevent deterioration of the epileptics.

The available services for epileptics at the present time are as follows:

1. Neuropsychiatric outpatient and inpatient units within a general hospital, Medical City, Basrah, Mosul, Kirkuk and Rasheed Military Hospitals.

2. Epileptic Center, Baghdad, which deals also with mentally retarded patients on an outpatient basis.

Apart from these centers, various outpatient clinics all over the country manage the epileptics. Investigations are not available except at the Neuropsychiatric Unit in the major hospitals.

RECOMMENDATIONS

With the anticipated industrialization and westernization of life in Iraq, it is urgent that preparation be started so that those afflicted with epilepsy can be treated in a reasonable and humanitarian manner. A great deal of work must be done to cope with the growing need:

1. Education of the people in their own language as to the understanding of their own illness, the importance of taking their medication regularly, the jobs they are allowed to take, and counseling with regard to marriage and pregnancy.
2. Saturation of all medical services with antiepileptic drugs.
3. Establishment of epilepsy centers so that patients can visit regularly for follow-up.
4. Instruction of general practitioners all over the country to counsel, support, and advise the epileptics; to supply them with the appropriate medicines; and to be aware of the side effects, idiosyncrasies, and intoxications of the various antiepileptic drugs.
5. Education of patients so that they can understand their chronic illness and learn to live with it.
6. Investigation of the hypothesis that since the nervous system is the medium through which the person relates to his environment, the interaction between the patient and his environment might ameliorate or aggravate his epilepsy.
7. Equipment of people dealing with epilepsy with sound knowledge about seizures and the pharmacology of antiepileptic drugs. Even after knowledge of the disease is widespread, the optimal care of epileptics can be accomplished only within the framework of high-quality medical, social, and rehabilitative services.

SUMMARY

It seems that the causes and clinical expressions of the epilepsies in Iraq differ in no respect from those elsewhere. More patients are being identified because of reasons mentioned. The services available for the epileptics are not sufficient to cope with the need. More efforts are needed to deal with the increasing demands.

REFERENCES

Andreas, F. D., and O'Doherty, D. S. (1961): An analysis of convulsive disorder in a general hospital. *Georgetown Med. Bull.,* 14:172–178.

Dada, T. O., and Odeku, E. L. (1966): Epilepsy in the Nigerian patient. A review of 234 cases. *West Afr. Med. J.,* 15:153–163.

Levy, L. F., Forbes, J. I., and Parirenyatawa, T. S. (1964): Epilepsy in Africans. *Cent. Afr. J. Med.,* 10:241–249.

Piraux, A. (1961): *Epilepsies in Central Africa,* pp. 95–99. First Pan-African Psychiatric Conference, Western Nigeria Government Printer.

Rose, S. W., Penry, J. K., Markush, R. E., Radloff, L. A., and Putnam, P. L. (1973): Prevalence of epilepsy in children. *Epilepsia,* 14:133–152.

Saffar, G., and Hamdi, T. I. (1968): The incidence of toxoplasmosis in a group of idiopathic epilepsy in Iraq. *Folia Parasitol. (Praha),* 15.

Taher, Y., Mousa, A. H., and Behery, N. (1973): Excerpta Medica International Congress Series No. 296, Amsterdam. Abstract No. 168, p. 58.

Tsiminakis, J. C., and Divolia, A. (1973): Excerpta Medica International Congress Series No. 296, Amsterdam. Abstract No. 171, p. 59.

Epilepsy, The Eighth International Symposium,
edited by J. K. Penry. Raven Press, New York
© 1977.

Problems of Epilepsy in Rhodesia

Laurence F. Levy and William C. Auchterlonie

University of Rhodesia, Salisbury, Rhodesia

Epilepsy is a common and serious disorder in Rhodesia. Every year, about 250 patients are admitted to Harari Central Hospital, Salisbury, with epilepsy or convulsions as the first diagnosis. Last year, epilepsy accounted for 1.2% of all admissions. Furthermore, approximately two patients are admitted to our hospital each month with burns sustained by falling into their traditional open fires during seizures.

It is difficult, however, to estimate the incidence of this disorder among our people. In 1964 we (Levy et al., 1964) published the results of a field study undertaken in a rural part of the country near Bulawayo known as Semokwe. This area had a population of 17,500 African people, the majority of whom were women and children. In this group of people 130 epileptics were discovered, an incidence of 0.7%. We believe, however, that the true incidence is considerably higher. One of the problems in making such a study is that the disorder has to be recognized by the sufferer or his relatives, and the researchers are entirely dependent on this. The educational, social, and cultural level of many rural people is such that many young children suffering transient episodes of loss of consciousness may not be remarked on and treatment may not be sought. For example, in the field study, only 6 patients out of the 130 were reported to have minor seizures; a comparable group of European epileptic patients matched for age revealed three times as many. Likewise, a greater percentage of young European patients are referred to our EEG department and are admitted to the hospital with epilepsy or convulsions as a first diagnosis than African patients (after correction for population age grouping difference). It is our belief that the existence of minor seizures, especially in the young, is frequently not noted, and therefore the incidence of 0.7% is falsely low. This overlooking of disease, however, applies to all sorts of conditions, not only to epilepsy. Some years ago we did another interesting study that illustrates this point well. Over 3,000 rural people were examined for the presence of disease by two fourth-year medical students. The subjects were villagers who were approached by the students and offered a small sum of money to permit a simple physical examination. Over a thousand of these had some disorder that was obvious to the students and was of a nature that would certainly have taken any Dubliner to see his doctor. When asked why they had not sought medical assistance, most answered that they were not bothered by the disorder; a few said that they could not afford to go to a hospital. The fact is that disease of all sorts is immensely tolerated among rural and uneducated people.

This rural study revealed how much epilepsy is untreated or maltreated. Of the 130 patients reviewed in Semokwe, only 1 had been to a hospital, although 118 patients had been to Ngangas or traditional herbal doctors and had been given various medications. This is understandable, considering that 60% of these rural patients, when questioned, considered their epilepsy to be due to bewitchment, and our traditional colleagues claim to be able to cure this. We do not. Of the 118 patients, 80 stated that the treatment given had had no effect. As far as we know, none of these medications contains any ingredients of an anticonvulsant nature. Thus, most of the patients have not attended formal westernized practitioners for treatment and have not been exposed to genuine anticonvulsant therapy. We have also been told that another reason for nonattendance at the European doctors is that the latter do not state the cause of the trouble, whereas the traditional doctors do give a cause—even if an incorrect and mystical one— and this satisfies the patient. The severely incapacitated rural patient naturally goes to the Nganga first because he is, after all, the equivalent of the general practitioner in the village as well as being the pastor and mentor of the social group. The thought here would be for us to attempt to influence the traditional doctor and cooperate with him; up to the present, however, such efforts as have been made have been sporadic and unsuccessful. An informed campaign is needed to draw people's attention to this disorder and the possibilities offered by treatment.

The African population that comes to the central hospitals is somewhat different from that investigated at Semokwe. Townspeople are more sophisticated and more dependent on staying free of attacks than their rural counterparts. In a comprehensive study of 100 consecutive patients who presented at Harare Hospital complaining of seizures, there were 88 males and 12 females and only 26% were under 20 years of age. The sex and age difference must in the main be attributed to the large number of men who have migrated to town to seek work and to the fact that the women who stay at home would be less vulnerable to social or job pressures aggravated by epilepsy. However, this cannot be the whole story because even in the Semokwe study there were still 73 males to 57 females, and there one would have certainly expected a reversal of the figures.

These 100 patients were investigated by routine clinical examination, plain X-rays, EEG, arteriography, pneumoencephalography, routine blood counts and chemistries, and urine and stool examination. In this study, 16 showed cerebral atrophy, 7 had an unquestionable posttraumatic basis and 1 a known birth injury, and 3 were judged due to encephalitis and 3 to chronic meningitis. Seven patients were found to be suffering from generalized cysticercosis. Twenty-six had abnormal EEGs but no other abnormality. Thirty-eight had no cause found. In this group there were no cases of cerebral neoplasia. We found that 15% of all these patients had active bilharzial infection. Although we do not suggest that bilharzia commonly causes epilepsy, we believe that it can do so either by irritative foci of ectopic ova in the cortex or as a result of the chronic ill-health which can be produced by this parasite, exaggerating an underlying seizure tendency. Although we acknowledge that bilharzia, cysticercosis, and tuberculosis play an etiological role in some of our cases of epilepsy, the eradication of these three diseases involves a public health program to educate and raise the standard of hygiene in the community.

The hospital study showed that the most important tests to be performed in an adult epileptic in this country are a good clinical examination, blood, urine and stool analyses, plain X-rays of skull and chest, and examination of the CSF. Only when these are abnormal need other investigations be undertaken, although we do EEGs and ultrasound scans on all patients. Investigation of patients with sophisticated equipment is of course possible only in the major hospitals, and most of the patients have to be treated symptomatically and on a clinical basis, and it is here that we see our greatest problem. Furthermore, very few of the patients, except those severely afflicted or whose jobs are in jeopardy, are willing to take continuous anticonvulsant therapy. Not unnaturally, perhaps, patients seem to expect that a course of pills will cure them and they find it difficult to understand that the action of the medication is only to suppress the attacks. Some understand the necessity for this treatment but may default because of expense or distance to be traveled to the hospital to collect the pills regularly. The greatest boon that we can see would be the development of a long-acting injectable anticonvulsant. Many patients have great faith in the power of the injection needle and are likely to attend once a month for such an injection. This problem has been discussed with a number of drug companies without any success in the development of such a method of therapy. It surely cannot be beyond the bounds of man's ingenuity to develop a depot type of phenobarbital, for example. We can assure any drug company that a fortune awaits them in Africa if they are successful in this regard (Levy, 1970).

An interesting observation that we have made, although possibly one with no validity, is that the majority of African patients who take continuing medication require only phenobarbital and rarely require phenytoin or other anticonvulsants as well. We rarely see the spectacle that we observe among some of our European patients of someone taking three or even four different types of medication. There could be many other variables in this situation, of course, but it is one that needs investigation. Unfortunately, we do not yet have the facilities of measuring blood levels of the various drugs, and this would be an essential prerequisite to such an investigation as we see it. If this were so, it might be an additional reason to develop a depot type of phenobarbital preparation.

It seems to us that there may be a subtle difference between the EEGs of European and African epileptics. If we compare the EEGs of 1,164 European epileptics with those of 1,396 major African epileptics—comparable from the age standpoint and excluding posttraumatic and focal epilepsies—we find that there is a significant increase in the amount of slowing, spike activity, and/or paroxysmal activity in the European group compared to the African group. Furthermore, the paroxysmal response to eye closure and the photoconvulsive responses are significantly less common in the African group. Similarly, the photoconvulsive response has not been seen in African patients with minor epilepsy.

Does this, together with the apparently lesser quantities of drugs required to produce seizure freedom, mean that the African brain is less prone to seizure than the European brain? We have to follow up these points, possibly by doing a large number of EEGs on casual asymptomatic persons of both races, by measuring anticonvulsant blood levels in patients, and by trying to eliminate other possible variables by using larger groups of patients.

REFERENCES

Levy, L. F. (1970): Epilepsy in Rhodesia, Zambia and Malawi. *Afr. J. Med. Sci.,* 1:291–303.
Levy, L. F., Forbes, J. I., and Parirenyatwa, T. S. (1964): Epilepsy in Africans. *Cent. Afr. J. Med.,* 10:241.

Subject Index

Absence epilepsy, EEG recordings in, 157, 158
Accident rates of epileptic drivers, 308–309, 310
Adrenal cortical function, phenytoin and carbamezapine therapy and, 210
Africa; *see also* Developing countries
epilepsy; *see* Epilepsy in Africa
medical services, 365–366
Age; *see also* Age of onset of epilepsy; Middle-aged persons
of epileptics in Africa, 367–368
frequency of seizures and, 1
at lobotomy, survival and, 31
at onset of carbamazepine therapy, 35
at onset of epilepsy
effects of, 223
epilepsy type and, 257–258
intellectual function and, 294
in Iraq, 394, 395
lobectomy outcome and, 29
at onset of Lennox-Gastaut syndrome, 64
at temporal lobe resection, 329
Amygdalotomy, 25
Anterior temporal lobectomy, follow-up studies of, 27–34
Antiepileptic drugs; *see also* individual names, e.g., Carbamazepine; Clonazepam; Sodium valproate
adverse effects and dosages of, 41
aphasia in childhood and, 305–306
automated analysis of EEG recordings and, 152
behavioral disturbances and, 226
and carbamazepine-10,11-epoxide, 143–146
cerebral cortex content of, 103–107
cerebrospinal fluid cyclic AMP levels and, 313–315
cessation of, relapses and, 18
chromosomal damage and, 87–93
determination of levels in body fluids; *see* Monitoring of antiepileptic drug levels
dosages for children, elimination rates and, 191–196
driving and, 309

EEG findings and, 157–158
in Lennox-Gastaut syndrome and slow spike-and-wave syndrome, 65–66
long-term combination therapy with phenytoin and phenobarbital, 77–79
long-term use of, 81
need for long-acting, 375
in personality traits in epilepsy study, 259
physicians' use of, 272–273
progressive suppression of, 70–74
research, 3
secondary psychiatric disturbances and, 231–232
seizure control and, 17–20
side effects of; *see* Side effects of antiepileptic drugs
sodium valproate and clonazepam comparison, 182
toxicity reduction with, 46
use of, in developing countries, 356, 371–372, 396
Aphasia
in childhood epilepsy, 305–306
in epilepsy, 295–303
Arterial occlusion, epilepsy after, 13
Astatomyoclonic petit mal; *see* Lennox syndrome
Ataxia; *see also* Side effects of antiepileptic drugs
clonazepam and, 161
in sodium valproate and clonazepam comparison, 183
sulthiame and, 121

Behavior characteristics; *see also* Behavioral disturbances
carbamazepine and, 49–52
chronic cerebellar stimulation and, 338
Behavior modification therapy for epilepsy, 231–232, 253–254
operant conditioning of institutionalized retarded children and, 285–290
seizure control and, 239–243
Behavioral disturbances in epileptic children, 225–227, 245–249
intellectual function and, 292–294

Benign epilepsy, with rolandic EEG
  paroxysms
  CAT findings in, 8
  partial sleep seizures in, 348
Biofeedback, seizure control and, 241
Blood counts, carbamazepine therapy and,
  61, 62
Blood diseases, CAT findings in, 13–14
Blood serum; *see* Serum
Bourneville, syndrome of, CAT findings in,
  13
Brain; *see also* Brain atrophy; Brain edema;
  Brain lesions; Brain tumors; Cerebral
  cortex
  cyclic AMP content, epilepsy and, 315
  gray and white matter, antiepileptic drug
    levels in, 103–107
Brain atrophy
  age and duration of epilepsy and, 6
  CAT findings in, 15
  secondary generalized epilepsies and, 6–7
  status epilepticus and, 9–11
Brain edema
  CAT findings in, 15
  status epilepticus and, 9–11
Brain lesions
  CAT in partial epilepsies and, 7
  posttraumatic, CAT diagnosis of, 12
Brain tumors
  CAT diagnosis of, 11, 12
  epilepsy and, 20, 22
Brief Psychiatric Rating Scale, car-
  bamazepine therapy and, 49, 52
Bronchial secretions, clonazepam and, 178

Calcium deposits, brain lesions with, 13
Calcium metabolism, antiepileptic drugs
  and, 23
Campotomy, 25
Carbamazepine (CBZ); *see also* Carbamazepine therapy
  half-life in children, 196
  structural formula of, 47
Carbamazepine therapy
  adverse effects of, 40–43, 53
  blood counts and, 60, 61, 62
  discontinuation of, 60
  dosages for, 57, 58
  duration of seizure control and, 39–40
  EEG findings and, 60
  elimination in children and, 191–196
  endocrine function and, 209–212
  in generalized epilepsies, 37–39
  grand mal seizures and, 59
  increase in psychomotor seizures and,
    59–60
  leukocyte chromosomal damage and,
    87–93

leukocyte counts and, 53
long-term study in hospitalized epileptic
  patients and, 47–55
long-term use of, 35–43, 57–62
with other drugs, 39, 58
in partial epilepsies, 37, 38
patients treated with, 36
phenobarbital and, in Lennox-Gastaut
  syndrome, 136
psychomotor attacks and, 58–59
psychotropic effects of, 47–55, 226
reasons for withdrawal of, 42
Carbamazepine-10,11-epoxide
  antiepileptic effects of, 143–146
  elimination in children, 191–196
Cardiac arrhythmia, EEG and EKG monitoring and, 112
Case histories; *see also* Case reports
  of patients with seizures increased by so-
    cial stress, 252–253
  of personality disorders with epilepsy,
    253–354
Case reports
  aphasia with bilateral spike-wave dis-
    charges, 305–306
  behavior disorders in epileptic children,
    227–228
  chronic cerebellar stimulation, 333–339
  of operant conditioning for eating training
    of mentally retarded epileptic child,
    286–287
Cassette recorders, for prolonged EEG
  monitoring in ambulatory patients,
  109–110, 112
Computerized Axial Tomography (CAT) in
  epilepsy, 5–15
  and benign epilepsy with rolandic EEG
    paroxysms, 8
  and diagnosis of posttraumatic epilepsy,
    12
  and etiology of epilepsies, 11–14
  and grand mal generalized epilepsy of late
    onset, 8
  hemiconvulsion-hemiplegy-epilepsy syn-
    drome and, 8–9
  partial epilepsies and, 7
  postinfectious epilepsy and, 13
  postischemic epilepsy and, 13
  primary generalized epilepsy and, 5, 6
  proportion and type of cerebral lesions
    and, 5–11
  secondary generalized epilepsy and, 6–7
  status epilepticus and, 9, 11, 14–15
  tumors and, 11, 12
Cerebellar stimulation, chronic; *see* Chronic
  cerebellar stimulation
Cerebral cortex, antiepileptic drug levels
  ratio to plasma levels, 103–107

Cerebral lesions, CAT diagnosis of, 5–11
Cerebrospinal fluid, cyclic AMP content in epilepsy, 313–315
Cerebrovascular disease, epilepsy and, 356
Childhood epilepsy
  behavior disturbances related to type of, 245–249
  carbamazepine elimination in, 191–196
  education of teachers and, 364
  intellectual function study in, 291–294
  parental treatment of, 225–227; see also parent-child relations
  phenytoin-induced IgA deficiency and, 204
  preventive rehabilitation in, 265–268
  progressive aphasia in, 295–303
  psychological intervention with parents of, 235–238
  refractory, sodium valproate and, 187–190
  retardation and, operant conditioning for behavior modification in, 285–290
  seizures during sleep in, 345–353
  temporary aphasia in, 305–306
Children, with febrile convulsions, 199–201; see also Childhood epilepsy
Cholesterol; see Serum, cholesterol
Chromosomal damage, antiepileptic drugs and, 87–93
Chronic cerebellar stimulation, 333–339
  cerebellar electrode implant procedure for, 334
  effect of, 336–338
  insertion of receivers for, 336
  procedure for, 336
Circadian sleep patterns, EMGs and, 111
Clonazepam
  compared with sodium valproate in intractable epilepsy, 181–186
  effect on EEG findings, 173
  intractable epilepsy and, 169–175
  posttraumatic epilepsy and, 177–179
  severe epilepsy in infancy and childhood and, 159–162
  side effects of, 161, 162, 165–166, 173–174, 178, 183
  trial in chronic epilepsy, 163–168
Cognitive functioning, chronic cerebellar stimulation and, 337–338
Complex partial seizures; see Psychomotor seizures
Computerized axial tomography; see CAT
Connective tissue, antiepileptic drugs and, 24
Consanguinity, epilepsy in India and, 362
Copenhagen Study Group of Side Effects of Antiepileptic Drugs, 209
Cortisol metabolism, phenytoin and carbamazepine and, 210

Cyclic AMP, cerebrospinal fluid levels in epilepsy, 313–315

Developing countries; see also Epilepsy in India; Epilepsy in Iraq; Epilepsy in Nigeria; Epilepsy in Rhodesia
  epilepsy in, 355–357
  epilepsy care and health care in, 379–383
Development quotient, brain atrophy and, 6
Developmental Disability Services and Facilities Construction Act, 3
Diazepam (DZ), in Lennox-Gastaut syndrome, 132–137
Digital recorder; see EEG digital cassette recording system
Diphenylhydantoin (DPH); see also Phenytoin
  leukocyte chromosomal damage and, 87–93
  monitoring serum levels of, 18
  serum cholesterol and triglyceride levels and, 215–218
Dipropylacetate; see sodium valproate
Doctor:population ratio, in Africa, 365–366
Domiciliary status, of middle-aged posttraumatic epileptics, 83
DPH; see Diphenylhydantoin
Driving
  epilepsy in Israel and, 307–310
  middle-aged posttraumatic epileptics and, 84
  seizure-free patients and, 73
Drowsiness; see also Side effects
  clonazepam and, 161, 165–166
  sodium valproate vs. clonazepam and, 183
Dysphasia, 227–228
DZ; see Diazepam

Eating training, operant conditioning of retarded epileptic child and, 286–287
Education, epilepsy in India and, 361–362
Electroencephalograms (EEGs)
  aphasia in epilepsy and, 295–297, 298, 299, 300
  behavioral patterns and, 245–249
  with bilateral spike-wave discharges, aphasia and, 305–306
  in chronic cerebellar stimulation, 334, 335–336, 337
  classification of epilepsy and, 258
  clonazepam therapy and, 166, 173, 174–175, 178
  diagnosis of posttraumatic epilepsy and, 12
  diagnosis of seizures and, 242
  diagnosis of temporal lobe epilepsy and, 326
  driving competence and, 309, 310

Electroencephalograms (EEGs) (*contd.*)
  epilepsy diagnosis in underdeveloped nations and, 382–383
  epilepsy secondary to tumor and, 12
  of epileptics in Iraq, 395
  of European and African epileptics, comparison of, 403–404
  in hemiconvulsion-hemiplegy-epilepsy syndrome, 8
  HL-A antigens and, 317–323
  interictal, slow-spike-wave discharges in; *see* Slow spike-and-wave syndrome
  monitoring of; *see* Monitoring of EEGs
  in multiple sclerosis with seizures, 342
  in nonepileptic paroxysmal nocturnal behavioral manifestations, 349
  normal, in epileptics, 22
  paroxysmal abnormalities, clinical state and, 153–158
  in posttraumatic epilepsy, 82
  with rolandic or midtemporal spikes, partial sleep seizures and, 348
  seizure frequency and, 270–272
  telemetered, 97
EEG digital cassette recording system, 97–98
EMI scanner; *see* Computerized Axial Tomography
EMIT, 223, 224
Employment of epileptics, 2, 21, 231, 281–282, 360–361
Encephalopathy, involutional or arteriopathic, grand mal generalized epilepsy of late onset and, 8
Endocrine function, phenytoin and carbamazepine and, 209–212
Enzymes, phenytoin metabolism and, 140–141; *see also* Liver enzymes
Epidemiologic studies of epilepsy, 355–356
Epilepsy; see also entries under various types of epilepsy, e.g., Benign epilepsy; Focal epilepsy; Generalized epilepsies; Temporal lobe epilepsy
  antiepileptic drugs and; *see* Antiepileptic drugs
  carbamazepine treatment of, 35–43
  computerized axial tomography (CAT) in, 5–15
  chronic cerebellar stimulation in, 333–339
  clonazepam and, 163–168
  in developing countries, 355–357; *see also* Developing countries
  diagnosis of, 109–113, 371
  distribution of types of, 63–64
  driving and; *see* Driving
  EEG recordings in; *see* Electroencephalograms
  employment and; *see* Employment of epileptics

  epidemiologic studies of, 359–361, 366
  etiology of, 1, 396
  factors causing psychiatric disorders in, 226, 227
  HL-A antigens and, 317–323
  impotence and, 209–212
  intractable, 169–175, 181–186
  legislation on, 1–3
  long-term control of seizures in, 17–25
  long-term follow-up studies of, 27–34
  long-term intensive monitoring of, 125–129
  long-term seizure-free, 69–74
  in middle-aged persons, 81–85
  mortality rates in, 326–327
  multiple sclerosis and, 341–343
  pathogenesis of, 356
  patient attitudes toward, 22–23
  patient and family attitudes toward in India, 388–391
  personality problems and, 251–252
  personality traits in, 257–262
  refractory, in children, 187–190
  relationship between quantitative EEG measurements and, 153–158
  secondary to brain tumor, 11, 12
  self-diagnosis of, 270
  severe, carbamazepine therapy in, 57–62
  severe in infants and children, clonazepam and, 159–162
  social stress and, 277–278
  triggered by fever, phenobarbital and, 199–201
Epilepsy in Africa, 365–376
  etiology of, 368–370
  incidence and prevalence rates, 366–371
  management of, 371–374
  prevention of, 373
  social problems and, 372–373
  types of, 370–371
Epilepsy care, 20–25
  case report of, 20, 22
  diagnosis and etiology in, 20, 22
  group psychotherapy and, 278–284
  of hospitalized patients, carbamazepine and, 47–55
  immediate and long-term consequences of, 22–24
  of institutionalized patients, 45–46
  in Iraq, 397–398
  long-term, 20–25
  medical management by physicians and, 269–275
  patterns of, 269–275
  phenytoin dosage adjustment and, 139–141
  phenytoin and phenobarbital therapy and, 77–79
  progressive suppression of medication and, 70–72

Epilepsy care (*contd.*)
  rehabilitation and; *see* Rehabilitation
  in Rhodesia, 401–402
  surgical treatment and, 24, 25
Epilepsy in India, 359–364
  sociocultural and economic implications
    of, 385–391
Epilepsy in Iraq
  incidence and facilities, 394
  sex incidence of, 394–395
Epilepsy research in United States, 1, 3
Epilepsy in Rhodesia
  etiology of, 402–403
  incidence of, 401–402
Epilepsy type
  behavior disturbances related to, 245–249
  carbamazepine therapy and, 36
  in India, 362–363
  personality traits and, 257–262
Epileptic children; *see* Childhood epilepsy
Epileptic encephalopathy, during slow sleep,
  349, 353
Epileptic myoclonus
  during sleep, 346
  on falling asleep, 345–346
Epilim®; *see* Sodium valproate
Erythrocytes, carbamazepine therapy and,
  61
E.S.E.S.; *see* Subclinical epileptic status
Ethosuximide
  adverse effects of, 41
  monitoring serum levels of, 18–19
Extinction techniques, for seizure control,
  241

Fahr syndrome, CAT findings in, 13
Family studies, of epilepsy and HL-A antigens, 317–323
Febrile seizures
  daily phenobarbital and, 199–201
  etiology of epilepsy and, 369
Fetus, effects of maternal anticonvulsant
  drugs on, 23
Focal epilepsy
  cerebral cortex antiepileptic drug levels
    and, 103–107
  clonazepam and, 167, 170
  multiple sclerosis and, 341
Follicle-stimulating hormone (FSH), phenytoin and carbamazepine treatment and,
  211

Gas chromatography
  antiepileptic drug level determinations
    and, 116, 117, 223–224
  plasma antiepileptic drugs in Lennox-
    Gastaut syndrome and, 132
Gastrointestinal symptoms, sodium valproate vs. clonazepam and, 183

Generalized epilepsies; *see also* Generalized
  seizures
  carbamazepine therapy and, 37–39
  clonazepam and, 163–168
  grand mal of late onset, 8
  in infants and children, clonazepam and,
    159–162
Generalized seizures
  on morning awakening or arousal from
    sleep, 346–347
  multiple sclerosis and, 341
Gingival hyperplasia, 231
  phenytoin-induced, 203–206
Grand mal epilepsy
  carbamazepine therapy and, 57–62
  CAT in primary generalized epilepsy and,
    6
  clonazepam and, 170
  personality traits and, 257–262
Group therapy, 278–284
  operant conditioning of mentally retarded
    epileptics and, 287–288
  for parents of epileptic children, 235–238

Habituation, seizure control and, 241
Head injuries, epilepsy study in middle-aged
  persons and, 81–85; *see also* Post-
  traumatic epilepsy
Headaches, sulthiame and, 121
Health care in underdeveloped nations,
  373–374, 379–383
Hemiclonic seizures, CAT findings in, 8
Hemiconvulsion-hemiplegy-epilepsy
  (H-H-E) syndrome
  CAT findings in, 8–9
  occlusion of sylvian artery and, 13
Hemispherectomy, 25
Heredity, epilepsy and, 1
Hirsutism, antiepileptic drugs and, 231
Histocompatibility system, in primary
  generalized epilepsy, 317–323; *see also*
  HL-A antigens
HL-A antigens, in primary generalized
  epilepsy, 317–323
Hypersalivation, clonazepam and, 178
Hyperthermic clonic seizures, CAT findings
  in primary generalized epilepsy and, 6
Hypnosis, seizure control and, 240

IgA, serum and secretory deficiency,
  phenytoin-induced, 203–206
IgM, phenytoin-induced IgA deficiency and,
  206
Immune disorders, phenytoin-induced,
  203–206
Immunoglobulins, phenytoin-induced deficiency of, 203–206
Impotence, effect of antiepileptic drugs on
  endocrine function and, 209–212

India, epilepsy in; *see* Epilepsy in India
Infantile myoclonic encephalopathy; *see*
  West syndrome
Infants, severe epilepsy in, clonazepam
  and, 159–162; *see also* Childhood
  epilepsy
Infectious disease
  of central nervous system, epilepsy and,
    369
  epilepsy in developing countries and, 356
Intelligence, epilepsy and, 229–230, 264,
  291–294; *see also* Mental status
Intensive monitoring; *see also* Monitoring
  benefits of, 99–100
  EEG digital cassette recording system for,
    97–98
  objectives of, 99
  of patients with intractable seizures,
    95–101
  simultaneous, 98–99
  telemetered EEG and, 97
  videotape recording and, 95–97
International Bureau for Epilepsy, 2
International classification of the epilepsies,
  5, 8, 63–64
International League Against Epilepsy, 1,
  383
Iraq, epilepsy in; *see* Epilepsy in Iraq
Isle of Wight survey, 245
Israel, epileptic drivers in, 307–310

Joint family concepts, epilepsy care in India
  and, 362
Juvenile myoclonic epilepsy, personality
  traits and, 257–262

17-Ketosteroids excretion, phenytoin and
  carbamazepine treatment and, 211

LC-Partigen immunodiffusion plates, 204
League Against Epilepsy, 237
Left hemisphere, acquired aphasia of childhood and, 300–301
Legislation on epilepsy, 1–3
Lennox-Gastaut syndrome (LGS)
  in adults
    age at onset of, 64
    diagnostic criteria for, 67–68
    incidence of, 64
    types of seizures in, 65
  antiepileptic drugs and, 65, 66
  CAT findings in, 6, 7
  etiology of, 66–67
  long-term monitoring of antiepileptic
    drugs in, 131–137
  tonic seizures during sleep in children
    with, 347–348

Lennox syndrome, clonazepam and, 170
  172, 173
Leukocyte chromosomes, antiepileptic
  drugs and, 87–93
Leukocyte counts, carbamazepine therapy
  and, 53, 61
Leukopenia, carbamazepine therapy and, 53
Life expectancy, of middle-aged posttraumatic epileptics, 84
Life table methodology, 200
Liver carbamazepine clearance in children,
  191; *see also* Liver enzymes
Liver enzymes
  diphenylhydantoin and barbiturates and,
    215
  function, in endocrine function and an-
    tiepileptic drugs study, 210
  phenytoin and carbamazepine treatment
    and, 212
Lobectomy, 82
  follow-up studies of, 27–34
Luteinizing hormone (LH), phenytoin and
  carbamazepine treatment and, 211

Malignant epileptic encephalopathies; *see*
  Lennox-Gastaut syndrome; West syndrome
Malnutrition, epilepsy and, 356
Marital status, of middle-aged posttraumatic
  epileptics, 83
Marke-Nyman scale, personality traits in
  epilepsy study and, 258–262
Meniére disease, in epilepsy and personality
  traits study, 258–262
Menkes syndrome, CAT findings in, 14
Menopause, seizure frequency and, 83
Mental retardation
  epilepsy and, 159
  in myoclonic epilepsy, 170
Mental status
  brain atrophy and, 6
  clonazepam and, 174
  of epileptics in India, 363
  of middle-aged posttraumatic epileptics,
    84–85
  sodium valproate therapy in children and,
    188, 189–190
Mentally Retarded Facilities and Construction Act, 2–3
Mesodiencephalon, Lennox-Gastaut syndrome and, 66–67
Middle-aged persons, epilepsy and, 81–85
Milan Collaborative Group for Studies on
  Epilepsy, 131
Minnesota Multiphasic Personality Inventory, in evaluation of epileptics, 262
Monitoring of antiepileptic drug levels,
  11–20, 23, 78, 79, 98, 223–224

Monitoring of antiepileptic drug
    levels (*contd.*)
  assay methods and, 115–118
  in Lennox-Gastaut syndrome, 131–137
  in phenytoin and phenobarbital combina-
    tion therapy, 78, 79
  reliability of, 115–118
  seizure control and, 17–20
Monitoring of electroencephalograms; *see
    also* Intensive monitoring
  in ambulatory patients, 109–112
  automated analysis of, 151–152
  long-term, 125–129, 151
  relationship between clinical state and,
    152–158
  use of, 274
Monitoring of seizures, group therapy and,
    283
Moray House scores, of epileptic children,
    292–294
Mortality
  reduction of, in institutionalized persons,
    46
  temporal lobe resection and, 28–34, 327
Multiple sclerosis, epilepsy and, 341–343
Myoclonic epilepsy
  clonazepam and, 170, 172
  in infants and children, clonazepam and,
    159–162
  sleep in children and, 345–346

Narcolepsy, prolonged electroencephalo-
    graphic monitoring and, 111
National Institute of Neurological and
    Communicative Disorders and Stroke, 3
National Institutes of Health, 1
Neuropsychological assessment, in aphasia
    and epilepsy, 298, 299, 300, 301
Nigeria, doctor:patient ratio in, 365–366; *see
    also* Epilepsy in Africa
Night sleepwalking, compared with
    epilepsy, 349
Norway, epilepsy in, 229

Occupations, of epileptics in India, 361; *see
    also* Employment of Epileptics
Operant conditioning, behavior modification
    for retarded epileptic children and,
    285–290
Overprotection of epileptic children, 266–
    268

Parent-child relations, childhood epilepsy
    and, 225–227, 235–238
  overprotection and overindulgence and,
    265–268
  preventive rehabilitation and, 265–268

Partial epilepsies
  carbamazepine therapy and, 37, 38t, 144–
    146
  CAT findings in, 7
  hemiconvulsion-hemiplegy-epilepsy syn-
    drome, 8–9
  suppression of medication in, 70, 71, 72
Partial sleep seizures, 348–349
  in benign epilepsy syndrome with rolandic
    or midtemporal spikes, 348
Pavor nocturnus, compared with epilepsy,
    349
Personality changes, sulthiame and, 121, 122
Personality traits of epileptics, 22, 257–262,
    363, 386–391
Petit mal seizures
  CAT in primary generalized epilepsy and,
    6
  clonazepam and, 169, 172
Phenobarbital
  adverse effects of, 41
  and carbamazepine, in Lennox-Gastaut
    syndrome, 136
  cerebral cortex levels of, 104–105
  cortex:plasma ratio of, 106–107
  febrile seizures and, 199–201
  and phenytoin, long-term therapy with,
    77–79
  serum clonazepam and, 166
  serum phenytoin and, 147–149
Phenozone metabolism, in antiepileptic
    drugs and endocrine function study, 210
Phenytoin
  adverse effects of, 41
  blood counts and, 62
  cerebral cortex levels of, 104–105
  clonazepam and, 178
  dosage adjustment with, 139–141
  endocrine function and, 209–212
  -induced salivary IgA deficiency and ging-
    ival hyperplasia, 203–206
  intoxication, 226
  monitoring serum levels of, 18, 19
  phenobarbital and, long-term therapy
    with, 77–79
  primidone metabolism and, 150
  serum levels of, 119–123, 139–141
  sulthiame and, 119–123
Physicians, management of epilepsy by,
    269–275
Plasma antiepileptic drug levels
  in Lennox-Gastaut syndrome, 131–137
  ratio to cerebral cortex levels, 103–107
Plasma carbamazepine
  and carbamazepine-10,11-epoxide, sei-
    zures and, 145, 146
  in childhood epilepsy, 194
  long-term therapy and, 40

Plasma phenytoin and phenobarbital, effect of seizure type and co-medication on, 219–221
Postinfectious epilepsy, CAT findings in, 13
Postischemic epilepsy, CAT findings in, 13
Posttraumatic epilepsy
  CAT findings in, 12
  clonazepam and, 177–179
  EEG in clonazepam-treated patients with, 178
  long-term study of, 82–85
Pregnancy, antiepileptic drugs in, 23
Preparative ultracentrifugation, in phenytoin-induced IgA deficiency study, 204
Primary generalized epilepsy
  CAT diagnosis of cerebral lesions in, 5, 6
  HL-A antigens in, 317–323
  prognosis for, 22
  seizures on morning awakening in, 347
  suppression of medication in, 70–72
Primidone
  adverse effects of, 41
  leukocyte chromosomal damage and, 87–93
  metabolism, phenytoin and, 150
Progressive muscle relaxation, seizure control and, 240
Psychomotor seizures
  carbamazepine and, 58–60
  personality traits and, 257–262
Psychophysiological techniques for seizure control, 241
Psychotherapy, seizure control and, 240–241; see also Group therapy
Psychotropic effects of carbamazepine, 42–43, 47–55

Rabbits, electrically-induced convulsions in, cerebrospinal fluid cyclic AMP and, 313–314
Race, epilepsy incidence and, 367, 370
Radiotelemetry, monitoring ambulatory patients with, 109–112
Rajotte's Scale, carbamazepine therapy and, 49–51
Rehabilitation of epileptics; see also Behavior modification; Therapy
  behavior modification and, 225–232
  in India, 360–361
  long-term casework support and, 251–255
  operant conditioning in institutionalized retarded children and, 285–290
  preventive, in childhood, 265–268
  theme-centered interaction groups and, 278–284
Rehabilitation Act, 2
Reid Report, 269

Retarded language ability, epilepsy and, 227–228; see also Aphasia
Reward management, in behavior modification for seizure control, 239–240
Rey-Osterreith test, chronic cerebellar stimulation and, 337–338
Rhodesia, epilepsy in; see Epilepsy in Rhodesia
Rivotril®; see Clonazepam
Rolandic EEG paroxysms
  benign epilepsy with, 8
  epilepsy with symptoms due to, 7
Rorschach test, evaluation of epileptics with, 262

S-Partigen IgA immunodiffusion plates, 204
Salivary antiepileptic drug levels, 224
Salivary IgA deficiency, phenytoin-induced, 203–206
Second Workshop on the Determination of Antiepiletic Drugs in Body Fluids (WODADIBOF II), 115
Secondary generalized epilepsy
  CAT findings in, 6–7
  suppression of medication in, 70–72
Seizure frequency; see also Seizures
  carbamazepine and, 49, 54
  chronic cerebellar stimulation and, 336–337
  clonazepam and, 165
  EEG findings and, 270–272
  group therapy and, 283f
  operant conditioning of mentally retarded epileptics and, 289–290
  in personality trait study, 259–260
  psychological factors in, 225
  social stress and, 251–253
  in sodium valproate vs. clonazepam comparison, 184, 185
Seizures; see also Epilepsy triggered by fever; Febrile seizures; Grand mal seizures; Hyperthermic clonic seizures; Petit mal seizures; Seizure frequency
  age and, 1
  antiepileptic drugs and; see Antiepileptic drugs
  behavior therapy for control of, 239–243
  brain antiepileptic drug levels and, 105, 106
  carbamazepine therapy and, 43
  cerebral cortex antiepileptic drug levels and, 103–107
  cerebrospinal fluid cyclic AMP levels and, 313–315
  clonazepam in posttraumatic epilepsy and, 178
  duration of control with carbamazepine, 39–40

Seizures (*contd.*)
  EEG monitoring during, 111–112
  epilepsy care of institutionalized patients and, 45–46
  epilepsy type and, 257–258
  five-year remission of, status of patients in, 45–46
  intractable, intensive monitoring and, 95–101
  long-term control of, 17–25
  multiple sclerosis and, 341–343
  performance and, 24
  plasma antiepileptic drug levels in Lennox-Gastaut syndrome and, 132–137
  plasma phenytoin and phenobarbital levels and, 219–221
  in posttraumatic epilepsy, 82–83
  precipitating factors in, 363
  in primary generalized epilepsy, 6
  psychological aspects of, 241–243
  relapses of, progressive suppression of medication and, 70–72
  serum sulthiame and phenytoin and, 119–123
  during sleep in children, 345–353
  social status and, 20, 21
  sodium valproate in children with refractory epilepsy and, 187–190
  surgical techniques and, 25, 328
  types of, clonazepam and, 172
  types of, driving and, 308–309
Self-control, in behavior modification for seizure control, 240–241
Serum
  antiepileptic drug levels; *see* Monitoring of antiepileptic drug levels
  cholesterol and triglyceride, diphenylhydantoin and, 215–218
  clonazepam, seizures and, 166
  IgA deficiency, phenytoin-induced, 203–206
  lipids, effect of diphenylhydantoin on, 215–218
  phenytoin, dosage adjustment and, 139–141
  phenytoin and carbamazepine, in endocrine function study, 210
  phenytoin and phenobarbital, 147–149
  sulthiame and phenytoin levels, seizure control and, 119–123
  testosterone, phenytoin and carbamazepine treatment and, 211
  triiodothyronine and thyroxine, phenytoin and carbamazepine treatment and, 211, 212
Sex
  behavioral problems in epileptic children by, 248

carbamazepine effects on blood cell counts by, 60–62
epilepsy prevalence in developing countries by, 356
of epileptics in Africa, 367–368
intellectual function of epileptic children by, 293–294
multiple sclerosis with seizures by, 343
Side effects; *see* also Headache, Impotence; and entries under individual antiepileptic drugs
  as cause of psychiatric symptoms, 231
  of clonazepam, 161, 162, 165–166, 173–174, 178
  phenytoin-induced salivary IgA deficiency and gingival hyperplasia, 203–206
  of sodium valproate therapy in children, 188–189
  of sodium valproate vs. clonazepam, 183
  of sulthiame, 121–123
Skin rash, carbamazepine therapy and, 40, 41
Sleep, nonepileptic paroxysmal behavioral manifestations during, 349
Sleep seizures, with complex symptomatology, 348–349
Slow sleep, epileptic encephalopathy during, subclinical epileptic status and, 349, 353
Slow spike-and-wave syndrome; *see* also Lennox-Gastaut syndrome
  in adults, 63–68
  antiepileptic drugs in, 65, 66, 68
  multi-ictal and uni-ictal, types of seizures and, 65
Social adjustment of epileptics
  long-term casework support and, 251–255
  middle-aged, 83, 84
  seizure-free, 72–73
  in theme-centered interaction groups, 281–282
Social class, temporal lobe epilepsy and, 329
Social evaluation, in epilepsy and personality traits study, 258-259
Society, attitudes toward epilepsy, 1, 362, 372–373
Sodium valproate
  adverse effects of, 41, 183
  compared with clonazepam in intractable epilepsy, 181–186
  dosage in childhood epilepsy, 187–190
  monitoring serum levels of, 19
Solidity, in personality traits and epilepsy study, 261, 262
Somnambulism, compared with epilepsy, 349
Speech retardation, 227–228; *see* also Aphasia
Stability, in personality traits and epilepsy study, 261, 262

Status epilepticus
  care of institutionalized persons with, 46
  CAT findings in, 9, 11, 14–15
  clonazepam and, 171, 173
  subclinical epileptic status and, 349, 353
Steroid metabolism, antiepileptic drugs and, 23
Stress, epilepsy and, 82, 277–278
Sturge-Weber-Crabbe syndrome, CAT findings in, 13
Subclinical epileptic status, EEG sleep recording and diagnosis of, 349, 352–353
Sulthiame
  adverse effects of, 41
  phenytoin and, 119–123
  serum level studies of, 119–123
  side effects of, 121–123
Surgery for epilepsy
  in Africa, 372
  outcome of, 25
  unilateral temporal lobe resection, indications for, 325–330
Sylvian artery, epilepsy after occlusion of, 13

T₃test; see Triiodothyronine resin uptake test
Tegretol®; see Carbamazepine
Telemetry, long-term EEG monitoring and, 97–98, 125–129
Television viewing, seizures and, 363
Temporal lobe epilepsy
  behavioral patterns and, 245
  impotence and, 209
  indications for surgery in, 325–330
Temporal lobe resection, indications for, 325–330
Temporal lobectomy, 25, 27–34
Third International Workshop on the Determination of Antiepileptic Drugs in Body Fluids (WODADIBOF III), 223–224
Thrombocytes, carbamazepine therapy and, 61

Thyroid gland, phenytoin and carbamazepine treatment and, 211, 212
Tomography, computerized axial; see CAT
Tonic-clonic seizures
  carbamazepine and carbamazepine-10,11-epoxide and, 143–146
  clonazepam in infants and children with, 160
  during sleep, 347–348
Torticollis, EMG monitoring in, 111
Treatment Emergent Symptoms Scale, carbamazepine therapy and, 53
Tri-Partigen IgA immunodiffusion plates, 203–204
Triglycerides; see Serum, triglycerides
Triiodothyronine resin uptake test, phenytoin and carbamazepine treatment and, 211–212

Unilateral epilepsy, suppression of medication and, 70–72

Videotape recording of epileptic seizures, 95–97
Vinland National Center for Handicapped Individuals, 4

Wechsler Intelligence Scale for Children
  chronic cerebellar stimulation and, 337
  epilepsy and, 291–294
Wechsler Logical Memory subtest, chronic cerebellar stimulation and, 337
Weight loss, sulthiame and, 121
West syndrome
  CAT findings in, 6
  clonazepam and, 170, 172
White House Conference on Handicapped Individuals, 3–4
Wilcoxon test for pair differences, 210, 211
World Health Organization, 355, 356–357, 383